Atopic Dermatitis - Eczema

Kilian Eyerich • Johannes Ring

Atopic Dermatitis - Eczema

Clinics, Pathophysiology and Therapy

Second Edition

Springer

Kilian Eyerich
Department of Dermatology and Venerology
Medical Center, University of Freiburg
Freiburg, Germany

Johannes Ring
Department of Dermatology and Allergology Biederstein
Technical University Munich
Munich, Germany

ISBN 978-3-031-12498-3 ISBN 978-3-031-12499-0 (eBook)
https://doi.org/10.1007/978-3-031-12499-0

Translation from the German language edition: Neurodermitis - Atopisches Ekzem by Johannes Ring, Georg Thieme Verlag 2012

This Springer imprint is published by the registered company Springer Nature Switzerland AG
The registered company address is: Gewerbestrasse 11, 6330 Cham, Switzerland

Foreword to the First Edition

Atopic dermatitis is a common and troublesome inflammatory skin disease, especially during childhood. For those affected and their families, this condition presents an extreme burden of personal suffering, impaired quality of life, and high direct and indirect costs.

While clearly described in the nineteenth century, atopic dermatitis continues to present a complicated puzzle for researchers, doctors, and patients. Even more so than asthma and hay fever, the "sister" diseases in the atopic triad, the pathomechanisms are considerably more complex. In addition to the epidermal barrier dysfunction and the Th2-deviated inflammatory and immune responses, the frequent IgE-mediated allergic reactions, neurogenic inflammation, pruritus, and an imbalance in the autonomic nervous system seem to play a role.

This book covers the wide spectrum of atopic dermatitis from epidemiology, pathophysiology, and clinical aspects to modern diagnostics and therapy. It is written by one person, namely Professor Johannes Ring, a dermatologist who has focused particularly on the puzzling relationship of allergy and irritancy in eczematous skin reactions.

He has been coeditor and editor of two editions of *Handbook of Atopic Eczema* and given lectures on national and international congresses both in dermatology, pediatric dermatology, and allergy. He was a friend and participant in George Rajka's international symposia on atopic dermatitis and has become president of the International Society of Atopic Dermatitis (ISAD) organizing the valuable research conferences which foster participation and knowledge exchange from many nations. He has also been active in several scientific societies, serving as president of the European Academy of Dermatology and Venerology (EADV) and the Collegium Interationale Allergologicum (CIA) and has organized several outstanding events like the European Dermatology Congress in 2001 and the World Allergy Congress in 2005 both in Munich. More recently, he has hosted a series of international symposia "New Trends in Allergy" taking place every 5 years.

A single-author book has both advantages and disadvantages. One disadvantage is that no individual can have full knowledge of a complex condition like atopic dermatitis, resulting in a certain degree of subjectivity in the selection and accentuation of topics. Such weaknesses may well be offset by the advantage to the reader who will get one clear opinion of an expert without the distracting contradictions and redundancies often found in multiauthor books.

Although I personally do not share every opinion of Johannes Ring—and we have a long history of debating our often-varied concepts—I enjoy reading his views such as those presented in this book. He provides a well-planned and comprehensive description of this complex disease, combining basic scientific knowledge and good clinical pragmatism for practitioners, be they primary care physicians, pediatricians, dermatologists, or allergists.

Department of Dermatology
Oregon Health and Science University,
Portland, OR, USA
November 2015

Jon Hanifin

Preface

Atopic Dermatitis/Atopic Eczema (AD/AE) is the most common non-communicable inflammatory skin disease characterized by strongly itching eczematous lesions.

Due to the individual suffering and also with respect to socioeconomic consequences, this disease represents a major challenge for most industrialized countries.

Yet this disease probably is not new. Early descriptions date back into antiquity; scientific descriptions can be found in the early nineteenth century.

While AD was rather rare in the 50s of the twentieth century, it has without doubt increased in prevalence over the last decades, with estimates ranging from 10 to 20% of preschool children and 3 to 5% of adults affected.

The pathogenesis of AD is characterized by the trias barrier dysfunction, disturbed microbial colonization of the skin, and a Th2 immune dysbalance; also psychosomatic involvement is clinically evident.

Recently, there has been a tremendous progress in the elucidation of pathophysiological mechanisms. This involves the complex genetic trait of AD. Mutations of relevant proteins forming the skin barrier—for example, filaggrin and protease inhibitors—have been discovered and found to be associated with AD. Also the genetic and epigenetic components of the immune deviation toward Th2 with increased interleukin 4 and interleukin 13 cytokine secretion and formation of specific immune globulin E-producing plasma cells have become largely elucidated. Furthermore, the pathogenic role for microbials such as *S. aureus* has been extensively studied. Also potential autoantigens and immune mechanisms beyond Th2 immunity are well investigated.

With regard to the psycho-neurogenic inflammation, the molecular basis is still not well understood.

Based on this new knowledge regarding pathophysiology, novel treatment options have appeared in the last years. At the moment, there are more than 150 clinical trials registered worldwide to study new therapeutic substances for AE.

Nevertheless, at the moment topical therapy with emollients and mild topical anti-inflammatory therapy with either glucocorticoids or calcineurin inhibitors are in the center of guideline recommendations. Treatment follows—with some differences between countries—the recommendations of various national and international guidelines. Severe AD can nowadays be treated with systemic therapies, either biological neutralizing Th2 response or small molecules such as JAK inhibitors.

A major problem in dealing with affected patients is the shortage of time. The complexity of the disease and of the therapeutic strategies is not explained in 5–10 min—the average time of a dermatological consultation in many countries. Therefore, educational programs ("Eczema School") have been developed and found to be effective in randomized prospective trials. In some countries, they are reimbursed by insurances.

All these aspects will be dealt with in our book which wants to be precise, scientifically in depth, practically usable and understandable to all physicians—and maybe patients—interested.

We want to thank Danielle Rogner and Alexander Zink for valuable help in preparing the text and searching the literature as well as Eleonora Enderlein and Brigitte Engelmann for secretarial assistance, also we want to thank Dr. Kleemann from Springer, Heidelberg, as well as Priyadharshini Aruchamy for excellent support during lecturing and book production.

Munich, Germany
December 2022

Kilian Eyerich
Johannes Ring

Preface to the First Edition

Atopic dermatitis (atopic eczema, eczema, endogenous eczema, Besnier's prurigo, neurodermitis constitutionalis, etc.) is one of the most common—in childhood the most common—noncontagious inflammatory skin diseases. Although easily recognizable by the experienced physician, the disease poses a variety of problems and difficulties in diagnosis due to its diversity and variability, with poorly defined morphology.

Affected individuals suffer considerably, not only from the disfigurement when face and hands are involved, but especially from the excruciating and tormenting itch. This sensation causes sleeplessness, fatigue, reduction of daily achievements, and a considerable impairment in quality of life not only for the patient but also for his familial and social environment.

Many physicians are helpless and talk about an "incurable" disease. There are only few other fields in medicine where so many "alternative," "complementary," or "unconventional" procedures are used as in atopic dermatitis. Many affected individuals can report an odyssey of visits to doctors and healers in search of a "miracle" ointment or pill!

The disease is frequent: 10–20% of 5–6-year-old children are affected, and this is the case in many countries of the world. This was different 50 years ago, when in high school I first heard about this condition, and later as a medical student from the unforgettable Professor Alfred Marchionini in Munich. Early epidemiological data from the 1950s reported a prevalence of ca. 1–2%.

The disease is part of the atopic triad, together with bronchial asthma and hay fever; however, it differs in essential aspects especially with regard to the understanding of the mechanisms involved in pathogenesis, which are better established in hay fever and allergic asthma.

For the dermatologist, atopic dermatitis does not belong to the classical diseases with a very characteristic, ideally pathognomonic, typical "beautiful" skin lesion as primary lesion—as for example in psoriasis as red, scaly, and sharply margined patches, or hexagonal slightly elevated red papules as in lichen planus or grouped vesicles as in herpes simplex. Atopic dermatitis shows a rather diffuse morphology with unprecise lesions, mostly characterized by secondary changes due to bouts of scratching for strong itch.

It is understandable that 40 years ago the interest in dermatological research in this disease was not very pronounced. Other fields of dermatology were more attractive for research, which holds true even today in many countries.

At the World Congress for Dermatology (Congressus Mundi Dermatologiae), which takes place every 5 years—since recently every 4 years—in various places in the world, in 1977 in Mexico City, among 1000 presentations, there was only one "workshop" dealing with "atopic dermatitis," chaired by the masters Jon Hanifin and Georg Rajka together with 12 participants. Most of these became famous personalities in the field of atopic dermatitis later on and are still good friends.

The interest in this disease obviously has increased tremendously in recent decades, in parallel with the increase in prevalence.

What attracted me to become engaged in this disease? In Germany, the majority of allergists are originally dermatologists, followed by pediatricians, ENT specialists, pneumologists, and other physicians. I was already an established immunologist, having written a PhD thesis on anaphylaxis due to dextran infusions for volume substitution or horse-anti-human lymphocyte globulin (ALG) for immunosuppression in the Institute for Surgical Research (Prof. Walter Brendel). Then I continued research with a stipend from the Deutsche Forschungsgemeinschaft in the laboratory of Prof. Eng Tan at Scripps Clinic and Research Foundation in La Jolla, California.

I already had decided to join—after returning to Germany—the Department of Dermatology at Ludwig Maximilian University of Munich (Prof. Otto Braun-Falco). So in La Jolla, Prof. Eng Tan sent me to the library to find a topic on which it was worthwhile to do 2 years of research, aimed at connecting the previous work in immunology and allergy with the future in dermatology. I wrote a short research grant on the role of vasoactive mediators in atopic dermatitis and started—not knowing that I would be caught by this disease for decades over my professional life. In the 1970s, the progress in the field was very slow. It was not like jumping onto a moving train into a glorious future! It required high frustration tolerance to keep going. One motivation was the surprising and obvious increase in the prevalence of this disease all over the world.

As representatives for many others, I would like to thank the above-mentioned teachers, as well as my predecessors as directors of the Allergy Department (Prof. Karlheinz Schulz) and the Department of Dermatology at the University Hospital Eppendorf (Prof. Theodor Nasemann) and the Department of Dermatology and Allergy, Biederstein (Prof. Siegfried Borelli) at the Technical University Munich.

When a researcher is asked to write or edit a book on his favorite topic, this means work and fun at the same time. The field is so extensive and rich that it would be easy to edit a new edition of a handbook—as we have done in the past involving over 50 authors!

However, I personally like books that have been written by one person as responsible author; there one can see a red thread, unnecessary repetitions are avoided, and contradictory statements will be rare. Of course, this goes along with the disadvantage of less actual objectivity. I believe that it is attractive for the reader not only to find, as in an encyclopedia, a collection of the newest publications but rather a painting of the whole disease with its many facets, and how it became apparent in the experience of a researcher and physician over decades. Thus, I apologize and ask the reader, as though he/

she is traveling on holiday, to trust my more or less experienced guidance with all its subjectivity in the selection and accentuation of various facts, hypotheses, and arguments, in the hope that the reader may not be bored!

It is obvious that many other distinguished individuals could have written this book equally well or probably better; therefore, it makes sense—here and now—to say thank you to people who have helped me on the long and difficult path of dealing with atopic dermatitis/eczema.

There is in the first place my experimental teacher Walter Brendel who brought me to transplantation research, immunology, and via antilymphocyte serum toward allergic skin reactions. Eng Tan from Scripps Clinic in La Jolla should be thanked for the openmindedness with which he supported my humble start in eczema research.

I thank my respected clinical teacher Otto Braun-Falco for his masterly education in dermatology and for the absolute freedom he gave me in research, which was quite different from the structured hierarchy in clinical responsibilities of a university department.

I thank my predecessor as founder and director of the Biederstein Department of Dermatology, Siegfried Borelli, for his early work in atopic dermatitis ("neurodermitis") and his manifold support for the activities in Davos, Switzerland. Without my friend Bernhard Przybilla as co-resident on the children's ward and longtime co-worker in allergy, many things would have been impossible. Thomas Bieber was a case of good luck for dermatology and allergy, and I am proud that I was allowed to superficially guide him for some time and carry out research with him. It is wonderful that this research has been continued by Andreas Wollenberg. Along with Dieter Vieluf and Barbara Kunz from Hamburg, it was Ulf Darsow and Knut Brockow who brought the eczema research to our department in Munich. At this juncture, Heidelore Hofmann, Dietrich Abeck, and Christina Schnopp should also be mentioned for holding up the flag of pediatric dermatology, together with Claudia Kugler in Munich and Martina Premerlani, Daniela Münch, and Matthias Möhrenschlager in Davos for excellent care for children with eczema and for the development of the "eczema school."

Without Torsten Schäfer and Ursula Krämer, the epidemiology of atopic dermatitis in various parts of Germany would not have been written. Marcus Ollert as master of in vitro allergy diagnosis and Bernadette Eberlein in skin physiology have contributed considerably.

Real research in a clinical department is only possible with good cooperation with an experimental unit. This was the case and the good luck we had at the Biederstein campus in cooperation with the newly established Zentrum Allergie und Umwelt—ZAUM (Center for Allergy and Environment) founded in 1998 by Heidrun Behrendt and directed by her until 2010, then later by Carsten Schmid-Weber; here, the experimental immunologic–allergologic together with dermatologic research allowed real progress and was connected to the names of Thilo Jakob, Martin Mempel, Claudia Traidl-Hoffmann, Johannes Huss-Marp, Florian Pfab, Jan Gutermuth, Kilian and Stephanie Eyerich, Stefan Weidinger, Wen-Chie Chen, Jeroen Buters, and many others.

I want to thank Andreas Mauermayer for the excellent clinical photographs, and Brigitte Engelmann, Eleonora Enderlein, Daniela Bolocan, and Sybille Walter for excellent secretarial work.

No research group can stand on its own; among the attractive things in research are the national and international contacts and friendships which refresh thinking and which via the exchange of experiences but also materials lead to new paths. In this sense, I want to thank Thomas Platts-Mills in Charlottesville/Virginia, Donald Leung in Denver, Jon Hanifin in Portland, Ikutaro Yoshida in Nagasaki, Hirohisa Takegawa in Matsumotu, Matsutaka Furue in Kumamoto, Hideyoki Ogawa in Tokio, José Caraballo in Bogota, Yoshiky Miyachi in Kyoto, Kenji Kabashima in Kyoto, Jean-Hilaire Saurat in Geneva, Brunello Wüthrich in Zürich, Alain Taieb in Bordeaux, John Harper in London, Agostin Alomar in Barcelona, Alberto Gianetti and Stefania Seidenari in Modena, Carlo Gelmetti in Milano, Kristian Thestrup-Pedersen and Mette Deleuran in Aarhus, Georg Stingl in Vienna, Alexander Kapp and Thomas Werfel in Hannover, Margitta Worm and Torsten Zuberbier in Berlin, Uwe Gieler in Giessen, Yves DeProst in Paris, Anne Broberg in Goeteborg, Carla Bruijnzel in Utrecht, Jan Bos in Amsterdam, Peter Schmid-Grendelmeier in Zürich, and many others.

I would also like to thank Georg Rajka, who created the tradition of international symposia on the disease "atopic dermatitis" which contributed considerably to progress in the field. It is reassuring that these ideas are taken up and still alive in the regular organization of these symposia under the International Society of Atopic Dermatitis (ISAD).

Finally, I want to thank Dr. Engeli from Thieme, Stuttgart, who gave the permission for an English version of this book, and Mr. Klemp from Springer Science who made the contract. Finally, I want to thank Mrs. Kayalvizhi for her excellent lecturing and final work in the book production.

Whenever medical doctors try to write something in an understandable way, this often does not mean that many people—even physicians of other specialties—will really understand. Yet I hope that this book may find readers also among individuals affected by atopic dermatitis and their caregivers, who might find interesting information for dealing practically with this difficult disease.

Munich, Bavaria, Germany Johannes Ring
December 2015

Contents

1 General Introduction and History . . . 1
1.1 Introduction . . . 1
1.2 History . . . 3
1.2.1 First Descriptions . . . 3
1.2.2 Milestones in the History of Allergy and Eczema . . . 4
1.2.3 Summary . . . 6
1.3 Terminology . . . 6
1.3.1 The Term "Atopy" . . . 6
1.3.2 The Role of Immunglobulin E . . . 7
1.3.3 Definitions of Atopy Given by EAACI and WAO . . . 7
1.3.4 Our Definition of Atopy . . . 8
1.3.5 The Term Eczema . . . 9
1.3.6 Summary . . . 9

2 Epidemiology of Atopic Eczema . . . 11
2.1 Prevalence of Atopic Eczema in Childhood . . . 11
2.2 Causes for Increase in Prevalence . . . 15
2.2.1 Own Investigations in Comparing East and West Germany after Reunification in 1990 . . . 16
2.3 Atopic Eczema Over Lifetime . . . 18
2.3.1 Atopic Eczema in Adulthood . . . 18
2.4 Clinical Course and Prognosis . . . 20
2.4.1 Intrinsic Versus Extrinsic Eczema . . . 21
2.4.2 Gender Differences . . . 22
2.4.3 Ethnicity . . . 22
2.4.4 Genetic Predisposition (See Also Chap. 5) . . . 22
2.4.5 Socioeconomic Status . . . 23
2.4.6 Psychosomatic Influence . . . 24
2.4.7 Pregnancy . . . 24
2.4.8 Hygiene, Infectious Disease, and Vaccinations . . . 24
2.4.9 Nutrition (See Also Chap. 8 "Prevention") . . . 26
2.4.10 Polyunsaturated Fatty Acids and Probiotics . . . 26
2.4.11 Peanut Oil . . . 26
2.4.12 Skincare . . . 26
2.5 Lifestyle . . . 26
2.5.1 Living on a Farm . . . 26
2.5.2 Pet Keeping . . . 27

2.5.3 Environmental Pollutants 27
2.5.4 Prognostic Factors 28
2.5.5 Summary 28

3 Burden of Disease in Atopic Eczema 31
3.1 Personal Burden and Individual Suffering 31
3.2 Financial Burden 32
3.3 Summary 33

4 Clinical Symptomatology of Atopic Eczema 35
4.1 Actual Symptoms of Disease 35
4.1.1 Primary Lesion "Itch" 35
4.1.2 Infiltrated Erythema 37
4.1.3 Erosive, Excoriated Erythema 38
4.1.4 Lichenification 39
4.1.5 Prurigo-Type of Atopic Eczema 41
4.1.6 Differences in Various Ethnic Populations 41
4.2 Minimal Manifestations 43
4.2.1 Minimal Manifestations in the Head Area 43
4.2.2 Minimal Manifestations on the Trunk and Extremities 45
4.2.3 Variants and Special Forms 48
4.2.4 Special Localizations 50
4.2.5 Summary 52
4.3 Stigmata of Atopy 54
4.3.1 Dry Skin (Xerosis, Sebostasis) 54
4.3.2 Ichthyosis Palms and Soles (Hyperlinearity of Palms and Soles) 54
4.3.3 Infraorbital Fold (Atopy Fold, Dennie-Morgan) 56
4.3.4 Periorbital Halo and Facial Pallor 56
4.3.5 Rarefication of Lateral Eyebrows (Hertoghe) 56
4.3.6 Low Temporal Hairline, "Fur Cap Hair Growth" 57
4.3.7 White Dermographism 57
4.3.8 Delayed Blanch 57
4.3.9 Role of Stigmata in Diagnosis 57
4.3.10 Summary 59
4.4 Differential Diagnoses 59
4.4.1 Differential Diagnosis in Infants 59
4.4.2 Chronic Inflammatory Skin Diseases 60
4.4.3 Inflammatory Tumor Responses 62
4.4.4 Infectious Skin Diseases 62
4.4.5 Metabolic Diseases, Immunodeficiencies or Immunopathies 62
4.4.6 Malignant Diseases 63
4.4.7 Summary 63
4.5 Associated Diseases 63
4.5.1 Hereditary Dermatoses 63
4.5.2 Hair Diseases 65

4.5.3 Atopic Respiratory Diseases and Other Allergic Reactions . . . 65
4.5.4 Ocular Diseases . . . 66
4.5.5 Nephrotic Syndrome . . . 66
4.5.6 Vitiligo . . . 67
4.5.7 Photosensitivity . . . 67
4.5.8 Ear Disease . . . 67
4.5.9 Inflammatory Bowel Disease . . . 67
4.5.10 Neuro-Psychiatric Diseases . . . 67
4.5.11 Summary . . . 68
4.6 Complications of Atopic Eczema . . . 68
4.6.1 Bacterial Infections . . . 68
4.6.2 Fungal Infections . . . 70
4.6.3 Viral Infections . . . 70
4.6.4 Summary . . . 73
4.7 Diseases Rarely Associated with Atopic Eczema . . . 73
4.7.1 Diabetes Mellitus . . . 73
4.7.2 Rheumatoid Arthritis . . . 74
4.7.3 Psoriasis . . . 74
4.7.4 Melanocytic Nevi . . . 74
4.7.5 Atopic Eczema and Cancer . . . 74
4.7.6 Contact Allergy . . . 75
4.7.7 Debates on Association of Common Diseases with Atopy . . . 75
4.7.8 Summary . . . 75
4.8 Atopic Eczema: Diagnostic Criteria and Severity Scoring . . . 76
4.8.1 Diagnostic Criteria . . . 76
4.8.2 Evaluation of Severity of Eczema . . . 77
4.8.3 Objective Signs and Subjective Symptoms . . . 77
4.8.4 Quality of Life as Health Outcome Measure in Atopic Eczema . . . 79
4.8.5 Summary . . . 79

5 Etiopathophysiology of Atopic Eczema . . . 81
5.1 Pathophysiological Concepts . . . 81
5.2 Genetics of Atopic Dermatitis . . . 82
5.2.1 Genome-Wide Association Studies (GWAS) . . . 82
5.2.2 Filaggrin . . . 83
5.2.3 Protease Inhibitors . . . 84
5.2.4 Genes of Innate Immunity . . . 84
5.2.5 Antimicrobial Peptides . . . 86
5.2.6 Genes of Adaptive Immunity . . . 86
5.3 Epigenetic Changes . . . 86
5.4 Skin Barrier . . . 89
5.4.1 The Skin in Evolution . . . 89
5.4.2 Anatomical Structure of the Skin . . . 90

5.4.3 Microbial Barrier 91
5.4.4 Chemical Barrier 91
5.4.5 Physical Barrier 92
5.4.6 Corneocytes 92
5.4.7 Corneodesmosomes 92
5.4.8 Desquamation 92
5.4.9 Summary 93
5.5 Changes in the Microbiome 93
5.5.1 Summary 94
5.6 Excursion into a New Concept for Classification of Pathogenic Immune Reactions in Noncommunicable Inflammatory Skin Diseases 94
5.6.1 Lichenoid Pattern (Pattern 1) 95
5.6.2 Eczematous Pattern (Pattern 2a) 96
5.6.3 Bullous Pattern (Pattern 2b) 96
5.6.4 Psoriatic Pattern (Pattern 3) 97
5.6.5 Fibrogenic Pattern (Pattern 4a) 97
5.6.6 Granulomatous Pattern (Pattern 4b) 97
5.6.7 Summary 98
5.7 Type 2 Immunity, Allergy, and Its Consequences for Atopic Dermatitis 98
5.7.1 Definition and Occurrence of Type 2 Immune Cells . . 98
5.7.2 Functions of Type 2 Immune Cells in the Context of Atopic Dermatitis 98
5.8 Autoimmunity and Atopic Dermatitis 100
5.8.1 Summary 102
5.9 Itch and Neuroimmunology 102
5.9.1 The Itch Sensation 102
5.9.2 Itch Research 103
5.9.3 Measurement of Itch 104
5.10 Psychological Influences in Atopic Dermatitis 106
5.10.1 Psychology and Pruritus 107
5.10.2 Autonomic Nervous System Dysregulation 107
5.10.3 The Problem of an “Atopic” Personality (or “Atopic Eczema Personality”) 108
5.10.4 Parent-Child Relation (“Family Dynamics”) in Atopic Eczema 108
5.10.5 Stress and Atopic Eczema 110
5.10.6 Hormonal Influences 112
5.10.7 Summary 113
5.11 The Heterogeneity of Atopic Dermatitis Pathogenesis with Regard to Clinical Course (Acute Versus Chronic) and Ethnicity. 113
5.11.1 Summary 115

6 General Management of Patients with Atopic Eczema 117
6.1 Diagnostic Procedures 118
6.1.1 History 118
6.1.2 Skin Test Procedures 119

6.1.3 In Vitro Allergy Diagnostics 123
6.1.4 Oral Provocation Test in Food Allergy 123
6.1.5 Microbiological Diagnostics 125
6.1.6 Psychological Diagnostics 125
6.1.7 Summary 125
6.2 Use of Biomarkers in Diagnostics of Atopic Dermatitis: New Aspects 126
6.2.1 New Aspects in the Diagnosis of Atopic Dermatitis 126
6.2.2 New Aspects in Monitoring Severity of Atopic Dermatitis 128
6.3 Avoidance of Individual Provocation Factors 130
6.3.1 Avoidance of Unspecific Irritants 130
6.3.2 Aeroallergens 132
6.3.3 Summary 134
6.4 Basic Therapy of Disturbed Skin Barrier Function 134
6.4.1 General Considerations for Topical Dermatotherapy 135
6.4.2 Basic Skin Barrier Therapy in Atopic Dermatitis 136
6.4.3 Emollients Used for Basic Dermatotherapy 138
6.4.4 Summary 139
6.5 Practical Tips in the Treatment of Atopic Eczema in the Acute Flare 139
6.5.1 Practical Management of an Acute Eczema Flare 139
6.5.2 Anti-inflammatory Treatment 140
6.5.3 Antipruritic Treatment 140
6.5.4 Inpatient Treatment 140
6.5.5 Amount of Topicals 141
6.5.6 Summary 141

7 Special Therapeutic Options and Substances in the Treatment of Atopic Eczema 143
7.1 Glucocorticosteroids 143
7.1.1 Effects 143
7.1.2 Side Effects 145
7.1.3 Summary 148
7.2 Topical Calcineurin Inhibitors 148
7.2.1 Pharmacologic Effects 149
7.2.2 Side Effects 150
7.2.3 Summary 151
7.3 Antimicrobial Therapy 151
7.3.1 Antiseptics 151
7.3.2 Antimicrobial Textiles (Functional Textiles) 152
7.3.3 Antibiotic Therapy 152
7.3.4 Antimycotic Therapy 153
7.3.5 Antiviral Therapy 153
7.3.6 Vaccination and Atopic Dermatitis 153
7.3.7 COVID-19 Infection and Vaccination 154

7.3.8 Summary 154
7.4 Antihistamines 154
7.4.1 Effects of H1 Antagonists 155
7.4.2 Side Effects of Antihistamines 156
7.4.3 Other Anti-Allergic Substances 157
7.4.4 Opioid Receptor Antagonists 157
7.4.5 Summary 157
7.5 Other Antipruritic and Anti-Inflammatory Substances 157
7.5.1 Topical Antipruriginous Agents 158
7.5.2 Local Anesthetics 158
7.5.3 Polidocanol 158
7.5.4 Cannabinoid Agonists 158
7.5.5 Capsaicin 158
7.5.6 Tar Preparations 158
7.5.7 Adstringentia 159
7.5.8 Etheric Oils and Others 159
7.5.9 Summary 160
7.6 UV Therapy 160
7.6.1 Heliotherapy 160
7.6.2 UVB Radiation 160
7.6.3 UVA Radiation 160
7.6.4 Photochemotherapy 161
7.6.5 Visible Light 161
7.6.6 Extracorporal Photophoresis 161
7.6.7 Summary 162
7.7 Allergen-Specific Immunotherapy 162
7.7.1 Results of Clinical Trials 162
7.7.2 Summary 163
7.8 Systemic Immunomodulatory Therapy 163
7.8.1 Conventional Systemic Immune-modulators 164
7.8.2 Modern Small Molecules 166
7.8.3 Phosphodiesterase Inhibitors 168
7.8.4 Biologics 168
7.9 Pre- and Probiotics and Polyunsaturated Fatty Acids 171
7.9.1 Summary 171
7.10 Psychosomatic Strategies 172
7.10.1 Exploration and Evaluation of Psychosomatic Involvement in the Disease 172
7.10.2 Therapeutic Modalities 173
7.10.3 Behavioral Therapy 174
7.10.4 Summary 175
7.11 Unconventional Methods 175
7.11.1 Evaluation of Some "Unconventional" Procedures . . . 177
7.11.2 General Recommendations for Dealing with "Alternative" Methods 179
7.11.3 Summary 180

8 Prevention 181
8.1 Primary Prevention 181
8.1.1 Risk Groups 181
8.1.2 Allergy Development 181
8.1.3 Avoidance Strategies and General Recommendations. 182
8.1.4 Nutrition and Dietary Recommendations 184
8.1.5 Summary 186
8.2 Secondary Prevention 187
8.3 Tertiary Prevention: Rehabilitation 187
8.3.1 Socioeconomic Impact 187
8.3.2 Summary 187
8.4 Climate Therapy in Secondary and Tertiary Prevention 188
8.4.1 High Altitude, North Sea, and Dead Sea 188
8.4.2 Summary 189
8.5 Educational Programs ("Eczema School") 190
8.5.1 Development of "Eczema School" 190
8.5.2 Contents 190
8.5.3 Evaluation 190
8.5.4 Practical Performance 190
8.5.5 Qualification of Trainers 191
8.5.6 Music Therapy 191
8.5.7 Summary 191

9 Outlook into the Future 193

10 Concluding Remarks: How To Live With Eczema/Atopic Dermatitis 195

References 197

Index 229

Abbreviations

ADCT	Atopic dermatitis control test
ADHS	Attention deficit hyperactivity syndrome
AEDS	Atopic eczema dermatitis syndrome
AESEC	Atopic eczema severity and emotional consequences
AIDS	Acquired immunodeficiency syndrome
APT	Atopy patch test
ASIT	Allergen-specific immunotherapy
BHR	Bronchial hyperreactivity
CFU	Colony-forming units
CLA	Cutaneous lymphocyte antigen
CMV	Cytomegalovirus
CNS	Central nervous system
COVID	Coronavirus infectious disease
DC	Dendritic cells
DLQI	Dermatology Life Quality Index
DMSO	Dimethyl sulfoxide
DNA	Desoxyribonucleic acid
DTH	Delayed type hypersensitivity
EAACI	European Academy for Allergy and Clinical Immunology
EBV	Epstein–Barr virus
ECP	Eosinophil cationic protein
EDC	Epidermal differentiation complex
ETFAD	European Task Force Atopic Dermatitis
FcγRI	High-affinity receptor for immunoglobulin G
FcεRI	High-affinity receptor for immunoglobulin E
FDA	Food and Drug Administration
FPI	Freiburg personality inventory
GALT	Gut-associated lymphoid tissue
GINI	German infant nutritional intervention study
GM-CSF	Granulocyte monocyte colony-stimulating factor
GvHD	Graft-versus-host disease
GWAS	Genome-wide association study
HADS	Hospital anxiety and depression score
HIV	Human immunodeficiency virus
HOME	Health outcome measures in eczema
HPV	Human papillomavirus
HSV	Herpes simplex virus

IBD	Inflammatory bowel disease
IDDM	Insulin-dependent diabetes mellitus
IDEC	Inflammatory dendritic epidermal cell
Ig	Immunoglobulin
IL	Interleukin
IR	Index of reactivity
ISAAC	International Study of Asthma and Allergies in Childhood
KIGGs	Studie zur Gesundheit von Kindern und Jugendlichen in Deutschland….
LEKTI	Lympho-epithelial Kazal-type-related inhibitor
LTT	Lymphocyte transformation test
MHC	Major histocompatibility complex
MMF	Mycophenolate mofetil
MVA	Modified virus Ankara
ncISD	Non-communicable inflammatory skin disease
NMF	Natural moisturizing factor
NRS	Numerical rating scale
OR	Odds ratio
PAH	Polyaromatic hydrocarbons
PAR	Protease-activated receptor
PDE	Phosphodiesterase
PEG	Polyethylene glycol
PLD/E	Polymorphous light dermatosis/eruption
POEM	Patient-oriented eczema measure
PUFA	Polyunsaturated fatty acids
QOL	Quality of life
RAST	Radio-allergo-sorbent test
RECAP	Recap of atopic eczema
SALT	Skin-associated lymphoid tissue
SAWO	Schulanfänger (school beginners)-Studie West-Ost
SCF	Stem cell factor
SCID	Severe combined immunodeficiency
SCORAD	SCORing Atopic Dermatitis
SPINK-5	Serine peptidase inhibitor Kazal type 5
SPT	Skin prick test
STAI	State trait anxiety inventory
TCI	Topical calcineurin inhibitor
TDT	Transmission disequilibrium test
TEWL	Transepidermal water loss
TGF	Tumor growth factor
TLR	Toll-like receptor
TNF	Tumor necrosis factor
TRAC	Thymus and activation-regulated chemokine
VOC	Volatile organic compound
WAO	World Allergy Organization

General Introduction and History

1

1.1 Introduction

Allergic diseases are among the major health problems of our time. Especially the so-called atopic diseases, namely asthma, rhinoconjunctivitis (hay fever), and eczema (atopic dermatitis AD, atopic eczema AE) have increased in prevalence during the last decades dramatically [19, 613, 719, 895].

Atopic eczema as a skin manifestation of the atopic trait represents today the most common chronic noncontagious inflammatory skin disease in childhood [441, 454, 658].

Atopic dermatitis usually starts in childhood or early adolescence and is characterized by intense pruritus and disfiguring inflammatory skin lesions. The disease is associated with a dramatic impairment in quality of life. In times when economic reasons only consider mortality statistics measurable in Dollars or Euro, we have to be the advocates of our patients suffering from chronic skin diseases. The skin as the surface and frontier organ of the human organism is characterized by a multitude of physical, chemical, and biological functions important for the integrity of the human being (Table 1.1). Skin diseases lead to an impairment of self-confidence [267, 645]. When skin diseases start in childhood, they may influence the whole life span of a person in a long-lasting way inhibiting or preventing life achievements.

At the beginning of this book, we want to start with some very personal reflections: Since 1977, JR has been engaged scientifically and clinically with this disease, when he performed a postdoctoral fellowship with a grant from the Deutsche Forschungsgemeinschaft (DFG) at the Scripps Clinic and Research Foundation in La Jolla, California, USA, in the Division of Allergy and Immunology under the guidance of Dr. Eng M. Tan. When hearing that after this postdoctoral fellowship he most likely would join the Dermatology Department in Munich, Dr. Tan sent him to the library to decide in what field he would like to spend the 2 years.

In those days he realized that many other and markedly rarer diseases attracted more attention than atopic dermatitis in the dermatological community. So he decided to start here. Later his teacher in clinical dermatology, Prof. Otto Braun-Falco, tolerated this decision although he himself focused on psoriasis; he probably did not like atopic dermatitis so much, since the disease was morphologically too unprecise and "diffuse." However, he always gave freedom to follow the scientific interests, and he accompanied the progress of the work intensively and critically.

At the World Congress of Dermatology (Congressus Mundi Dermatologiae) 1977 in Mexico City, among a program with over a 1000 lectures and posters, there was only one workshop on the subject "atopic dermatitis" chaired by Professors Georg Rajka and Jon Hanifin with about 12 participants. Most of them stayed attracted to this disease in the following decades.

You cannot study atopic dermatitis without touching and questioning the phenomenon of

K. Eyerich, J. Ring, *Atopic Dermatitis - Eczema*, https://doi.org/10.1007/978-3-031-12499-0_1

Table 1.1 Functions of the skin

Frontier
Barrier
• Physical (mechanical, radiation, temperature)
• Chemical
• Biological
• Immunological
Metabolic organ
Immune organ
Organ to express psychologic reactions
Esthetic organ

allergy. In the meantime, the disease—most likely due to the rapid increase in prevalence—has attracted much more followers also in clinical research. Even if 50 years ago the majority believed that allergy does not play an important role in this disease, but dry skin and psychology are the major factors, it became clear that this "atopic" disease cannot be studied without basic knowledge of allergy.

Thus, in the first edition of his allergy book "Angewandte Allergologie" (Allergy in Practice) 1982, JR included a special chapter on atopic eczema. In 1991, the first edition of the "Handbook of Atopic Eczema" (Ruzicka, Ring, Przybilla, editors) appeared, and in 2006 the second edition (Ring, Ruzicka, Przybilla, editors). In 1993, the Minister of Health of the Federal Republic of Germany asked to write an expertise regarding the "health care and prevention in children with atopic eczema," which was finally published as a book in 1998 and gave the start signal to develop an educational program "Eczema School for Parents and Children."

KE is a mentee of JR. His primary interest was the interaction of infiltrating immune cells with resident epithelial cells in chronic inflammatory skin diseases, primarily in AD. When he started doing research in this field in 2001, the concept of Th1 versus Th2 cells started to be investigated in dermatology, in particular in AD. At that time, a switch from Th2 in early AD to Th1 in chronic AD was the most prominent hypothesis. A few years later, this hypothesis was enlarged after the discovery of filaggrin, and AD was more seen as a genetic barrier disease. Early microbiome studies suggested AD to be a disease primarily mediated by microbial dysbalance on the skin; finally, immunologists discovered Th17 and Th22 cells in addition to numerous antigen-presenting cell types. In parallel, genetic methods became more sensitive and genetic studies bigger and bigger, detecting numerous other predisposing factors for AD. The development of highly efficient biologics targeting Th2 immunity as well as advancing methods in immunology such as single-cell techniques subsequently drew a more complex picture of the pathogenesis of AD. Today, we can say that AD is a heterogeneous disease based on an enormously complex pathogenesis—and we are at the step toward realizing precision medicine, the biggest challenge in AD today. Thus, AD perfectly reflects the change and gain of knowledge in dermatology, from a traditionally descriptive toward a molecular discipline.

Why do we need another book on atopic dermatitis?

The state of the art has shown a tremendous increase in knowledge in molecular techniques and experimental dermatology and allergology during the last years. New concepts of individualized and targeted therapeutic approaches allow the vision of totally new treatment and management options.

Beside this progress, there is an urgent need of information for the many affected individuals and physicians as well as health personnel dealing with this disease; it is not enough just to write a prescription! These patients often are "exhausting," they need intense empathy together with ample information about and introduction to causes and individual provocation factors. There is neither a "miracle" injection, "miracle" ointment nor "miracle" pill which applied once will solve the problem forever!

On the other hand, there is no reason to become desperate; we want to fight against the so often used term "incurable" disease. It is true that there is a genetic predisposition with regard to barrier disturbance and hypersensitivity of the skin that gives rise to the formation of eczema, and which at the moment cannot be changed. However, eczema itself can be treated very well, and many patients are symptom-free over decades. They "grow out" of eczema.

Already today, considerable progress has been made in anti-inflammatory basic dermatological and targeted immunological therapies which unfortunately are not accessible to all patients, especially in low-income countries. To illustrate all these developments in a very practical way is one of the aims of this book.

1.2 History

1.2.1 First Descriptions

In most dermatology textbooks, historical reflections on the description of atopic eczema start with Robert Willan who in 1808 used the term "eczema" in a scientific morphological way [866]. The term "eczema" was coined in the sixth century AD by the Greek physician Aetios from Amida who described the boiling and bubbling (eczeo = to bubble up) as it can be observed in the kettle with a boiling soup (Aetios from Amida 1542). Aetios from Amida himself probably did not realize how illustratively he described the modern concept of pathophysiology of spongiosis in those times, namely the intercellular formation of edema starting in the dermis and reaching the epidermis, flooding it with lymph until the occurrence of blister formation [57].

Early descriptions can be found in the book of the Italian physician Girolamo Mercuriali "De morbis cutaneis" with a description of "lactumen" as crusty skin lesions on the scalp [507] which look like burnt milk in a pan and were later called "cradle cap" or—in German—"Milchschorf" (milk crust). Cradle cap is often regarded to be the first manifestation of atopic dermatitis in infants.

The first documented individual patient of history may have been emperor Octavianus Augustus (Fig. 1.1) from the Julian-Claudian emperor family [641] who, as we find in Suetonius' "De Vita Caesarum," was suffering not only from "catarrhal" at the time of spring winds and episodic "tightness of the chest," but also from "tormenting itch" with lichen-like skin changes (which he used to scratch on his back using a long instrument). Also in the Julian-Claudian emperor family, a positive family history (even according to today's standards) can be found with emperor Claudius with perennial rhinoconjunctivitis and Augustus' great-grad nephew Britannicus as a horse-allergic individual [641]. The diagnosis of "eczema" for Octavianus Augustus seems plausible. Unfortunately, the many statues and images are of no help, since they always were idealized and did not represent individual portraits (Paul Zanker, personal communication).

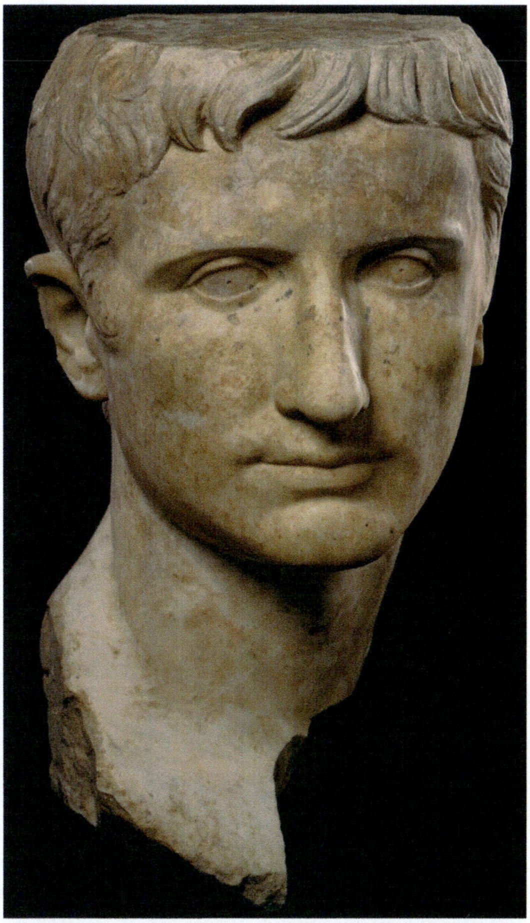

Fig. 1.1 Emperor Octavianus Augustus from the Julian-Claudian emperor family (with friendly permission of P. Zanker)

The great rival of Robert Willan, the French dermatologist at the hospital St Louis, Jean-Louis Alibert, described itchy and oozing skin changes in infants under the name "teigne muqueuse" where teigne, like “tinea,” just meant an inflammatory skin disease [784].

1.2.2 Milestones in the History of Allergy and Eczema

In Table 1.2 the most important milestones of history of atopic dermatitis are listed which also reflect the wide spectrum of names used for this disease.

Erasmus Wilson described in detail an “infantile eczema” and he also included skin changes without blisters as dry eczema. Ferdinand von Hebra, the great Viennese dermatologist, described a “constitutional prurigo” which we today would call prurigo type of atopic eczema.

The great breakthrough came with the French School and was connected with the names Vidal, Jacquet, Brocq, and Besnier. Besnier coined the term “prurigo diathésique“ (“dermatites multiformes prurigineuses chroniques exacerbantes et paroxystiques de prurigo de Hebra“) [60]. For a long time, the disease also was called “Prurigo Besnier.”

Brocq and Jacquet coined the term “neurodermite” [106], focusing on the dry lichenified skin lesions, and by enlarging the lichen simplex chronicus, Vidal gave a name for a similar, more localized eruption. In Germany the pediatrician Czerny coined the term “diathesis” as a concept [155]. Rost defined an “exsudative state,” “früh- bzw. spät-exsudatives Ekzematoid” (“early or late exsudative eczematoid”) [669]. Soon in Germany, the term “Neurodermitis” prevailed, while it was forgotten in France.

The discovery of transferability of allergy with serum by Prausnitz and Küstner [600] and the observation of a familial tendency for certain diseases with the definition of the term “atopy” by Coca and Cooke [142] in the USA led to the inclusion of allergic reactions in the description of this disease. In 1906 the Viennese pediatrician Clemens von Pirquet created the term “allergy” [595]. Today we see allergy as an environmental disease where, on the basis of a genetic predisposition, the organism reacts against environmental substances (Figs. 1.2 and 1.3). Allergy can be regarded as a specific alteration of immune reactivity leading to a hypersensitivity disease [637].

Many dermatologists have problems describing the morphology of this disease due to its wide spectrum and the difficulty to identify a classical primary lesion. Therefore, at national and international congresses, again and again intense debates arose about this disease. In 1933, the American dermatologist Marion Baldur Sulzberger—who had joined Joseph Jadassohn and Bloch in Switzerland—together with Wise, defined the unifying concept of infantile and

Table 1.2 Milestones in the history of allergy since 1870 [658]

Pollen: skin and provocation tests	Blackley	1873
Mast cell	Ehrlich	1877
Neurodermite diffuse	Brocq	1891
Prurigo diathésique	Besnier	1892
Patch test for contact allergy	Jadassohn	1895
Anaphylaxis	Richet and Portier	1902
Allergy	von Pirqueet	1906
Histamine effects mimic anaphylaxis	Dale and Laidlaw	1910
Immunotherapy (prophylactic inoculation)	Noon and freeman	1911
Transfer of hypersensitivity with serum	Prausnitz u Küstner	1921
Atopy	Coca and Cooke	1923
Reagins in atopy	Coca and Grove	1925
Allergic diathesis	Kämmerer	1928
Bronchial hyperreactivity	Tiffeneau	1945
Shock fragment	Hansen	1941
Autonomic nervous dysregulation	Korting	1954
Genetic basis	Schnyder	1960
Types of pathogenic immune reaction	Coombs and Gell	1963
Immunoglobulin E	Ishizaka et al. Johansson et al.	1966/67
House dust mite	Vorhoorst Spieksma	1967
Betablockade in asthma	Szentivanyi	1968
Fc-epsilon receptor	Metzger	1977
Th1-Th2 concept	Mossman	1987
Interleukin 4	Coffman	1988
Filaggrin mutation	McLean and Irvine	2006

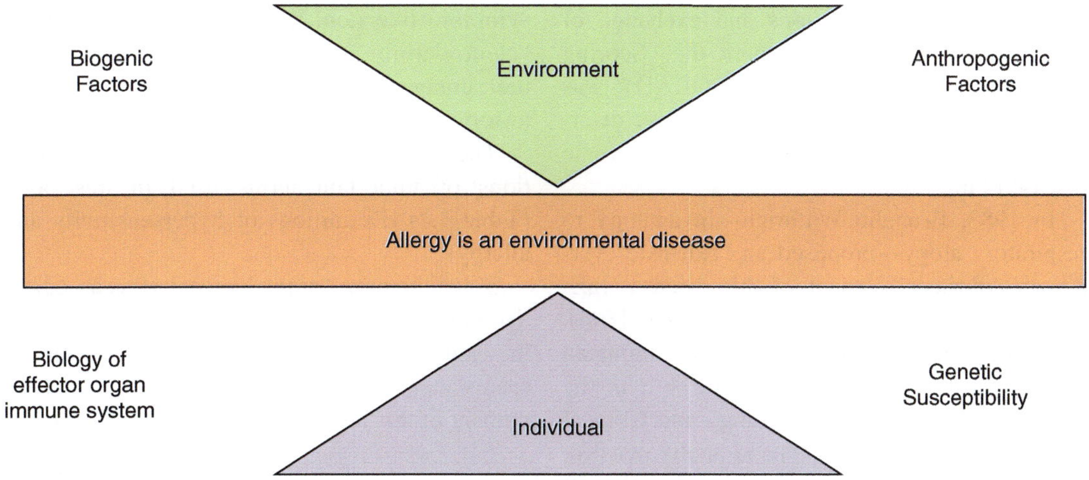

Fig. 1.2 Allergy as environmental disease (according to H. Behrendt)

Fig. 1.3 Not every impairment of feeling well by environmental factors is an allergy

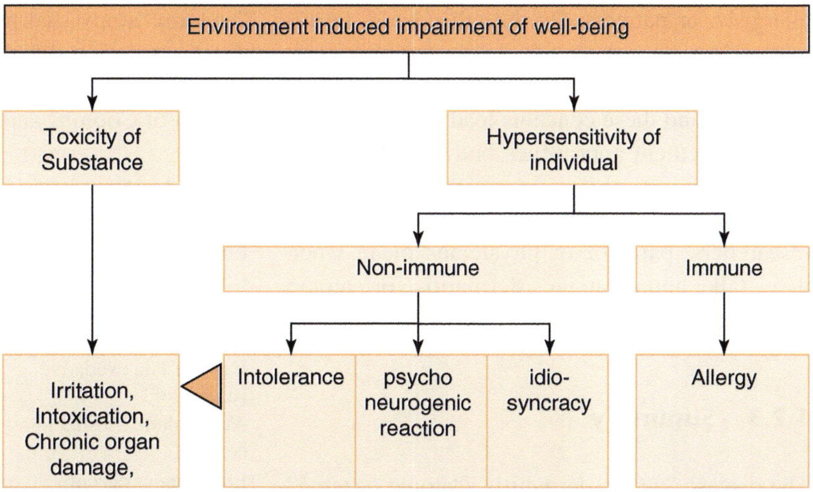

adult disease as atopic dermatitis or atopic eczema [872]. For a long time, this concept was neglected in Europe. Robert Degos in Paris liked the term "constitutional eczema" [175]. In the handbook chapter in the "Jadassohn-Ergänzungswerk," edited by Alfred Marchionini, Urs Schnyder and Siegfried Borelli wrote on "Neurodermitis diffusa constitutionalis sive atopica" [85]. Korting wrote his thesis on "endogenous" eczema where he focused on the abnormal reactivity patterns in the autonomic ("vegetative") nervous system not only affecting the skin but also provoking cardiovascular and even pupillar reactions with an increased cholinergic and decreased adrenergic reactivity [418].

Hans-Jürgen Bandmann was an allergist and dermatologist and a supporter of the term "Neurodermitis" [40]. The transatlantic differences were overcome by the pioneers Georg Rajka in Oslo and Jon Hanifin in Portland/Oregon who, at an international symposium organized by Georg Rajka focusing on atopic dermatitis, developed a consensus on diagnostic criteria which are used until today [305]. These symposia became the platform for researchers and clinicians all over the world interested in atopic dermatitis and a place for free discussions and exchange of information. It was there where the "Scoring System for Atopic Dermatitis (SCORAD)" was conceived and born, allowing an objective determination of various severity grades of this chronic disease [436].

In 1983, Brunello Wüthrich—in analogy to respiratory atopy—proposed an "extrinsic" versus an "intrinsic" variant of this disease (IgE-associated versus non-IgE-associated) [894]. Around the millennium, this conflict culminated in an intense nomenclature debate both in the European Academy of Allergology and Clinical Immunology (EAACI) [371] and finally in a task force of the World Allergy Organization (WAO) [370]. Today the debate on terminology is not led quite so emotionally by many dermatologists, allergists, or patients. On the other hand, terminology is not a matter of sophisticated pickiness, but rather of pathophysiological concepts hidden in names, and these concepts lead to quite different management approaches both in diagnostics and therapy.

Therefore, it is important to understand what researchers, patients, or physicians mean when they talk about atopic dermatitis or atopic eczema.

1.2.3 Summary

The disease "atopic dermatitis"/"atopic eczema" most likely is not new; the term eczema was coined around 600 AD. First descriptions of the disease can be found in the nineteenth century under various names, and only around 1900 the term "Neurodermitis" was clearly differentiated from other types of eczema. In 1933, Wise and Sulzberger proposed the name "atopic dermatitis" or "atopic eczema."

1.3 Terminology

As can be seen from Table 1.3 a variety of names have been used to describe this disease.

All these terms were based on a certain understanding of the disease and a specific emphasis on one or the other aspect, namely a symptom like itch, the nerve component (like "Neurodermite"), the constitutional aspect, and the connection to other allergic diseases (Atopy).

Therefore, it makes sense to give basic definitions of important terms used in this book (Table 1.4) (Definitions of hypersensitivity and allergy).

Since the term "atopy" is central as an adjective in the description of this disease—more than in asthma or rhinoconjunctivitis/hay fever—it seems adequate to briefly comment on the development of this term through the last 100 years.

1.3.1 The Term "Atopy"

The term "atopy" has provoked a variety of interpretations during the almost 100 years following its birth. Atopic diseases, according to the classification of Coombs and Gell, range among type I

Table 1.3 Atopic dermatitis/eczema: names in history

Eczema	Aetios from Amida
Eczema	Willan
Constitutional prurigo	Hebra
Neuroderrmite diffuse	Brocq
Prurigo diathésique	Besnier
Early or late exudative eczematoid	Rost
Atopic dermatitis/atopic eczema	Wise and Sulzberger
Endogenous eczema	Korting
Neurodermitis constitutionalis sive atopic	Schnyder and Borelli
Atopic eczema dermatitis syndrome (AEDS)	Johansson et al. EAACI
Eczema	Johansson et al. WAO consensus JACI 2004

Table 1.4 Definitions of terms in the description of allergy phenomena

Sensitivity	Normal response to a stimulus
Hypersensitivity	Abnormally strong response to a stimulus
Toxicity	Normal harmfulness of a substance
Intoxication	Reaction to normal pharmacological toxicity
Sensitization	Development of increased sensitivity after repeated contact
Allergy	Immunologically mediated hypersensitivity leading to disease

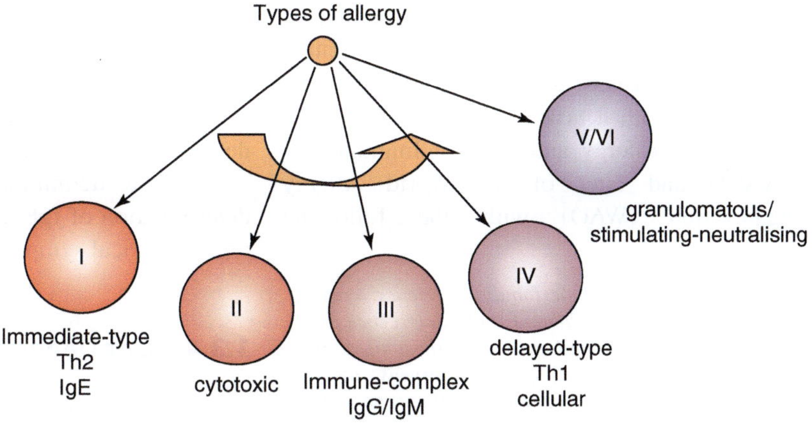

Fig. 1.4 Types of allergic reactions in the classification according to Coombs and Gell modified by Ring

(immediate-type) reactions (Fig. 1.4) with some aspects of type IV [146].

In 1923, Coca and Cooke coined the term "atopy" to describe an "inherited" hypersensitivity against environmental allergens which manifests as asthma or hay fever [142]. Different from other physicians who are not so critical, they knew their limits in philology and asked the Greek philologist Perry from Columbia University in New York to propose a term for this condition. Perry proposed "atopy," meaning "not on the right place, out of order" [57].

Two years later, Coca and Grove proposed the term "atopic reagins" for the substances in serum with which the hypersensitivity of the immediate-type can be transferred according to Prausnitz' and Küstner's experiments (Coca and Grove 1925) [143]. They added this characteristic to the term atopy. Translated into today's language, this means that IgE antibodies are an important part of atopy.

In 1933, Wise and Sulzberger also included the skin manifestations in this spectrum and called it "atopic dermatitis" or "atopic eczema."

In 1943, Coca modified his definition toward "atopy comprising a group of allergic diseases with a common hereditary influence and characterized by atopic reagins."

1.3.2 The Role of Immunglobulin E

After the discovery of immunoglobulin E (IgE) as a carrier of the immediate-type hypersensitivity by the groups of Ishizaka [358] and Johansson [369], atopy was identical with IgE-mediated disease for many authors [374].

However, it soon became apparent that this was too simple. There are individuals with IgE-mediated diseases without family background like IgE-mediated penicillin anaphylaxis or insect venom anaphylaxis [644].

In the 80s, it was J. Pepys who stressed the concept that all human beings or all organisms under certain conditions can form IgE antibodies against protein allergens either after heavy exposure or when they have the "atopic background" in abnormal concentrations.

On the other hand, there are clinically identical diseases also without elevated IgE levels.

According to clinical experience, the disease itself does not differ from "asthma bronchiale" or "non-infectious rhinoconjunctivitis," even if patients do not show IgE-mediated hypersensitivity reactions. Therefore, the term "intrinsic" or "non-IgE-associated" became popular in respiratory atopy and was also used for atopic dermatitis by Wüthrich [894].

1.3.3 Definitions of Atopy Given by EAACI and WAO

The new considerations of subpopulations "atopic" versus "non-atopic," based on the detection of IgE antibodies, were not problematic in respiratory diseases; however, in the description of the skin condition, absurd terms like "non-atopic atopic eczema" appeared. While this was never a serious nomenclature in dermatology textbooks, in international debates these discussions took place, and the necessity was felt to come up with a new atopy definition. This was then started with a task force of the European Academy of Allergy and Clinical Immunology (EAACI) and later of the World Allergy Organization (WAO) with the following definition:

> *Atopy is a personal or familial tendency, commonly starting in childhood and adolescence, to become sensitized and produce IgE antibodies after normal exposure against allergens, commonly proteins. In consequence, these persons develop typical symptoms like asthma, rhinoconjunctivitis or eczema* [370].

According to this definition, all patients with asthma, rhinoconjunctivitis or eczema without detectable IgE antibodies would not suffer from an "atopic" disease. In consequence, this terminology then would lead to an "atopic" versus a "non-atopic" "atopic dermatitis." Therefore, it became necessary to come up with a new name for the skin manifestations of atopy. The EAACI Nomenclature Task Force proposed "atopic eczema dermatitis syndrome AEDS" which aroused intense criticism and was not accepted, not least for lack of logic since the adjective "atopic" again was used for the definition of the atopic disease, and furthermore because of the association with the immunodeficiency syndrome AIDS.

Therefore, the task force of the WAO found consensus by defining the term "eczema" anew in a way that dermatitis is the headline and the term "eczema" defines the disease which before was called "atopic dermatitis" or "atopic eczema." So the adjective "atopic" would only be used when IgE antibodies could be detected [370]. In consequence, there would be an "atopic" versus a "non-atopic" eczema, similar to Wüthrich's extrinsic versus intrinsic variant of atopic dermatitis.

The future will show whether these definitions will be adopted by practicing allergists and dermatologists [88].

The root of the problem in terminology can be found in the endeavor to give ad definition of a clinical symptomatology and at the same time of a pathophysiological mechanism with one term.

Early definitions started with the clinical symptomatology of disease and later included the detection of IgE antibodies.

The WAO definition starts from the laboratory determination of IgE and only later includes the typical clinical symptoms.

1.3.4 Our Definition of Atopy

Our definition from the Handbook of Atopic Eczema starts with the clinical symptomatology:

> *Atopy is a familial tendency to develop certain diseases (rhinoconjunctivitis, asthma bronchiale, eczema) on the basis of hypersensitivity of skin and mucous membranes against environmental agents, associated with increased IgE production and/or epithelial barrier dysfunction.*

Previously, we used "altered nonspecific reactivity" [643]. Today, we want to stress the importance of the barrier problem in atopic diseases, especially in atopic dermatitis, but also in airway allergy.

Therefore, atopy describes on the one hand a subgroup of IgE-mediated diseases (Fig. 1.5), on the other hand, it is more.

With this definition, it is possible to describe intermediate states which can be found in the

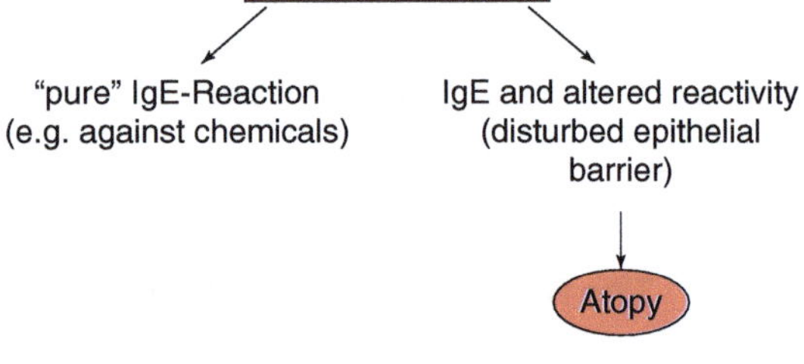

Fig. 1.5 Atopy as a subgroup of IgE-mediated allergy

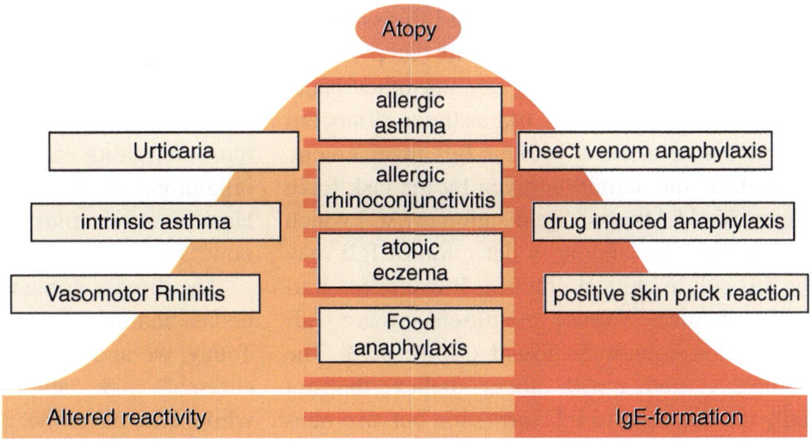

Fig. 1.6 Gaussian distribution of atopic reactivity

type of a "Gauß distribution" of atopic diseases which can be observed when comparing the two dimensions of "increased IgE production" with "epithelial barrier dysfunction" (Fig. 1.6). Where both parameters overlap, there is no doubt of an atopic disease. Toward both sides of the curves however the situation becomes increasingly unprecise with entities such as "latent atopy" (only detection of positive skin tests or IgE antibodies in serum without clinical symptoms) or so-called intrinsic variants of atopic diseases [644].

This dilemma only will be solved when the term "intrinsic" or "non-atopic" will not only be negatively defined by exclusion, but by measurement of a positive marker of this intrinsic variant.

In our experience, the atopy definition from our textbook seems to be more useful for clinical practice.

1.3.5 The Term Eczema

Finally, one also should give a definition of the term "eczema" which has been intensively discussed over the last 200 years since Robert Willan brought it to modern descriptive dermatology. On the basis of many illustrious dermatologists in the past and by intense discussions with colleagues we want to stick to the definition of eczema as given in the first edition:

*Eczema = a non-contagious epidermo-dermitis with typical clinical signs (erythema, papule, vesicle, scales, crusts, nodules, lichenifications *).*
and
characteristic dermato-histopathological changes like akanthosis, parakeratosis, spongiosis, lymphocytic infiltration.
mostly on the basis of skin hypersensitivity.

This definition also holds true for "dermatitis" as it is used nowadays, especially by American colleagues.

Among this definition, several types of eczema/dermatitis can be distinguished, like

Irritative-toxic contact dermatitis/eczema.
Allergic contact dermatitis/eczema.
Atopic dermatitis/eczema.
Seborrheic dermatitis/eczema.
Nummular dermatitis/eczema.
Unclassified dermatitis/eczema.

1.3.6 Summary

The term "Atopy" has been coined in 1923 by Coca and Cooke and since then has changed its meaning several times. The problem is the lack of a clear-cut biomarker. If one uses immunoglobulin E as marker, there are clear-cut IgE-associated diseases which do not belong to "atopy," e.g., insect venom anaphylaxis. On the other hand, there are atopic diseases like asthma, rhinoconjunctivitis or eczema without IgE involvement. Therefore, the definition given by the task force of the World Allergy Organization (WAO) which is based on the laboratory detection of IgE may be difficult in clinical practice. It excludes clinically identical disease conditions where IgE association cannot be found ("intrinsic"). The authors—together with others—believe that not only the tendency to IgE formation but also nonspecific alterations of the epithelial barrier represent a basic feature of "atopy."

The term eczema as a noncontagious epidermo-dermitis (inflammation) of the upper skin parts is around for 1500 years and also understood among the general population. The term dermatitis is actually broader—meaning inflammation of the skin—and less precise. However, it is mostly used in many countries now.

The disease nomenclature of AD is heterogeneous, and numerous terms have been proposed. Today, we and others see the two terms "atopic eczema" and "atopic dermatitis" equivalent, while eczema alone is not sufficiently precise [743].

2 Epidemiology of Atopic Eczema

There is no doubt that atopic eczema has increased in prevalence since the 60s of the twentieth century dramatically in the general population [489, 653, 689, 720, 843]. The reasons for this increase are yet unclear however there are hypothetical concepts (Table 2.1). Significant differences exist in reported prevalences all over the world which only can be partly explained by methodological differences.

Some studies just describe an increase in incidence in the patients of a clinical department or office, others use population-based studies with questionnaires, others require the diagnosis of a physician (dermatologist?). Some population-based studies with actual dermatologic examinations have been performed [696]. Most of these studies describe examinations in childhood; there are only a few data regarding the prevalence of atopic eczema in adults [516, 890]. Clinical examinations usually only represent a point prevalence, while questionnaires can detect cumulative prevalence rates over a lifetime.

Table 2.1 Hypothetical concepts to explain the increase in allergy prevalence

Increased awareness and improved diagnostics
Psychosocial influences (acceleration of daily life)
Allergen exposure
Lack of adequate immune stimulation in early life
Iatrogenic (medications)
Environmental pollution
Climate change

According to general estimations, approx. 3% of adults and 12% of preschool children are affected, with consistently changing numbers between 1% and 25% in the general population [762].

2.1 Prevalence of Atopic Eczema in Childhood

Atopic eczema is the most common noncontagious chronic inflammatory skin disease in childhood with a dramatic increase in prevalence in the last decades.

Early investigations from various countries in the years between 1939 and 1964 indicate a prevalence of 1.3–3.1% in various populations [643]. Studies between 1980 and 2005 show dramatically increased numbers ranging between 26% for questionnaire-based and 32% for actual investigations with dermatological inspections. The highest numbers were detected in the International Study of Allergy and Asthma in Childhood (ISAAC) [30]: in 90 centers, 256,410 children at the age of 6–7 years and 151 centers with 458,623 children at the age of 13–14 years were examined in 56 countries (Figs. 2.1 and 2.2). In these studies, there was a worldwide variation with rather low figures in Albania and Iran and exceeding 20% in the United Kingdom. Generally, the prevalence of atopic eczema seems to be higher in Australia and Northern Europe compared to Asia and Eastern Europe.

K. Eyerich, J. Ring, *Atopic Dermatitis - Eczema*, https://doi.org/10.1007/978-3-031-12499-0_2

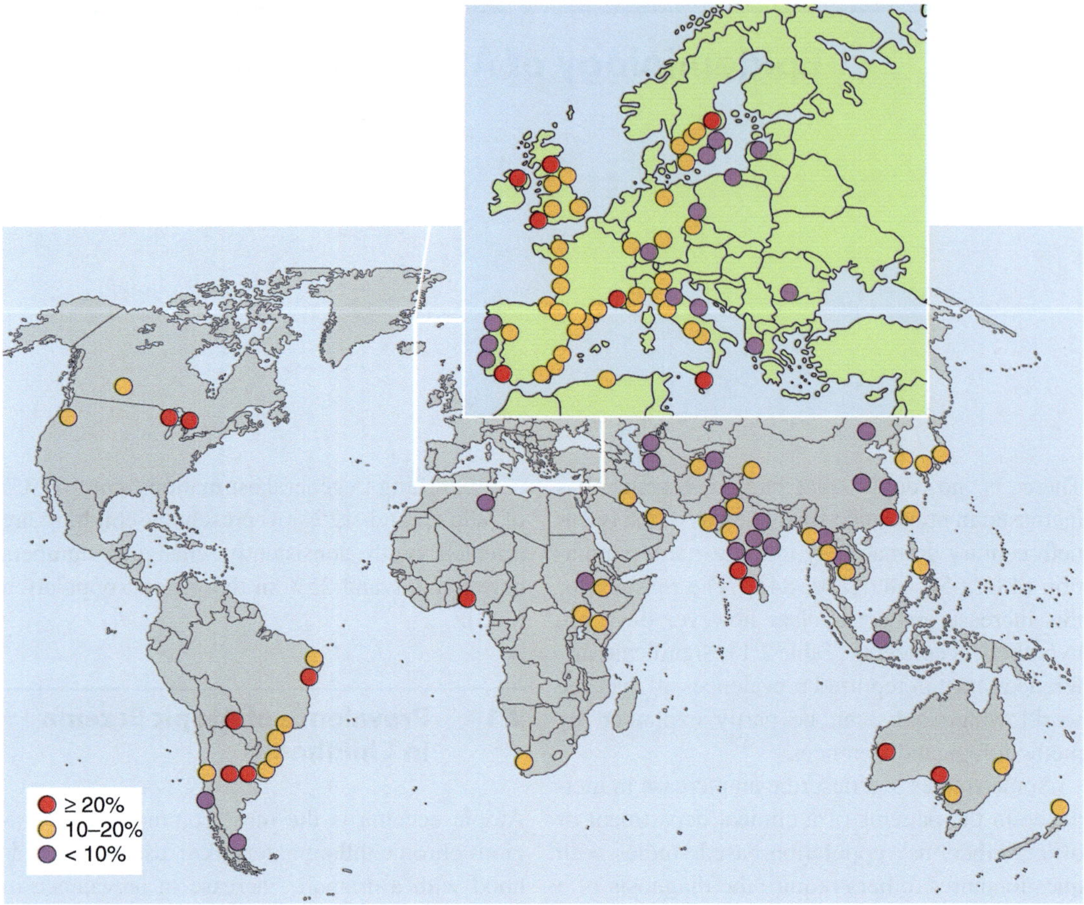

Fig. 2.1 ISAAC study, prevalence of allergic rhinitis worldwide in 13–14 year adolescents [357]

A systematic review showed a high variability of prevalence and incidence of atopic eczema globally with values of prevalence of up to 17% in adults and up to 22% in children [121].

Studies from Germany have been reported in the so-called KiGGS study (Kindergesundheits-Survey) [700] (Fig. 2.3). Contrary to hay fever and asthma [533, 535], atopic eczema showed a higher prevalence in Eastern Germany compared to West Germany (Table 2.2) [696].

Only few studies followed the prevalence rates over longer time periods with a consistent identical methodology: most of them show marked increases in prevalence (Fig. 2.4) [696]. Most of these studies have been performed in Europe. Some of these studies now show a plateau formation or even slight decreases in prevalence in some European countries.

In the KiGGS study (basics) 2003–2006 [404, 700] prevalence rates are given from 10% to 15%

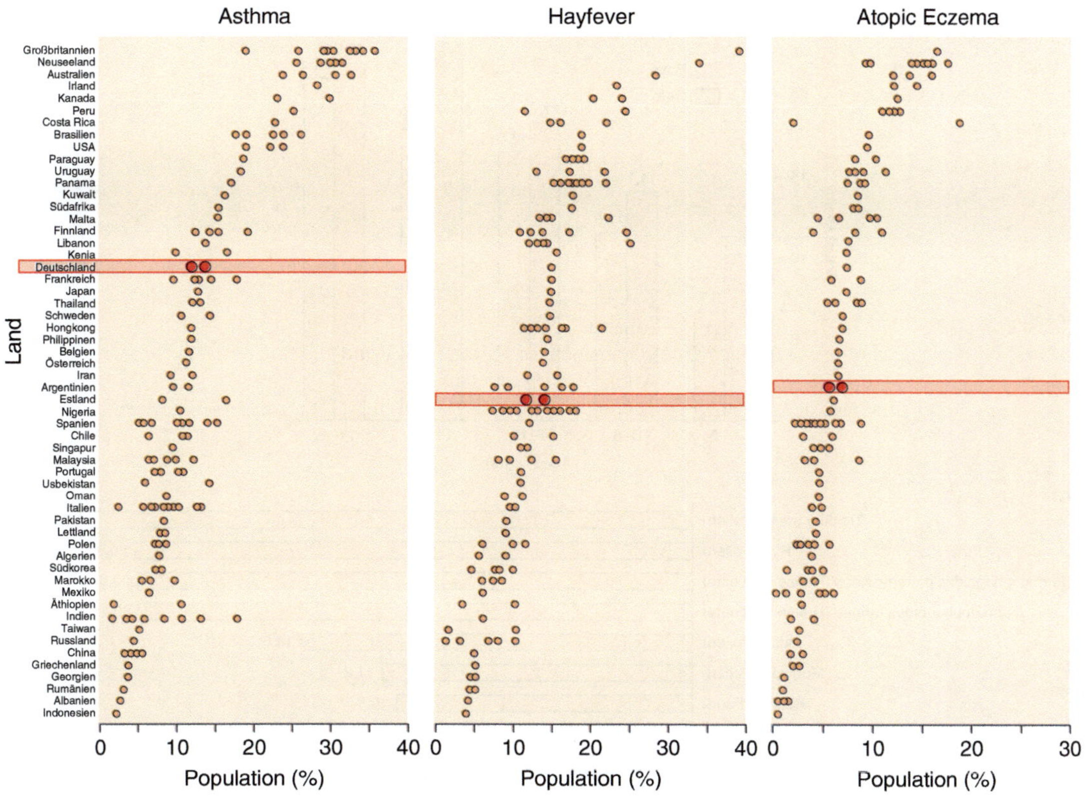

Fig. 2.2 Symptom prevalence of allergic diseases including atopic dermatitis in the ISAAC study in 14-year-old adolescents [356]

with higher values in boys below 2 years of age and in girls over 14 years of age.

In the same study prevalence rates of allergic contact dermatitis ranged between 2,2 and 9,3 in boys and 2,5 and 21,2 in girls, especially at the age of over 7 years of age.

Life-time prevalence rates for atopic eczema in adulthood were given in the DEGS 1-study 2008–2011 [404] from around 7% for young adults (18–29 years) to 1–2% in elderly people over 60. Interestingly, in the age groups of 30–39 years and 50–70 years, there was a significantly higher rate of atopic dermatitis in females within Europe.

Similar data can be found around the world, allergy is a global problem [6, 121].

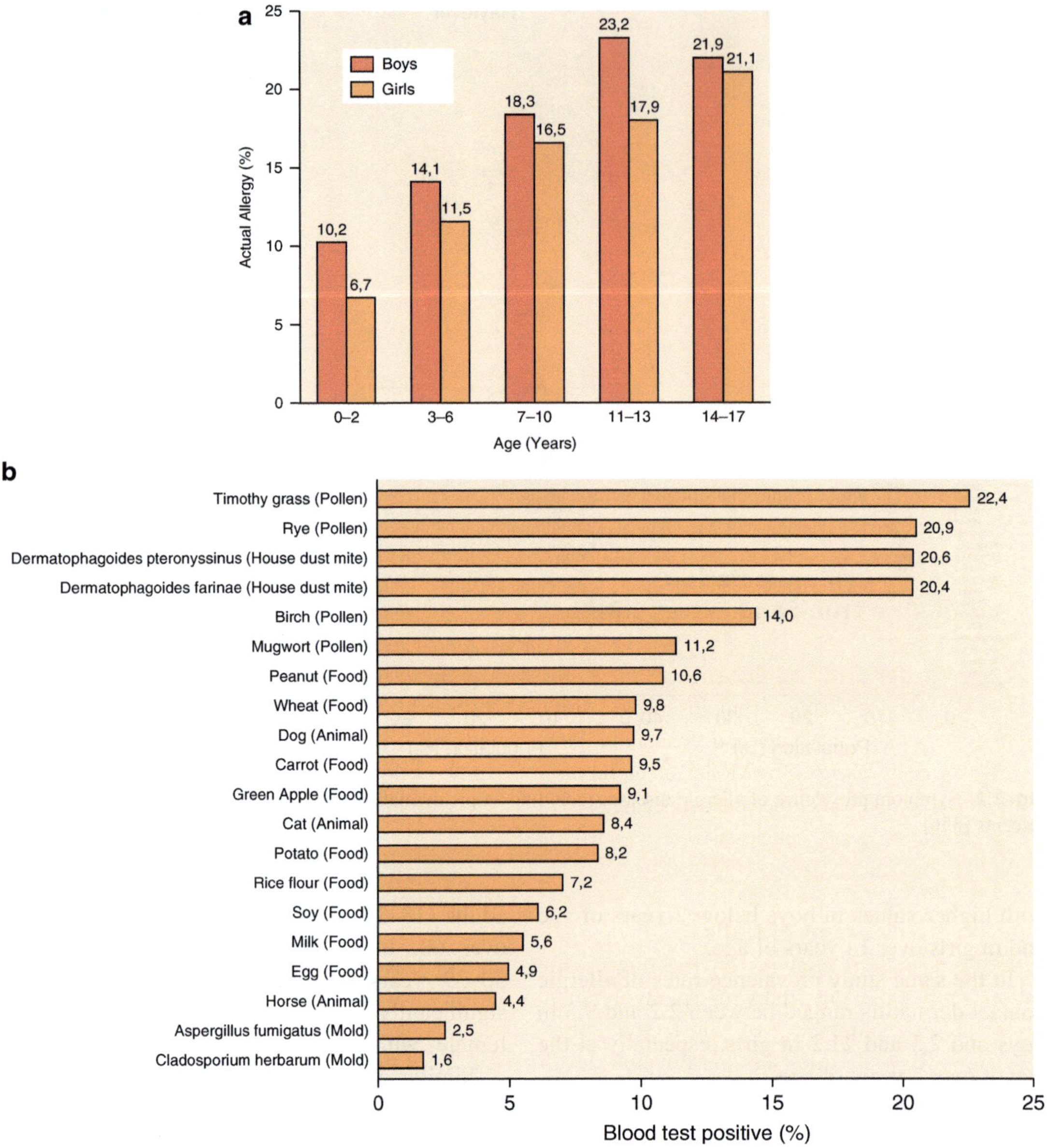

Fig. 2.3 Results of the KiGGs study (Kinder- und Jugendlichen-Gesundheitssurvey) of the Robert-Koch-Institut 2003–2006 in 17.641 children and adolescents (**a**) Doctor's diagnosis of atopic disease. (**b**) Prevalence of sensitization against 20 common allergens

Table 2.2 Prevalence of atopic dermatitis in East and West Germany (n = 1404 children) [694]

West	Prevalence (%)	East	Prevalence (%)
Essen	3.4	Osterburg	7.1
Duisburg North	4.1	Gardelegen	8.4
Duisburg South	6.2	Salzwedel	11.7
Borken	4.9	Halle/Saale	11.2
		Magdeburg	13.8

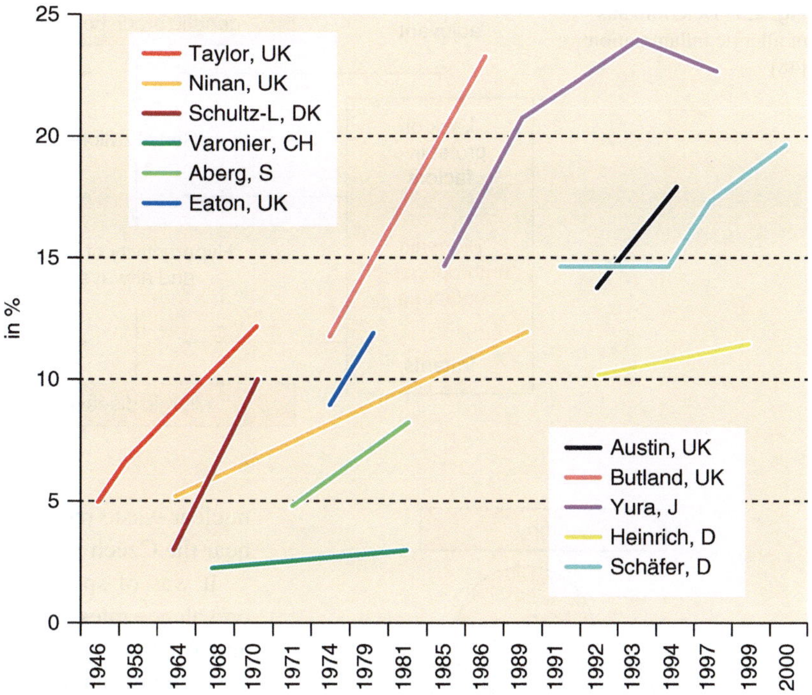

Fig. 2.4 Increase of prevalence of atopic dermatitis in various studies in the second half of the twentieth century [660]

2.2 Causes for Increase in Prevalence

The causes for the increasing prevalence of this disease are still largely unknown. However, there are hypothetical concepts trying to give an explanation (Table 2.1).

Allergic diseases have been increasing in prevalence over the last decades in a dramatic way. The increase started in the "Western World" but has now reached almost all countries around the globe. The first epidemiological studies investigating environmental influences on allergy prevalence were originating in Japan when the group around Terumasa Miyamoto reported that exposure to Diesel exhaust particles was associated with an increased prevalence of hay fever (allergy to Japanese cedar pollen).

Apart from the genetic predisposition with an immunological and an epithelial basis, environmental factors play a role in modulating allergy development in an enhancing or protective manner [48]. Allergen exposure may not be regarded as the only causal factor [27]. A variety of additional substances or factors from the environment can modulate allergy development, in the sense of an enhancement like traffic exhaust with fine or ultrafine diesel particles, tobacco smoke, volatile organic compounds [VOCs] or in a protective way, like infections in early childhood, microbial contacts, and nutrition [46, 48, 150, 201] (Fig. 2.5). Climate change with an increasing tendency toward global warming may additionally contribute to a further increase in allergy prevalence [46, 47].

Deficient training of the immune system by improved hygiene, less infection, and less parasite infestation (IgE antibodies in evolution provided the defense against large intruders) has been summarized under the term "jungle" or "hygiene" hypothesis [69, 324, 424, 769]. Though these hypothetical concepts may be interesting for scientific investigations, they are a debatable basis for practical recommendations. General statements like "dirt is allergy-protective" or "natural infection is healthier than vaccination" have no scientific basis.

The triad of atopic diseases shows large overlaps between eczema, asthma, and rhinoconjunctivitis (Fig. 2.6).

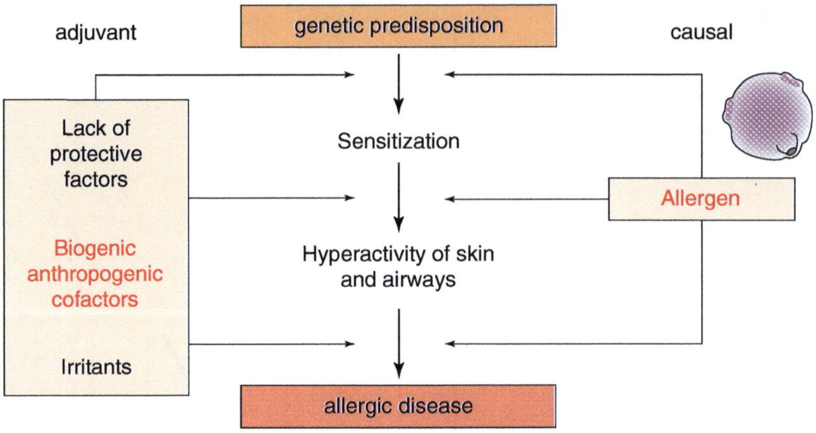

Fig. 2.5 Determinants of allergic inflammation [48]

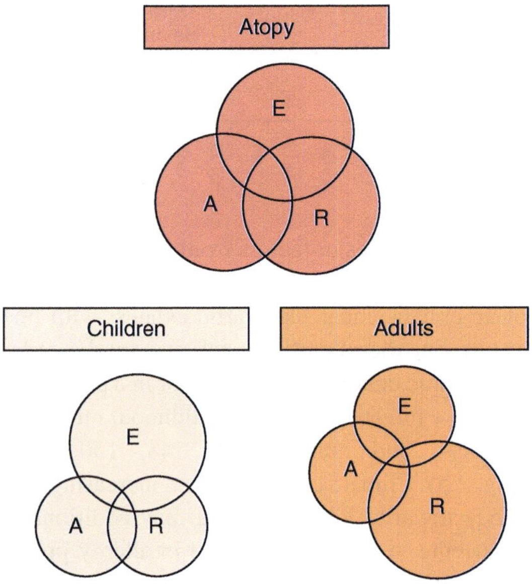

Fig. 2.6 Overlap of three atopic diseases according to lifetime in a Venn diagram

2.2.1 Own Investigations in Comparing East and West Germany after Reunification in 1990

In Germany first epidemiological studies were performed at the end of the 80s starting in North-Rhine-Westphalia where the effect of environmental factors on human health were investigated in the Medizinisches Institut für Umwelthygiene (MIU) in Duesseldorf and in Bavaria where the population was alarmed because of a planned nuclear waste recycling plant in Eastern Bavaria near the Czech border.

It was of special interest to compare allergy prevalence rates and manifestations between East and West Germany, when the iron curtain broke down at the end of 1989. Several groups used this "experimentum dictaturae" with different study designs and different geographical locations and age groups. All these studies however had the surprising result in common that hay fever (allergic rhinoconjunctivitis) was less frequent in East Germany compared to the West. Similar findings were observed in other European areas with a comparison between Estland and Sweden (Björksten).

At the Dermatology Department of the Ludwig-Maximilians-Universität (LMU) in Munich, later at the Department of Dermatology and Allergy at the University Hospital Eppendorf in Hamburg and then at the Department of Dermatology and Allergology at the Technical University Munich, together with the Medical Institute for Environmental Hygiene (now Institut für Umweltmedizinische Forschung IUF) at the Heinrich-Heine-Universität in Düsseldorf since 1988 we have studied over 40,000 children of the age of 5–6 years during the preschool medical examination; these investigations have been performed in various states of the Federal Republic of Germany both in former East and West parts (Bavaria, Northrhine Westphalia, Saxony, Saxony-Anhalt, Hamburg, Schleswig-Holstein) [427, 696, 809]. We found large differences between the different states in Germany, but especially between East and West Germany (Table 2.2) there was a clear-cut increase in the prevalence of hay fever with markedly increasing prevalence rates in East German children during the 10 years from 1991 until 2000.

The rate of atopic eczema was high already, in some parts even significantly higher than in West German children in 1991 [428].

In the following decade after 1990 several studies investigated the prevalence of allergy in allergic diseases in East and West Germany and found a steep increase in allergy prevalence in East Germany within the last decade of the second millennium.

Within these 10 years, allergy prevalence showed convergence between East and West in many aspects with some of the most striking differences disappearing in children who were born after reunification, while the differences were still present in the adult population.

A meta-analysis of total 14 cross-sectional epidemiological studies performed after 1989 and comparing allergy prevalence rates in West and East Germany was performed. The prevalence rates for West compared to East were calculated and compared, certain well-known risk factors were studied with regard to their effect on associations, e.g., exposure to outdoor and indoor pollutants, influences from early childhood with regard to nutrition and awareness.

These cross-sectional studies were done on ca. 120.000 children (8 studies) and 30.000 adults (6 studies). In order to recognize a risk factor as possibly responsible to explain the differences, it had to be

1. Influential in the East-West comparison,
2. more prevalent in exposure in the West compared to the East,
3. in a way that the prevalence rate of the risk factor should converge after reunification during the last decade of the millennium. When the data are individually adjusted for risk factor, the differences between East and West should disappear [428].

The most striking differences were found in pollen sensitization and hay fever in children. There was no difference and no conversions in grass pollen sensitization. In asthma and house dust mite sensitization the differences were smaller.

Both the prevalence of atopic eczema as well as the level of total serum IgE showed an opposite pattern of differences and trends than those observed for airway allergy (hayfever) and pollen sensitization. Atopic eczema and total IgE values were higher in East German children than in the West; these differences also slowly disappeared. In trying to find out which of the well-known risk factors could be responsible for the East-West differences the "explanatory power" was studied for outdoor and indoor air pollutant exposure, early childhood influences, nutrition as well as patient awareness.

In single studies, air pollution has been found as a risk factor. But the classical air pollution type (SO2, coarse particles) was not related to allergy or atopic sensitization. However, outdoor exposure to traffic exhaust was found to be associated with increased rates of airway allergy [428].

Indoor factors like carpets, duvets, and pet keeping were not responsible for the increase in allergy prevalence in East Germany in these studies.

However, single room heating with fossil fuels—so far not a known risk factor for airway disease—was found to be rather protective against allergy development.

Common risk factors discussed in many studies from early childhood—like preterm birth, birth weight, age of mother, absence of breath feeding—were not able to give an explanation for the East-West differences in possible conversion trends. A clear protective effect was found in larger families with more siblings and in children visiting early day-care centers ("Kinderkrippe") which had a lower risk for airway allergy, except an opposite trend for eczema.

Similar worm infestation seemed to be protective and showed a conversion pattern. In a single study pertussis vaccination was found to be protective since pertussis infection was a significant risk factor for the development of airway allergy and asthma.

Another lesson out of this East-West comparison studies is that the time in life seems to be crucial for the effect of environmental influences: effects observed in infants or very young children shortly vanished after reunification while they still prevail until today in adults.

2.3 Atopic Eczema Over Lifetime

One of the most common misconceptions when dealing with atopic dermatitis is the note that it starts "at birth." This is what mothers often say to us; only when we precisely ask "was the baby born with eczema?", the answer is "of course not!." This is a crucial question since there are skin diseases occurring at birth or in the very first days of life which however almost never represent atopic dermatitis. This disease starts later, classically after 3 months, sometimes maybe already after 4–8 weeks. Since the differential diagnosis in neonates is difficult, the term "infantile eczema" (eczema infantum) has been found useful. Apart from genodermatoses (see Chap. 4) and infectious disease, it is mostly seborrheic dermatitis making problems in the differential diagnosis.

Atopic eczema usually is the first manifestation of an atopic disease, later asthma and hay fever develop, also called the "atopic march" (Fig. 2.7).

In probably 80% of cases, atopic dermatitis starts within the first 2 years of life, yet there is an increasing number of patients showing or developing atopic dermatitis in adulthood.

With regard to the developing immune response over lifetime, the "miracle of tolerance" during pregnancy stands at the beginning, in the neonatal period Th2 predominates, during childhood the immune system is stimulated and trained to become mature. In puberty, hormonal influences may play a role (see Chap. 5).

During adulthood, our immune system lives from memory. The first organ to really go into senescence is the thymus which already begins to turn into fatty tissue around the 17th year of life. During senescence, the immune system suffers a loss of regulation and a tendency to develop autoimmune diseases.

2.3.1 Atopic Eczema in Adulthood

Several studies have been performed to determine the prevalence of atopic dermatitis in adulthood.

In 1980, Vickers published a prospective study on 2000 children from the pediatric dermatology department in Leeds with a follow-up of up to 21 years: in around 90% of the children, eczema

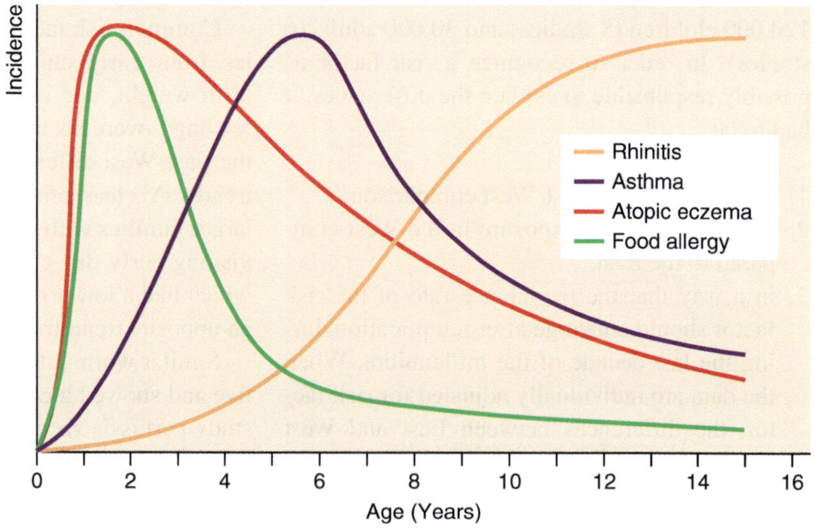

Fig. 2.7 Schematic representation of the course of allergic diseases in the "atopic march"

disappeared and they stayed in remission when they had reached the age of 10 [825]. However, there were critical comments to this study, since it was only one observer who designed the study and examined the children, also the definition of "remission" was not clear. Furthermore—and this is the most crucial critical issue—he also included "eczema infantum" which at first might have been seborrheic dermatitis (see above). Other studies showed a significantly worse prognosis with remission rates of only 10–70% [676]. A retrospective study in Australia in 2600 outpatients comprised 519 patients with atopic eczema; 47% had observed the new occurrence of atopic dermatitis at the age of over 20 years (adult onset, 158 women, 85 men) [41]. The peak of the age group was between 40 and 50 years, but also over 70 years, 10% of newly occurring eczema were found.

The largest study was performed in Berlin as a cross-sectional study involving 13,300 subjects randomly selected at the age of birth to 99 years and in the years 1999 and 2000. This study used telephone interviews and—if there was evidence of skin lesions—a dermatologic investigation. From 1739 answered questionnaires, there was a cumulative 1-year prevalence of atopic dermatitis of 8.4% and a point prevalence of actually existing skin lesions of 1.6% [890].

It is interesting that in the adult onset of persisting eczema, females are generally more frequently affected than males.

A similar study regarding airway allergy in a follow-up of the SAPALDIA population in Switzerland, a self-supported prevalence of allergic rhinitis in subjects over 60 years showed 13.0% for men and 15.4% for women; atopic sensitization had a prevalence of 26.2% in men over 60 years compared to 18.1% in women [896].

Own investigations: between autumn 1991 and spring 1992, an environmental epidemiological trial was performed in Hamburg as the "Project Bille-Siedlung" with a total of 739 persons living in a certain area possibly heavily polluted by chemicals from an industrial factory. In this study we found a point prevalence of 3.4% for atopic eczema in the whole population; in children aged below 14 years, the prevalence was 10.2% whereas adults showed 2.3% prevalence [693].

We found indirectly similar rates in the first epidemiological trials in Bavaria in the years of 1988–1991, where 988 5- to 6-year-old preschool children were investigated; 8.3% suffered from atopic eczema, while the respective mothers and fathers of these children only showed prevalence rates of 4.2, respectively 2.1%. This clearly showed that in the comparison of generations the children suffered twice as often from atopic eczema as their parents. We could observe similar findings for hay fever and asthma.

Manifestation of atopic eczema in adulthood:

When discussing adult atopic eczema, one has to distinguish between

- Persistent atopic eczema since childhood and
- Newly developing atopic eczema in adulthood ("late onset").

The study in Berlin investigating the population with telephone interviews and questionnaires even showed a 10% prevalence of atopic eczema in adulthood [890].

It can be concluded that newly developing atopic eczema in adulthood or even elderly individuals has been little regarded in the literature. Often these conditions may be misdiagnosed as "generalized eczema of unknown origin."

The clinical symptomatology of eczema in adulthood or in the elderly may differ in some way from the classical early-onset childhood atopic dermatitis [132]. A study from Turkey in 63 out of 376 patients with atopic dermatitis who had developed eczema only in adulthood showed that 22% did not fulfill the UK working party's diagnostic criteria, and that 11% had non-flexural involvement, 6% nummular, 3% prurigo-like, and 1.6% follicular patterns [575]. The diagnostic problems in adult atopic eczema were also discussed by Thyssen et al., who found that for severe cases the UK party criteria would work quite well, but there may be difficulties in mild cases or currently asymptomatic individuals [798]. Another study from Greece comparing adult and childhood atopic dermatitis, found that head and neck and hand are more commonly involved in adults, in elderly patients eczematous erythroderma may be common [386]. A study from Poland observed skin manifestations predominantly on the extensor sides of the upper extremities, the neck, and the face with significant lichenification [91]. In patients with low IgE, they found significant immune reactivity against staphylococcal enterotoxin superantigens.

In two-thirds of the patients there was concomitant respiratory atopy, like allergic rhinitis or allergic asthma.

Significantly more females were affected in the adults compared to males.

The majority of the patients suffer from mild to moderate atopic dermatitis; however, in the elderly, eczematous erythroderma may be a feature of atopic dermatitis.

In a large study, it was found that adult onset eczema is not as rare as presumed from the literature. Of adult-onset patients, only 38% had already been suffering from atopic dermatitis as children [4]. Also pathophysiologically there seem to be differences with a more pronounced role for IgE and filaggrin deficiencies in childhood eczema.

2.4 Clinical Course and Prognosis

The general public, but also many physicians believe that atopic eczema is a disease that mostly disappears during childhood ("the child will grow out of it"); however, this unfortunately only holds true for a part of the affected individuals (Fig. 2.8).

In studies following the long-term clinical course, variable rates of cure have been observed between 37% in Zurich [398] and 84% in a study by Vickers [825].

A very differentiated study by Kissling and Wüthrich showed that principally three types of clinical course of atopic eczema can be distinguished (Fig. 2.8):

- In one-third of patients, eczema will disappear in early childhood.
- In another third of patients, eczema is lost until puberty however will appear later again.
- One last third of patients will be affected from childhood into adulthood continuously by atopic eczema [398].

The prognostic factors are only poorly known. High IgE levels in serum, concomitant existence of atopic respiratory disease as well as strong psychosomatic involvement seem to be risk factors for a longer persistence of eczema.

Development of asthma: the more severe the atopic eczema in infants, the higher the risk of asthma development in childhood. In a study by Gustafsson et al. with 94 children with atopic eczema, 30% of children with mild eczema developed asthma and 25% allergic rhinitis, while children with severe atopic eczema developed asthma after 8 years in 70% and hay fever in 90% [289].

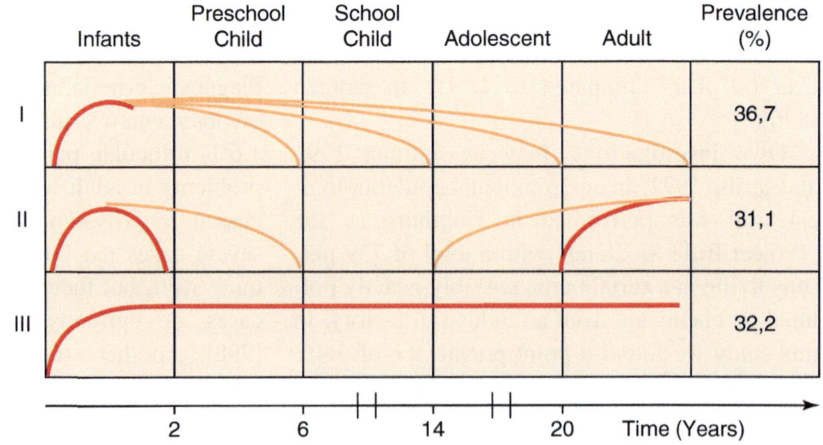

Fig. 2.8 Long-time observation of the clinical course of atopic dermatitis over 20 years (From Ref. [398])

Lauffer et al. elaborated three endotypes of atopic eczema patients with characteristic inflammatory markers; in the same study, they noted that certain clinical and molecular features seem to predict long-term persistence of eczema [446].

2.4.1 Intrinsic Versus Extrinsic Eczema

Intrinsic variant: for many physicians the detection of IgE-mediated sensitization is the crucial diagnostic step in the diagnosis of atopic eczema (see Chap. 1). However, there is no doubt that there are typical cases of atopic eczema without detectable IgE levels or specific IgE sensitization in blood or in skin prick test. This so-called intrinsic variant [517, 553, 701, 895] is not very well investigated. It might be that specific IgE antibodies are present in low concentrations, but not detectable because they are directed against allergens which are so far unknown, e.g., microbial allergens from S. aureus on the skin [552]. Another hypothesis is that these sensitizations only develop during lifetime. There are few studies regarding the exact prevalence of these two subvariants of atopic eczema [895].

The intrinsic variant is more common in children than in adults as generally estimated. In a study in the city of Augsburg (MIRIAM), we found significant differences with regard to gender: the intrinsic atopic eczema was significantly more prevalent in girls than in boys (Fig. 2.9) [517]. In East-West comparison of the large study comprising children just starting school (Schulanfängerstudie West-Ost, SAWO), the intrinsic variant was more common in East German children than in the West [427]. Taïeb observed that children with milder manifestations less often showed IgE-mediated reactions which were generally present in severe atopic eczema [783].

Many authors tried to improve the definition of the subpopulation of "intrinsic atopic eczema," but this was found to be difficult. Generally, it seems that intrinsic eczema begins later in life and shows a milder severity and less skin barrier disturbance—which is very surprising! Among the atopy stigmata, intrinsic eczema often shows Dennie-Morgan folds, but rarely ichthyosis vulgaris or palmar hyperlinearity. It was speculated that intrinsic eczema is triggered not so much by protein allergens and Th2 responses, but maybe other antigens play a role [800].

However, activation of all T cell subpopulations including Th2 has been found in a study comparing extrinsic and intrinsic atopic dermatitis in adult patients. In intrinsic atopic dermatitis, there was a higher activation of all inflammatory

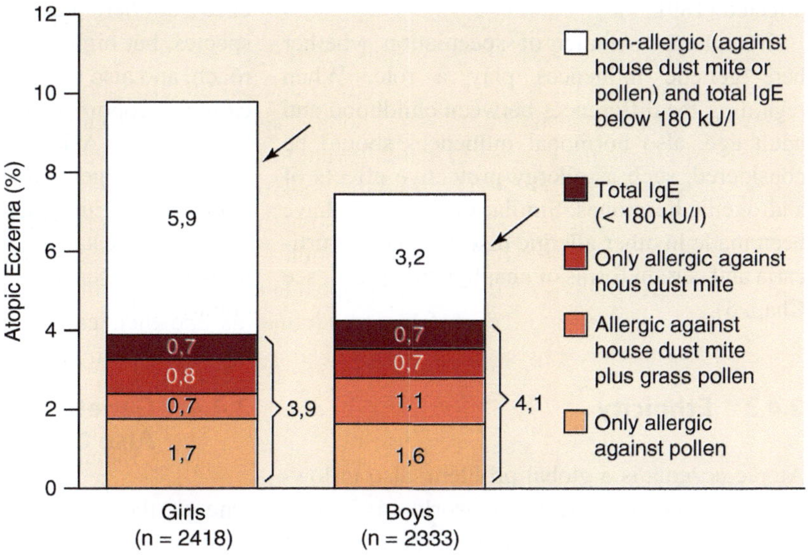

Fig. 2.9 Intrinsic and extrinsic atopic dermatitis in childhood: intrinsic variant is more common in girls than boys [517]

cells including Th2, but particularly Th17 and Th22 cells [774].

Gene expression studies using microarrays and protein-protein interaction (PPI) mapping from skin biopsies of extrinsic atopic dermatitis patients showed the following gene classes to be specially activated:

- Extracellular matrix and cell adhesion-related genes.
- ATP-, GTP-binding genes.
- Immune response genes.
- Proteolytic enzyme genes.
- Structural genes [468].

Thomas Bieber therefore postulated that atopic eczema always starts as an "intrinsic" condition, possibly on the basis of a disturbed skin barrier function (see Chap. 3, "Disturbance of Skin Barrier"), and that the IgE-mediated sensitizations only develop later in life [64, 241, 557, 558]. He believes that intrinsic atopic eczema in adult males is an absolute rarity.

2.4.2 Gender Differences

In adults, the female gender is slightly more commonly affected with estimated numbers between female to male of 1,1:1 till 2:1 [314, 715] In early childhood however boys seem to be more often affected [189].

It remains a matter of speculation whether here genetic influences play a role. When regarding the differences between childhood and adult age, also hormonal influences should be considered, such as allergy-protective effects of androgenic hormones. Similar observations have been made in other allergic diseases such as urticaria and certain forms of anaphylaxis ([136], see Chap. 5).

2.4.3 Ethnicity

Atopic eczema is a global problem, also in low-income countries around the world [447, 483, 772]. Of course in these countries, there are a lot of other problems with severe infections, e.g., leprosy or HIV. Yet in the daily life of practicing doctors, health medical officers, or nurses dealing with skin problems, atopic dermatitis is among the most time-consuming problems.

Although the diagnosis usually is no problem, based on clinics and history with regard to family or personal history of atopy, together with strong itch sensation, there are some obvious morphological—and maybe also pathophysiological—differences. A meta-analysis of 101 studies evaluating the prevalence and phenotype of AD all over the world came to this conclusion: "The most prevalent AD features were pruritus, lichenification, and xerosis." There were differences in AD characteristics by study region. Flexural involvement was less commonly reported in India, the Americas, and Iran. Studies from East Asia reported more erythroderma and truncal, extensor, scalp, and auricular involvement. Studies from Southeast Asia reported more exudative eczema, truncal involvement, lichenification, and prurigo nodularis. Studies from Iran reported more head, face, and neck involvement; pityriasis alba; and xerosis. Studies from Africa reported more papular lichenoid lesions, palmar hyperlinearity, ichthyosis, and orbital darkening. [902]. Typically, the epidermal involvement so characteristic for eczema in people of color is not red as in Caucasian skin, but grey ("ashy").

Also the immune signature may show differences, so there was much less IgE to Malassezia species, but higher levels for storage mite, cockroach, and also seafood in Moshi, Tanzania, indicating tropomyosin cross-reactivity [439]. Furthermore, Asian AD and African AD might have a stronger Th17 immune component as compared to European AD [154].

Still the established diagnostic scoring systems for measuring severity also work on skin of color [227].

2.4.4 Genetic Predisposition (See Also Chap. 5)

One of the most relevant risk factors for the development of atopic eczema is the genetic predisposition, which is so often manifest and already included in the definition of atopy [142].

In classical genetics, the risk increases with the number of parents affected: with only one parent atopic, there is an approximate risk of 30% for the child to develop eczema, with 2 parents atopic the risk is around 50%. If both parents are suffering from eczema, this leads to a further increase up to 70 or 80% (Table 2.3). This could also be in descendant family history (Table 2.4). Also, this illustrates that not only the pathophysiological phenomena like deviated immune response or epithelial barrier dysfunction are genetically determined but also the manifestation organ, namely the skin or the airways.

Numerous studies have found similar figures with different approaches and in different populations. Some found a more pronounced effect of maternal predisposition compared to paternal (Schaefer 2000), others could not observe this and found an equal influence of maternal and paternal atopic constitution upon the offspring.

More will be explained under the chapter "pathophysiology" (Sect. 5.1).

Table 2.3 Atopy prevalence in children and parental atopy [399] (percent in 12th years of life)

Parents	Atopy prevalence (%)
No atopy	10–15
One parent atopic	20–30
Two parents atopic (different manifestations)	30–40
Two parents atopic (same manifestation)	60–80

Table 2.4 Incidence of atopic eczema in children from families with atopic eczema in one or both parents [812]

Partners of patients with atopic eczema	N (families)	N (children)	Children with atopic eczema
Parents of partners non-atopic	164	321	180 (56%)
Atopic eczema	26	59	48 (81%)
Respiratory atopy	80	149	88 (59%)
Total	270	529	316 (60%)

2.4.5 Socioeconomic Status

The influence of socioeconomic status upon the development of atopic diseases has been investigated by several authors [182]. Usually, there was a positive linear correlation between the parameters "socioeonomic status" and "prevalence of hay fever or allergic asthma" or "atopic sensitization." Also, with regard to atopic eczema, there was a significant association with a higher socioeconomic status in affected adults.

A study from Hannover investigated 4219 children just starting school and found a significant correlation of atopic eczema to maternal education or paternal occupational categories [855]. The reasons for this influence of socioeconomic status on allergy development are unclear; some authors speculate about exaggerated hygiene procedures in these families (see below).

"Western lifestyle": It would be wrong to conclude from these data that atopic eczema is a disease of the "rich" only [867]. Own experiences in Central Sub-Saharan Africa as well as from inner-city slums in US-American metropoles observe a high incidence of atopic diseases and also of atopic eczema in children investigated [231, 702].

Western lifestyle seems to favor allergy-enhancing factors [47]. A study from a very remote island in Papua New Guinea showed that in the center of the island of Karkar where people still live in a very original way (no electricity, no houses, etc.) there are no allergies, while in villages closer to the sea, allergies are known, and in villages at the seashore with more Western influence, prevalence rates of 6–8% can be observed (Table 2.5) [323].

Also the number of children seems to influence the rate of atopy [569, 609, 769].

Table 2.5 Prevalence of atopic diseases in various villages on the island of Karkar (Papua New Guinea) [323]

		(%)
Center of island (naïve conditions)	Karmok	0
Between center and shore	Did	2.4
Shore villages (some Western influence)	Kurum	8.1
	Gaubin	7.7
	Kavailo	6.7

A conservative lifestyle (like, e.g., living on a farm, in an Amish or in an anthroposophical family) seems to protect against allergy development in children [21, 94].

Often socioeconomic aspects overlap with problems of ethnicity. People even talk about "structural racism" when they describe worse living conditions and elevated risks for diseases, also allergic diseases in ethnic minority groups [782]. In a large UK-based study exploring over four million people from databases there was a significantly increased risk for developing hay fever and atopic eczema in three ethnic minority groups, while there was no difference in asthma [775].

2.4.6 Psychosomatic Influence

One of many lifestyle factors also includes the psychosocial interaction which may influence the development of allergy and atopic eczema. The strong psychosomatic influence on clinical manifestation and course of this disease is reflected in the name of the disease in German-speaking countries, "Neurodermitis," although the term was originally derived from French dermatology (see Chap. 1).

There is no doubt that psychologic factors are able to influence considerably the clinical course of eczema, both in a positive and in a negative way [118, 266]; in families with parental disharmony (continuous quarreling, separation, divorce) the eczema rate is significantly elevated.

In an ongoing birth cohort study, also parameters of "life events" were investigated such as severe disease or death of a family member, unemployment, marital problems, or divorce of parents. There was a reduced risk for atopic eczema in families with other severely sick family members. At the same time, there was a significantly increased risk of developing atopic dermatitis when parents were separated or divorced (OR 3.59, CI 1.6–7.6) (Table 2.6) [75, 705].

Another study showed a clear-cut association of stress with symptoms of atopic dermatitis by increased expression of nerve growth factor-reactive cells in epidermis and dermis, and intensity of neuropeptide Y-positive cells as a parameter of anxiety and stress-inducing pruritus [565].

Table 2.6 Life events in the family and risk of atopic eczema in the offspring: results of the LISA birth cohort study [75]

Life event	Odds ratio (OR)	Confidence intervals (CI)
Severe disease of a family member	0.29	0.1–0.7
Separation/divorce of parents	3.59	1.6–1.7

Psychosomatic factors do not only influence the course of existing eczema but might also be of relevance in the early initiation and triggering of first symptoms. Social and psychosocial aspects influence the severity of the disease, in a way that depression both can be a consequence of eczema, but also act as a trigger or exacerbating factor [907].

2.4.7 Pregnancy

A study from Denmark reported that prolonged gestation periods go along with an increased risk of atopic eczema in children (over 40 weeks compared to 39–40 weeks; OR 1.32, CI 1.06–1.63) [570].

2.4.8 Hygiene, Infectious Disease, and Vaccinations

The general aspects of the so-called hygiene or jungle hypothesis (see above) are discussed elsewhere. The question of a possible benefit or risk of vaccination is controversially discussed.

2.4.8.1 Measles

In a large study from Denmark, 9744 children of age 3–15 years were investigated for the influence of measles. The majority of children (93.3%) had received measles vaccination. Five percent had suffered from a measles infection. In children who were vaccinated against measles, mumps, and rubella, there was an increased eczema incidence (OR 1.64; CI 1.24–2.16). On the other hand, the risk of atopic eczema was even higher in the group of those children who had suffered measles infections (OR 1.91; CI 1.04–3.51) [572]. Discordant results have been reported with regard to a measles infection leading to either an increase or a decrease in the incidence of atopic eczema [64].

2.4.8.2 Pertussis

In our own investigations comparing East and West German preschool children, we found that vaccination against Bordetella pertussis, which was obligatory in the 80s in the former East German Democratic Republic GDR, while it was only accepted by approx. 75% of West German parents, was a decisive factor. We found a significant protective effect against the development of atopic respiratory diseases, especially bronchial asthma [270]; after adjusting the East-West differences for the factor "pertussis vaccination," the East-West differences observed earlier in prevalence of respiratory airway disease disappeared. There was no influence of pertussis vaccination with regard to atopic eczema.

2.4.8.3 Smallpox (Variola Vera)

Until 35 years ago, the vaccination against smallpox with vaccinia antigen was considered a contraindication in individuals with atopic eczema because of the dramatic condition of "eczema vaccinatum" which represented a generalized blistering disease with possible life-threatening consequences. Therefore, it was impossible for many European young people to travel to the USA where smallpox vaccination was mandatory. In the late 70s of the twentieth century, the veterinary virologist A. Mayr, together with Helmut Stickl, the director of the Bavarian Vaccination Institute (Bayerische Landesimpfanstalt), developed a new vaccine against smallpox using an attenuated virus (modified virus Ankara MVA) which could be applied subcutaneously, while the classical smallpox vaccination had to be applied by scarification to the epidermis [332] and dated back to 1807, when Bavaria was the first country in Europe to install an obligatory vaccination program against smallpox.

Immunogenicity of this MVA vaccine was excellently measured by humoral and cellular immune responses against smallpox antigen. The safety was dramatically better. Among approx. 100,000 persons vaccinated with MVA only few severe side effects were observed [496]. With the declaration of the official eradication of smallpox at the end of the 80s (in 1987), smallpox vaccination was no longer necessary or recommended.

After September 2001, concerns of bioterrorism using still available smallpox strains (in high safety labs in the USA and Russia) gave rise to study the risk of smallpox vaccination for high-risk population groups (soldiers, medical personnel, especially dermatologists). In a prospective study in various volunteers with or without atopic diseases including atopic eczema, the MVA vaccine was found effective and safe in in vitro measurements [163].

2.4.8.4 COVID-19 Infection and Vaccination

At the moment there is little evidence that SARS-CoV-2 infection increases the risk for eczema development or exacerbations—although this would not be too surprising. Other inflammatory diseases have shown exacerbations after COVID-19 [253]. There are even case reports that SARS-CoV2 infection might ameliorate eczema [126]. The situation regarding COVID-19 vaccination is a matter of discussion among lay people. However, several societies have given clear recommendations and position statements on the risk of anaphylaxis or severe allergic reactions in patients with atopic eczema or other allergic diseases [35]. The message is that people with AE can well be vaccinated. Contraindications may be seen in patients with prior history of anaphylaxis to ingredients of the vaccine to be applied.

2.4.8.5 Vaccination Recommendations

Considering the actual controversial data and in the light of a rather high risk of certain infectious diseases, it makes sense to recommend the common vaccinations also for persons with risk of atopy [233, 855] (see also Chap. 8 "Prevention").

2.4.9 Nutrition (See Also Chap. 8 "Prevention")

When discussing the influence of nutrition, one has to differentiate between effects upon initiation of development on the one hand and triggering of exacerbations of eczema on the other.

2.4.9.1 Breast Feeding

Most studies are available with regard to the effect of breastfeeding [423]. A meta-analysis showed a significant preventive effect [258]. However, it should not be left unconsidered that there are studies which do not show this effect or even show a higher risk of atopic eczema in breastfed infants.

2.4.9.2 Maternal Nutrition and Baby Formula

Alterations of maternal diet during pregnancy or lactation has no significant effect on eczema prevalence as has been shown in a recent Cochrane review [425].

From the results of the German Infant Nutritional Intervention Study (GINI) it became obvious that there was a significant preventive effect of certain hypoallergenic formulas [54, 55] on the development of atopic eczema.

2.4.10 Polyunsaturated Fatty Acids and Probiotics

The role of polyunsaturated fatty acids (PUFA) has been studied in Australia where positive effects in the prevention of atopic eczema by addition of PUFA have been found [195], but omega-6 fatty acids may have an allergy-enhancing effect [892].

Already in early East-West European studies, the role of intestinal microflora has been stressed [70]. Recent interesting results show a preventive effect of prebiotics (oligosaccharides) [282]. The preventive effect of probiotics (e.g., Lactobacillus GG) has been studied mainly in Finland [359, 379] however has not been reproduced by other groups in a significant way.

2.4.11 Peanut Oil

A study from England supported the hypothesis that peanut allergy is enhanced by applying peanut oil contained in bath oils in young children [437]; however, there is no quantitative measurement of the specific skin care procedures with regard to the amount of peanut oil applied. Furthermore, one must know that in refined peanut oil there are no measurable concentrations of peanut protein and even less of peanut allergen which makes this hypothesis rather unlikely with regard to practical relevance [655].

2.4.12 Skincare

The hygiene hypothesis supports the concept that too much or too intensive procedures in baby care may contribute to eczema development by changing the cutaneous microbiome. However, the fact that pathogenic microbes like Staphylococcus aureus are colonizing atopic skin and probably can act as triggers of eczema also has to be considered (see Chap. 7).

There is agreement that contact with irritative effecets for the skin—like wool contact or too strong cleansing procedures should be avoided [877].

There is a controversy with regard to the effect of emollient application as primary prevention soon after birth since some studies have shown beneficial effects [870]; however, recent larger studies did not confirm these results [128] (see also prevention Chap. 8).

2.5 Lifestyle

2.5.1 Living on a Farm

The clear-cut protective effect for children growing up on a farm with regard to development of atopic diseases [94, 201, 532] is true for respiratory allergies and especially when the mother had been working on the farm or in the stable during pregnancy or the children had been drinking fresh warm milk directly from the cow. For atopic eczema, there is a study showing an effect with regard to the diversity of foods introduced during the first year of life, especially yogurt showing a preventive effect with regard to the development of atopic eczema [662].

2.5.2 Pet Keeping

In allergy textbooks, until the 90s was like a dogma "fur and feather bearing animals have to be avoided!" This only holds true today for the cat which still are regarded as risk factors. New studies have shown that dog keeping bears not so much risk or, on the contrary, even a protective effect, while cats are still regarded as a risk factor for the development of atopic diseases and atopic eczema. These studies were commented in lay newspapers with the headline "Snuffy the Dog found not guilty" (*"Freispruch für Schnuffi"*). It has to be mentioned that these data are still controversial and that in families genetically predisposed for atopy pet keeping is significantly less common; it may be possible that there is an effect of "reversed causality."

2.5.3 Environmental Pollutants

There is no doubt that exposure to air pollutants can influence the development of atopic diseases [685].

2.5.3.1 Environmental Tobacco Smoke

In the indoor air, it is mainly exposure to tobacco smoke which is of relevance. In an own large epidemiological trials, MIRIAM (Multicenter International Study On Risk Assessment of Indoor and Outdoor Pollution on Allergy and Eczema Morbidity) we could show that exposure to tobacco smoke (measured as cotinin in the urine of the children) was highly significantly associated with the development of atopic eczema, especially in families where one parent already was suffering from an atopic disease [426] (Fig. 2.10). This study supported earlier reports where we found that "smoking during pregnancy" was enhancing the atopy risk of children significantly [690].

2.5.3.2 Nitrogen Oxides

In the indoor air also nitrogen oxides are present, especially when gas is used for cooking or heating water; this could be shown in studies in East German children with a significantly elevated prevalence of atopic eczema associated with the use of gas indoors [427].

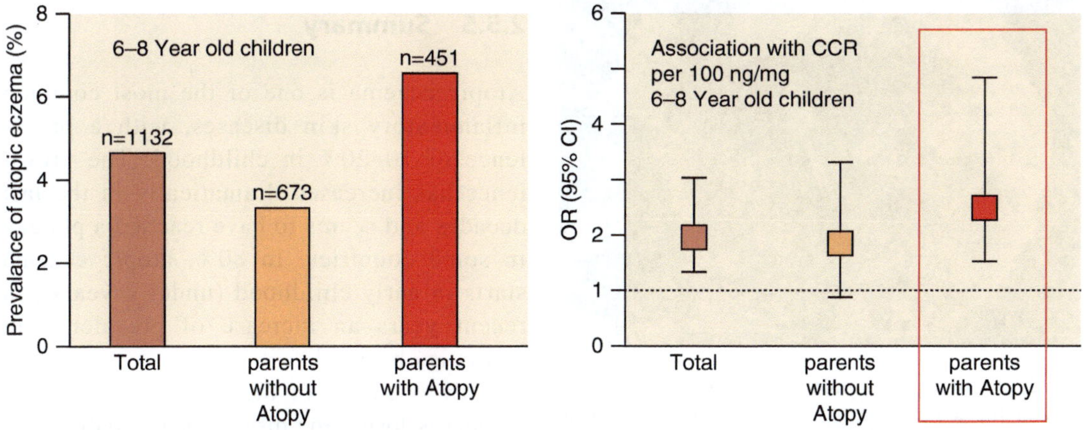

Fig. 2.10 Atopic eczema and tobacco smoke exposure measured by Cotinin-creatinin Ratio (CCR) in the urine of school beginners (MIRIAM study Augsburg 1996–1998), *OR* odds ratio, CI coincidence interval, Krämer et al. [426]

2.5.3.3 Traffic Exhaust

In the outdoor air, traffic exhaust seems to be the most important risk factor. Children growing up near a heavy-traffic road show significantly elevated incidence rates of atopic eczema (Fig. 2.11) [422]. Similarly, exposure to truck traffic showed the same effects [49, 850]. Experimental investigations by Behrendt et al [47] showed that pollutants in the outdoor air can lead to changes in the pollen surface and lead to the liberation of pollen grain constituents (Fig. 2.12) of possible relevance for allergy development.

A detailed study in the city of Munich showed a significant and dose-dependent increase in the prevalence of atopic diseases, also atopic eczema, in clear association to exposure to fine dust particles [522]. In animal experiments, allergic inflammation was enhanced over many days by pre-exposure to fine or ultrafine particles before allergen application [17, 790]. This effect was most likely due to oxygen radical formation by fine and ultrafine particles, since antioxidant treatment could diminish inflammatory changes in mice lungs [17].

A study from Korea showed a clear-cut association of traffic exposure, measured as NOx or Particles exposure to elevated rates of atopic eczema, marginally also for hay fever [511].

Taken together there are many environmental factors influencing the initiation and development until manifestation of atopic eczema which can be regarded as the "envirome" [116].

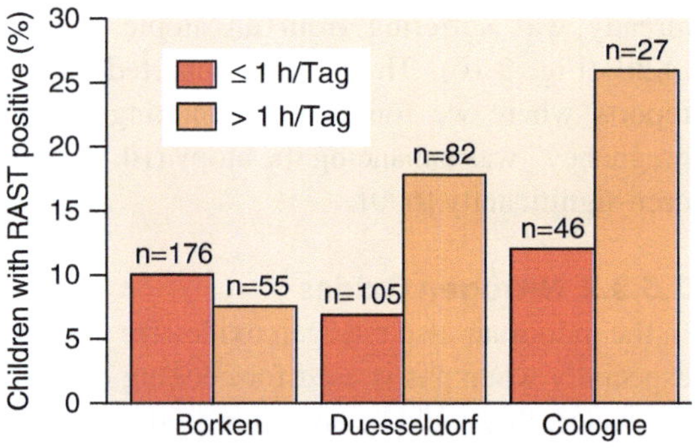

Fig. 2.11 The prevalence of allergic sensitization depends upon traffic exposure: investigations in 5–6 – year-old children in May 1988 [422, 424]

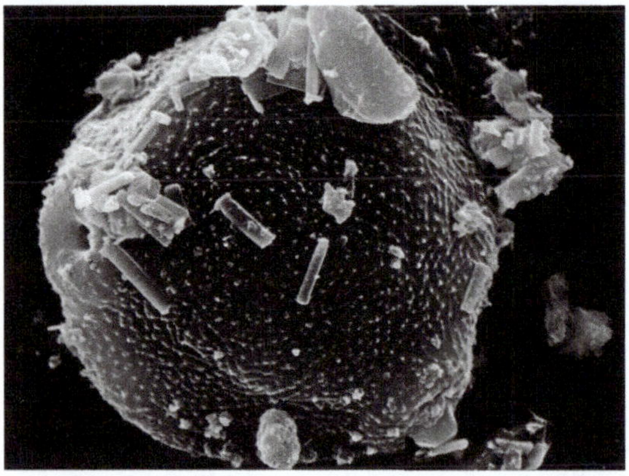

Fig. 2.12 Birch pollen grain covered by pollutant particles in the atmosphere of a West German city (with friendly permission of H. Behrendt)

2.5.4 Prognostic Factors

In a study from Switzerland, the following factors were correlated with a bad prognosis for children with atopic eczema [895]:

- Early onset (before the 6th month of life).
- Severe manifestation of eczema.
- Single child.
- High IgE concentration in serum.
- Concomitant manifestation of respiratory atopy.

2.5.5 Summary

Atopic eczema is one of the most common inflammatory skin diseases, with a prevalence of 10–20% in childhood. The prevalence has increased dramatically in the last decades and seems to have reached a plateau in some countries. In 80%, atopic eczema starts in early childhood (under 2 years), in recent years an increase of prevalence in adults is observed.

Only one-third of the children with atopic eczema is losing the disease before puberty; in two-thirds of the children affected it can be estimated that eczema stays or reoccurs in adulthood. Risk factors from epidemiologic studies are higher socioeconomic status (as measured as the educational level of parents), psychosomatic influences, alterations in the course of pregnancy, allergen exposure (especially pet keeping), as well as pollutant exposure (especially tobacco smoke in indoor and traffic exposure in outdoor air).

The attractive "jungle" or "hygiene" hypothesis, where stimulation of the immune system in early childhood seems to have a protective effect on the development of atopic diseases seems to be predominantly true for respiratory atopy and only to a lesser extent for atopic eczema.

3 Burden of Disease in Atopic Eczema

It is obvious that a disease like atopic eczema affects the life of patients, but also their families and their environment in a dramatic way. In a time where financial aspects are becoming increasingly important, it is good to stress this "individual and socioeconomic" burden in a quantitative way.

The individual burden for a patient with atopic eczema consists in

- Dysesthesia, especially intense itch sensation, but also pain.
- Loss of function (e.g., when hands or feet are affected) or when the patient is not able to work.
- Social stigmatization and disfigurement.
- Sleep loss and intense pruritus lead to loss of productivity and absenteeism at school or at work [270, 332, 458, 459].

The individual affection does not only manifest itself as a diminishment of quality of life as measured by instruments such as the Quality Of Life (QOL) and the Dermatology Life Quality Index (DLQI) [35, 233, 234]. Besides the DLQI, the HOME (Harmonizing outcome measures for eczema) initiative recommends either the RECAP or ADCT tool as well as measuring the most intense pruritus in an 11 point numeric rating scale at each visit [792]. All tools can be downloaded at HOME's website (www.homeforeczema.org).

Compared to other severe diseases, it is of interest that impairment of quality of life through atopic eczema is in the same or an even higher range of diseases like cancer, diabetes mellitus, or myocardial infarction (Biett). It also affects the life of caregivers [332].

3.1 Personal Burden and Individual Suffering

The personal burden of an individual affected by atopic eczema manifests itself differently during lifetime.

Infants only learn to scratch between the 3rd and 6th months of life; earlier they only can express their dysesthesia by a whimpering noise which often is not understood as itch. The lack of scratch marks cannot be regarded as a sign of absence of itch!

Psychologic consequences for lifetime are often underestimated when a young human being never knows the feeling of normal skin, but only a hypersensitive, rough, and destroyed skin surface with intense itch. The lack of understanding of many adults expressing itself in admonitions like "Stop scratching yourself once and for all!" leads to additional isolation. Emotional changes

K. Eyerich, J. Ring, *Atopic Dermatitis - Eczema*, https://doi.org/10.1007/978-3-031-12499-0_3

can trigger itch crises; this can change the emotional life of a human being. Anger can lead to scratch attacks. In families sometimes this is used as a "weapon" by the child which makes educational procedures difficult.

In kindergarten or at the latest in school, stigmatization is a major factor for eczema children; even in our modern and reasonable society, archaic reflexes of 3000 years ago are still prevalent which associate any skin disease with contagion, and postulates like "Put the contagious leppers out of town!" In Munich, the first skin patients were treated at the Gasteig outside East of the city walls, on the right side of the river Isar [831].

Sleep loss and intense itch lead to diminished concentration and achievements in school, but also to conflicts with teachers. Maybe this is one of the reasons often "hyperactive" syndromes are diagnosed when eczema children just cannot remain seated because of the intense pruritus.

Attention deficit and hyperactivity syndrome ADHS and eczema show interesting overlaps: in a large study it has been shown that sleep loss is a major factor in the development of ADHS, and sleep loss due to intense itch occurring in early childhood in eczema children may also lead to a higher prevalence of ADHS in atopic eczema [704].

Also, an association with autism disorder has been observed in several studies [804] (see also comorbidity).

Special dietary requirements—sometimes not indicated—in the case of concomitant food allergy, together with the requirement for time-consuming skincare procedures, or selection of certain textiles for clothing make life additionally difficult for eczema children.

In adolescence, young people are suffering tremendously by the stigmatization when their skin is not "smooth and pure," as can be seen in TV advertising around the clock, and their skin shows red patches, scales or eyelid edema or halo formation. Social stigmatization leads to isolation and makes friendships or partnerships more difficult.

When the genital area is involved, which often occurs in the lichenified manifestation, problems in sexual life are obvious. Few people and also—unfortunately—physicians can openly discuss these very important problems of many eczema patients.

In most studies dealing with the burden of atopic dermatitis financial aspects are the focus of interest. In a large European study together with patient organizations (EFA—European Federation of Allergy) a total of 1198 adult patients from nine European countries were participating and asked to describe their individual suffering and problems with the disease. The patients had been selected by dermatologists as suffering from moderate to severe atopic eczema. Apart from interviews with professional interviewers, the following instruments were used to assess the severity of the disease and quality of life:

- Patient-oriented-eczema measure (POEM),
- Dermatology life quality index (DLQI),
- Hospital anxiety and depression scale (HADS-D), and,
- Atopic eczema score of emotional consequences (AESEC).

Despite up-to-date medical treatment including systemic immunosuppressants almost half of the patients still had actual moderate to severe atopic eczema as measured in the POEM. In the AESEC 57% were suffering from emotional burdens with feelings like, e.g., "trying to hide the eczema," "feeling guilty about eczema," having "problems with intimacy," and others. Patients actually suffering from severe eczema stated in 88% that their eczema sometimes compromised their ability to face life. The authors concluded that in spite of modern medicine patients with atopic eczema are suffering more than what would be acceptable [660]. Similar findings have been observed in patient-reported analyses [107].

3.2 Financial Burden

In addition to the impairment in quality of life, rather high financial costs have to consider not only for drugs and medical aids but also for a variety of other aspects of daily life which are necessary for affected individuals [35, 266, 706].

These direct and indirect costs can be measured and estimated to be about 3–5 × 10^9 Euros per year in Germany [205].

There is a high degree of variability with regard to the yearly costs of atopic dermatitis when only doctor's visits or drug prescriptions are counted or when also indirect costs for the patient are included.

In the outpatient sector, the introduction of an "office fee" for outpatients in Germany in January 2004 led to a marked reduction in visits of patients with atopic dermatitis in the dermatologist's office. At the same time there was a steep increase of "alternative," "unconventional" treatments as well as no evidence-based treatment of eczema with systemic glucocorticosteroids especially in patients with rare doctor visits [707].

The financial burden of eczema is difficult to measure; there are different estimates from different countries. The direct costs of atopic eczema in childhood have been estimated to be 47 mio GBP per year in the United Kingdom, in the Netherlands to 71 mio Euros per year. Indirect costs have been estimated to be between 0.9 and 3.8 × 10^9 USD per year in the USA [210]. A study from Australia showed similar figures with 1140 AUD in mild eczema up to 6999 AUD for patients with severe eczema per patient and year [389].

The costs for atopic eczema have been studied in Germany by different authors. Yearly total costs for patients to be paid by insurance have been estimated to be 1600 Euros. In addition, there are costs to be paid by the patient himself, as well as indirect costs adding up to a total of 6200 Euros per year (Table 3.1).

Table 3.1 Average costs (per patient and year) of disease for patients with atopic dermatitis [83]

Sum of direct costs (doctor and medications)	2229.46	Euro
Indirect costs (for living, clothes, diets, etc.)	4257.90	Euro
Total	6487.36	Euro
Other skin diseases compared		
Psoriasis	6169.86	Euro
Chronic urticaria	4321.74	Euro
Acne	1342.55	Euro

These costs can be explained by about 70% direct costs, 20% for drugs, 35% for outpatient treatment, 12% for inpatient treatment, and 3% for rehabilitation. In addition, 30% of indirect costs for invalidity (8%) or absence from work (22%) [169].

In addition to direct and indirect costs for insurance and society, there are considerable out-of-pocket costs to be paid by the patients themselves [909].

3.3 Summary

Atopic eczema not only is characterized by individual suffering but also affects families and society with a considerable socioeconomic burden. Direct and indirect costs in Germany have been estimated to reach 3–5 × 10^9 Euros per year, 70% for direct costs, drugs, outpatient and inpatient treatment, and rehabilitation. Thirty percent can be estimated as "indirect" costs for daily life expenses regarding nutrition, clothing, and others.

4 Clinical Symptomatology of Atopic Eczema

Describing the clinical symptomatology of this skin disease is more difficult than in other dermatoses. Maybe this is why the big masters of morphology in dermatology preferred other skin diseases like psoriasis, bullous diseases, or lichen planus with clear-cut primary lesions and well-described secondary skin changes.

Atopic dermatitis often presents as a "diffuse" skin condition. The definition of the whole disease seems to be as imprecise as the borders of affected skin areas. Sometimes the term "involved" skin is questionable, especially when the dermatohistopathological investigations used to show signs of inflammation also in clinically "uninvolved" skin areas.

The susceptibility to environmental influences, especially on the psychosocial level, underlines the strong variability of this dermatosis. Each crisis can elicit attacks of rage. Rage can elicit attacks of itch and scratching. In addition, this disease manifests itself differently in different age groups and different body regions.

For logic didactic reasons, this chapter will describe the clinical symptomatology of atopic dermatitis in the following order:

- Actual symptoms of disease.
- Minimal manifestations.
- Stigmata of atopic constitution.
- Possible complications.

However, it is clear that these four phases often exist simultaneously and are variable over time even with regard to stigmata.

This variability also reflects the role of various pathophysiological reaction patterns involved in the clinical course of atopic dermatitis [221].

This will be followed by aspects of differential diagnosis, associated diseases, and criteria for diagnosis and severity scoring.

4.1 Actual Symptoms of Disease

4.1.1 Primary Lesion "Itch"

Normally dermatologists in the description of a skin disease start with the "primary lesion." There is no consensus with regard to the primary lesion of atopic eczema; it is described as erythema, papule, and seropapule. Some authors, starting with Jacquet [363] and the French School, stress the symptom "pruritus." According to good tradition, the authors state, together with Saint John the Evangelist or Johann Wolfgang von Goethe (Faust): "In the beginning there was the itch!" [613, 637].

Rarely it is possible to observe the acute development of an eczematous skin lesion in atopic dermatitis directly; however, sometimes—e.g., with your own children or under provocation tests in the hospital—it is possible.

K. Eyerich, J. Ring, *Atopic Dermatitis - Eczema*, https://doi.org/10.1007/978-3-031-12499-0_4

From this experience, it can be concluded that human beings, who never before have shown any signs of eczematous skin changes, triggered by some environmental or psychologic factors suddenly develop itch and start scratching on apparently normal skin. Only hours later the typical clinical manifestations of atopic dermatitis develop. These phenomena are especially common in the areas most affected such as elbow, knee flexures, or eyelids. It is a pity that there is little scientific documentation with regard to these early manifestations in the individual initial phase. Many colleagues, parents, and patients have made this experience.

Itch as "dermatose invisible" is the primary lesion of atopic dermatitis which, via the scratch reaction, then gives rise to the characteristic morphologic skin changes (Fig. 4.1a,b). Besides, it is possible that primarily skin changes occur which go along with increased itch. The borders are fluent. Typical atopic eczema without itch is extremely rare, if not inexistent. Since the French School at the beginning of the twentieth century, the central importance of itch for atopic dermatitis has been stressed by many authors [96, 396, 410, 613, 658, 763].

Itch is the most agonizing symptom of the manifest disease and often is perceived as "incurable." It leads to sleep loss, nightly scratch attacks with bloody bedding, a feeling of "powerlessness," because it cannot be stopped voluntarily [852, 854]. Unfortunately, this symptom is not

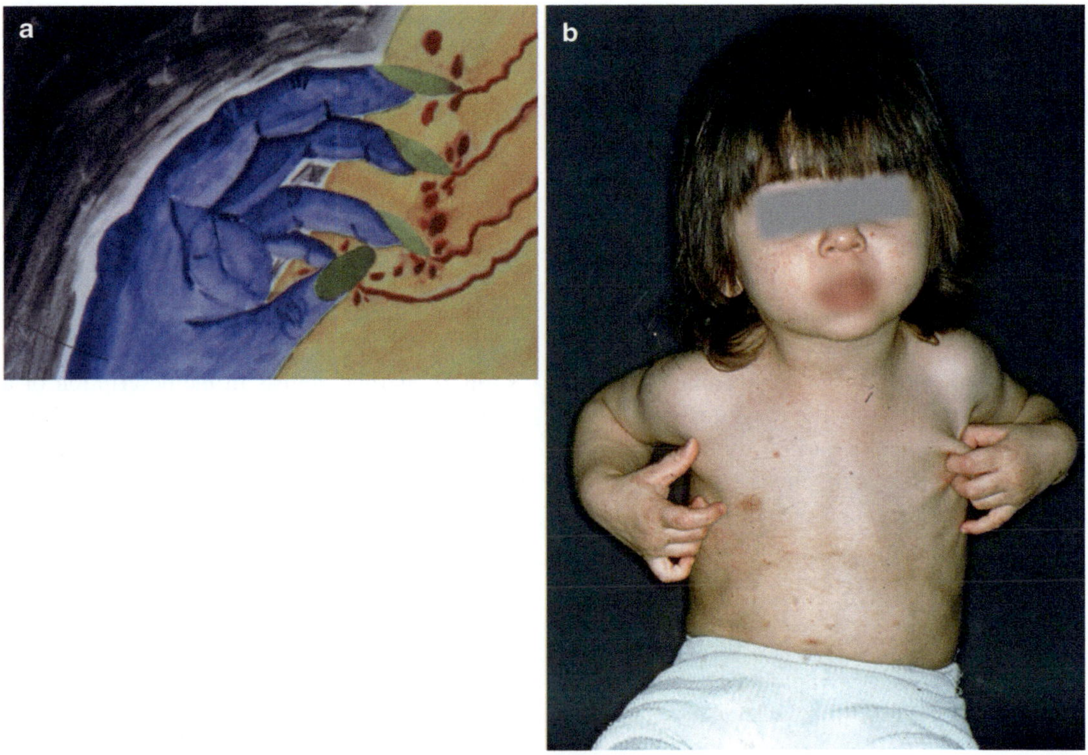

Fig. 4.1 (**a**): Itch sensation painted by a 9-year-old girl suffering from atopic dermatitis. (**b**): The primary lesion "itch" leads via scratch effects to the typical skin changes of atopic dermatitis

yet taken seriously by many physicians and the society, contrary to the other main subjective symptom "pain." Regarding the latter, everybody is full of compassion [763]. We personally know patients who wanted to commit suicide because of severe itch, a fact also observed by other authors [186].

The old sentence "It is not the rash which itches, but the itch that rashes" [216] illustrates the situation. Early attempts of treatment 80 years ago quite brutally used procedures like fixation of children in bed or applying plaster to their extremities, so that scratching became impossible. Lesions in unreachable skin areas were indeed healing faster. Pathophysiologically this indicates that by scratching pro-inflammatory substances may be released (see Chap. 5 "Pathophysiology").

Today, mildly elastic tube bandages—sometimes together with wet wraps—are a more humane variant of scratch protection and the prevention of direct scratch effects by mechanical procedures using these tube bandages plays a central role (see Chap. 6). The treatment of itch is the focus of the management of atopic dermatitis.

4.1.2 Infiltrated Erythema

Mild cases or the beginning of an exacerbation become manifest in flat, mildly infiltrated, erythematous patches with only little epidermal involvement—yet clearly different from an urticarial wheal—which in the course can be excoriated and change to oozing crusting areas (Fig. 4.2).

In the severity scoring of the SCORAD (see below section) criteria not only "erythema," "edema and papule," but also "lichenification" are enlisted.

It is important to stress that there are these manifestations since they are not clearly mentioned in many textbooks.

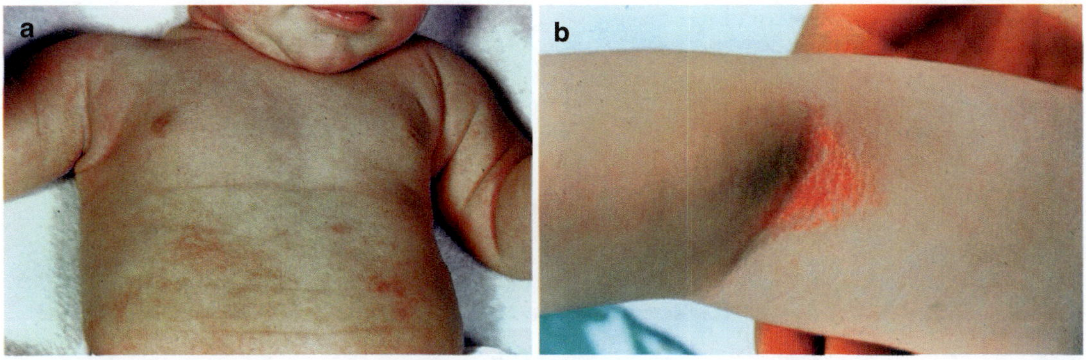

Fig. 4.2 Infiltrated erythema. (**a**) on the trunk in an infant. (**b**) in the elbow of a 1-year-old child

4.1.3 Erosive, Excoriated Erythema

Especially in childhood, often patchy or punctate erosive or excoriated erythematous skin changes with mild scaling are observed, going along with intense itch (Fig. 4.3).

Histologically these lesions are characterized by spongiotic changes in the epidermis. This

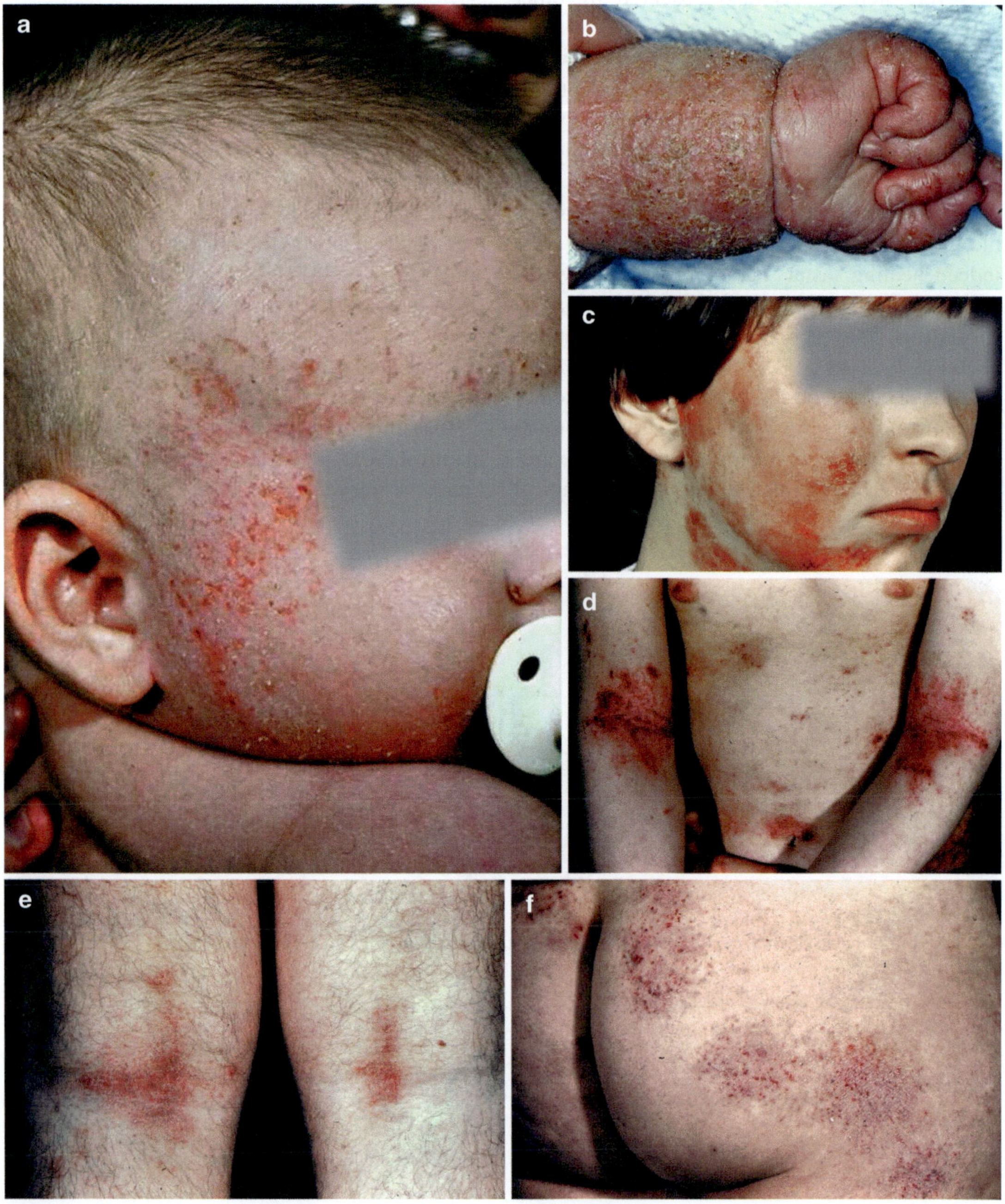

Fig. 4.3 Erosive excoriated eczematous skin changes in atopic dermatitis. (**a**) Facial eczema in an infant. (**b**) Scaling hand and forearm eczema in an infant. (**c**) Diffuse erythematous excoriations in the face. (**d**) Marked erythematous flexural eczema in the elbow. (**e**) Punctate erosive and excoriated skin changes in the knee joints. (**f**) Diffuse, partly nummular appearing erythemata with punctate erosions on the buttocks. (**g**) Massive facial eczema in an infant. (**h**) Facial eczema in an infant. (**i**) Facial eczema in a small child

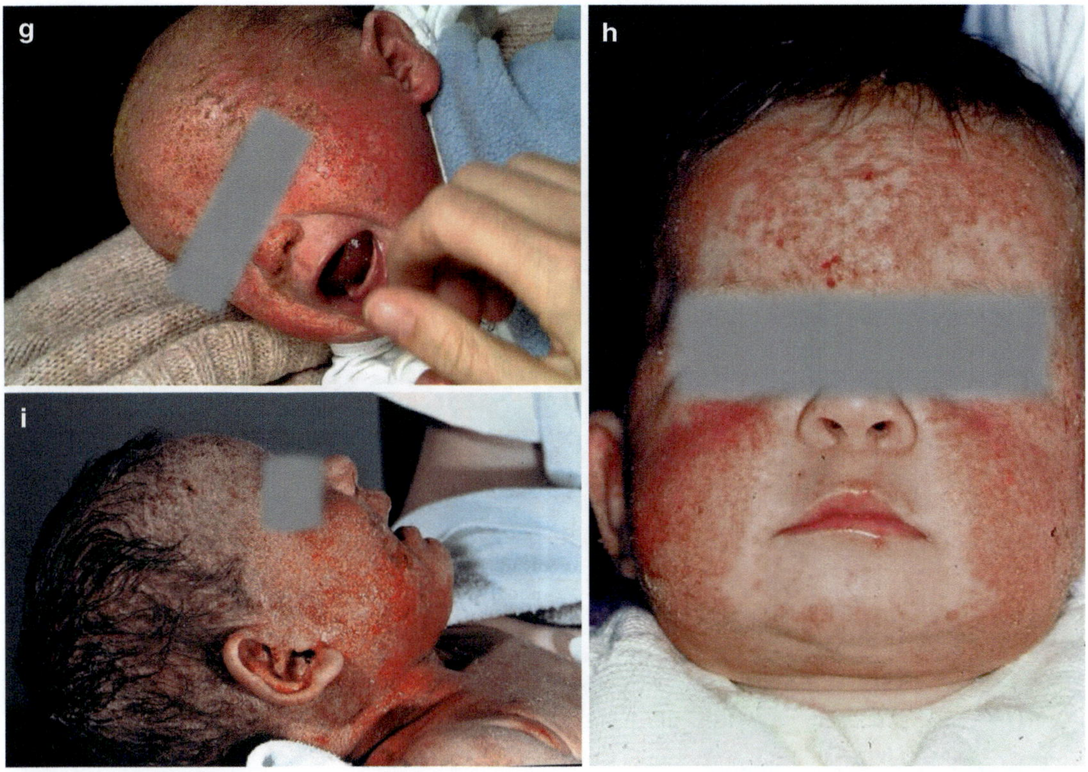

Fig. 4.3 (continued)

form often has been called "eczematoid type" in the restricted sense. This may have contributed to dissatisfaction with the name "eczema" for the whole disease and may be a reason for the terminology debate and preference of the unprecise term "dermatitis."

In the broader definition of eczema (see above), it becomes clear that in the local and timely course the polymorphy of symptoms in eczema also includes other morphologies like lichenification, prurigo-type excoriated papules, etc.

Maybe strongly oozing and crusty skin changes in childhood represent signs of superinfection with, e.g., Staphylococcus aureus.

This morphology also can be observed in circumscribed skin lesions with nummular variants (see below). Whether nummular eczema in childhood represents an own identity is still to be discussed. In the opinion of the authors, this nummular variant is a subtype of atopic eczema in childhood [78].

4.1.4 Lichenification

The more chronic the skin changes, the more they show a tendency to lichenification. This means a coarsening of skin signs with thickening of the skin and livid red color "purple." These skin changes occur predominantly in the flexures of the big joints (elbow, knee flexure), but also as large plaques on the dorsum of hands and feet. They also represent most likely the consequence of long-lasting scratch effects (Fig. 4.4).

The entity of lichen simplex chronicus (Vidal) or "circumscribed neurodermatitis" can be regarded as a subgroup of localized variants of atopic eczema; however, this is a matter of discussion.

Lichenification can be provoked by scratching as could be shown in classic experiments with the use of a scratch machine with a pressure of 75 g on the skin. After 60–90 h lichenification could be provoked [273].

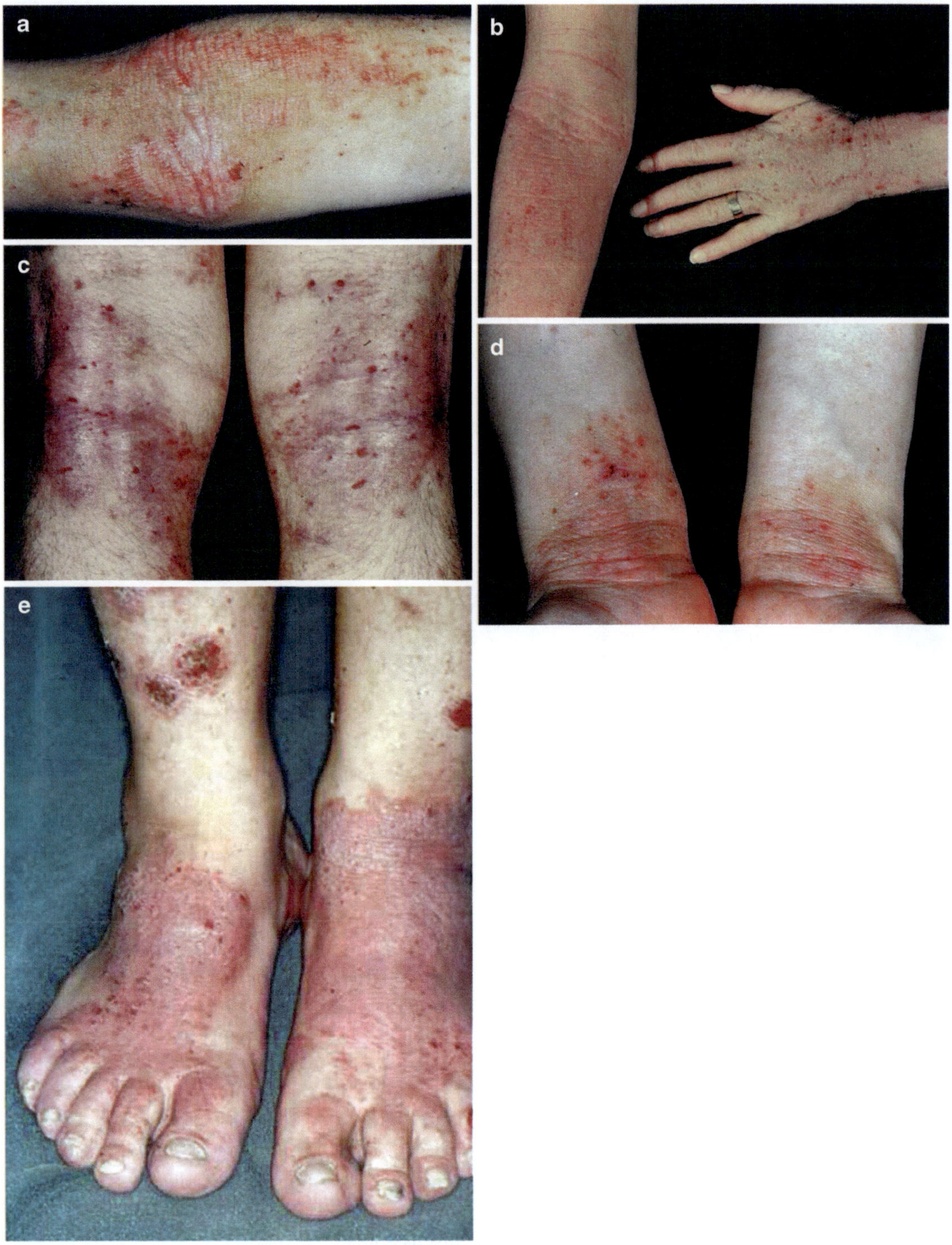

Fig. 4.4 Lichenification in chronic atopic dermatitis. (**a**) Lichenified flexural eczema in the elbow. (**b**) Lichenified eczema on the wrist. (**c**) Lichenified eczema in the knee joints. (**d**) Lichenified skin areas on the wrists. (**e**) Massive lichenification on the dorsum of the feet in an adult patient with atopic dermatitis

4.1.5 Prurigo-Type of Atopic Eczema

When the follicular affection in chronic courses is prominent especially in adults, a variant can be observed which shows the clinical symptoms of prurigo; it is relatively marked by strongly itching papules or nodules with a diameter of 0.5–3 mm and central excoriation and crusting. This variant most likely gave rise to the term "prurigo Besnier," and can be found commonly in the severe manifestations in adults (Fig. 4.5). Recently, the term chronic prurigo has been established to define several subtypes of chronic and pruritic nodules, among them variants of AD [588].

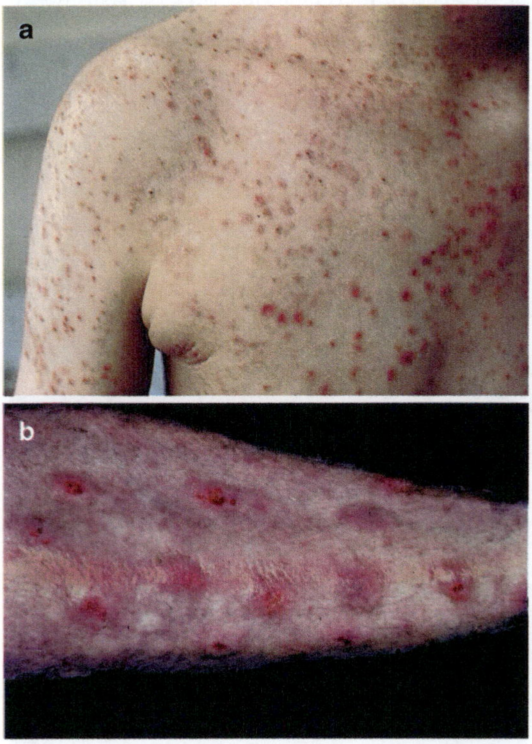

Fig. 4.5 Prurigo type of atopic dermatitis. (**a**) Extremely itchy excoriated papules on the trunk. (**b**) Centrally excoriated and crusted papules and nodules in a 17-year-old girl with severe atopic dermatitis

4.1.6 Differences in Various Ethnic Populations

Although the diagnosis of AD usually is no problem in ethnic populations around the world—based on clinics and history with regard to family or personal history of atopy, together with strong itch sensation—there are some obvious morphological, and maybe also pathophysiological differences. A meta-analysis of 101 studies evaluating the prevalence and phenotype of AD all over the world came to this conclusion: "The most prevalent AD features were pruritus, lichenification, and xerosis. There were differences in AD characteristics by study region. Flexural involvement was less commonly reported in India, the Americas, and Iran. Studies from East Asia reported more erythroderma and truncal, extensor, scalp, and auricular involvement. Studies from Southeast Asia reported more exudative eczema, truncal involvement, lichenification, and prurigo nodularis. Studies from Iran reported more head, face, and neck involvement; pityriasis alba; and xerosis. Studies from Africa reported more papular lichenoid lesions, palmar hyperlinearity, ichthyosis, and orbital darkening" [902] (Fig. 4.6). Typically, the epidermal involvement so characteristic for eczema in people of color is not red as in Caucasian skin, but grey ("ashy").

Also, the immune signature may show differences, so there was much less IgE to Malassezia species, but higher levels for storage mite, cockroach, and also seafood in Moshi, Tanzania, indicating tropomyosin cross-reactivity [439]. Furthermore, Asian AD and African AD might have a stronger Th17 immune component as compared to European AD [154].

Still the established diagnostic scoring systems for measuring severity also work in skin of color [227].

Furthermore, there may be differences in ethnic populations with regard to itch perception. This may be due to biologic factors like

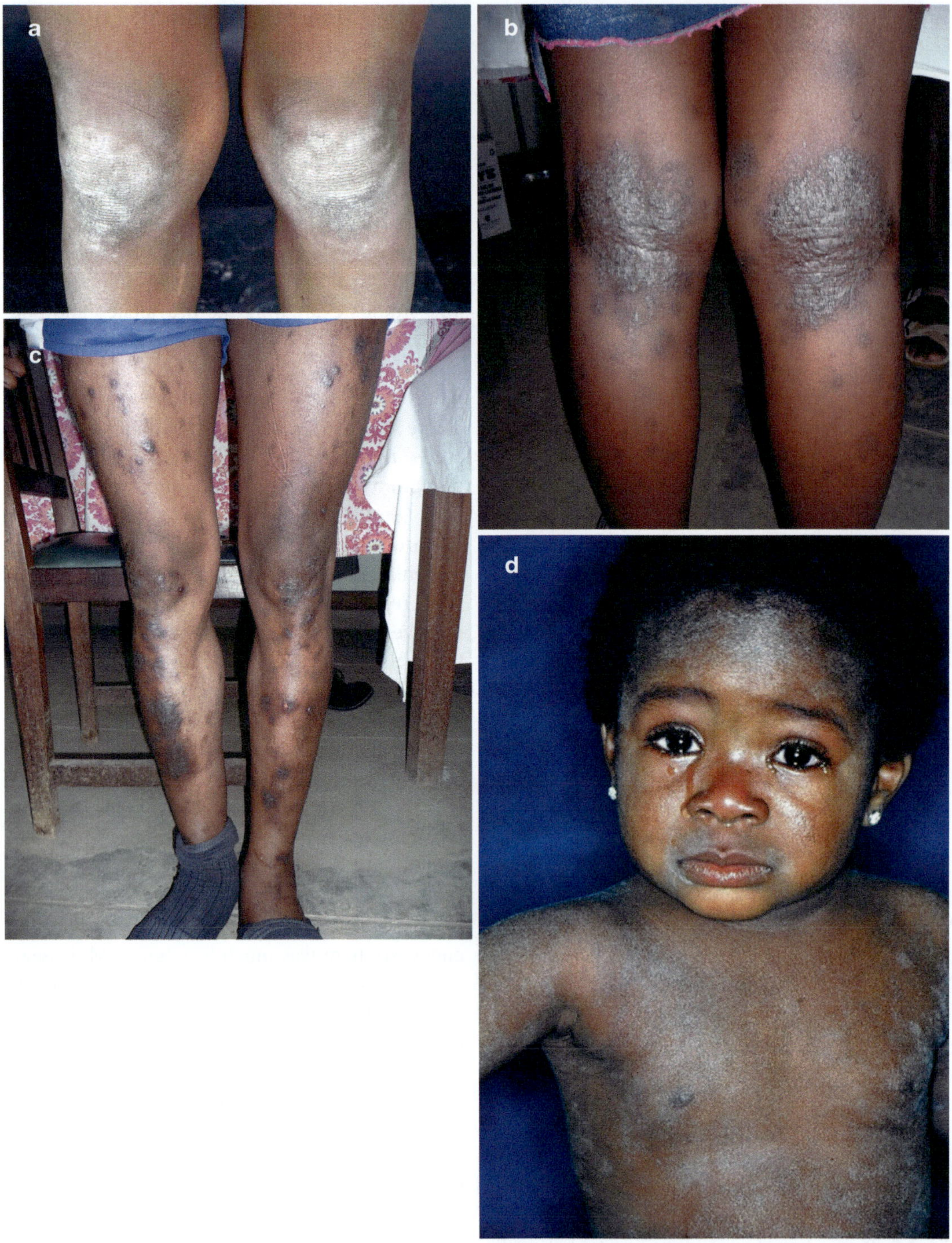

Fig. 4.6 Patchy pityriasiform lichenoid eczema as a special variant of atopic dermatitis appearing on the extensor sides of the joints. These skin changes are particularly common in dark skin. (**a**) Lichenoid papules and plaques on the extensor side of the knee. (**b**) Atopic dermatitis of the knee joints in an African patient from Tanzania. (**c**) Atopic dermatitis (nummular pattern) on both legs in an African patient from Tanzania. (**d**) Facial eczema in an African child (with friendly permission of P. Schmid-Grendelmeier)

genetic predisposition to certain diseases like, e.g., amyloidosis, or prurigo pigmentosa, which is more common in Asian individuals [791], or intrahepatic cholestasis of pregnancy, which seems to be more common in Latin America [627]. Also, genetic polymorphisms in the interleukin-31 receptor may play a role. In Africans, a common condition is chloroquine-induced itch and primary bilharziosis [791].

Also, the response to capsaicin, a substance known to destroy sensory nerves and usually induce an initial burning sensation, is different between ethnic groups: African Americans do not suffer the same degree of acute hyperalgesia and neurogenic inflammation as people from Spain or East Asia [791]. Also, psychosocial and lifestyle factors may be involved in the itch process.

4.2 Minimal Manifestations

Atopic eczema can change in course and localization and also in morphology over lifetime. There are certain localizations, where so-called minimal manifestations are typical: they can occur alone or sometimes in combination with other skin changes [325]. The affection of very small skin areas can lead to severe impairment of quality of life.

4.2.1 Minimal Manifestations in the Head Area

4.2.1.1 Facial and Lid Eczema

While face involvement is characteristic in children, this is different in adults with common involvement of the big flexures and extremities; however, in some patients only the face is involved. Unfortunately, there are little data describing the exact distribution of adult eczema skin lesions over the body in a larger number of patients; there are estimates of 20% face involvement [742].

Lid Eczema

Sometimes only eyelids are affected, especially in cases where aeroallergens play a causal role, sometimes also in food-induced reactions. The more chronic the course, the more difficult the treatment. Already very little contact elicits eyelid itch. Through the itch-scratch cycle, a vicious cycle develops with continuous deterioration (Fig. 4.7).

4.2.1.2 Cheilitis Sicca and Perlèche

Dry lips—sometimes also with a median fissure of the lower lip—are characteristic signs of atopic eczema (Fig. 4.8), going along with fissures at the lateral angles of the mouth (Perlèche) and often superinfection (Candida albicans) [684].

Sometimes, in the area surrounding the red part of the lip, there is an irritative eczema caused by increased lip licking (lip lick eczema) (Fig. 4.9), in infants sometimes also called suck eczema with a perioral inflammatory reaction.

4.2.1.3 Infranasal Erosion

In persons with concomitant respiratory allergy such as rhinoconjunctivitis and chronic nasal secretion or itch, sometimes erythema and fissures on the nasal entrance develop. This has to be differentiated from seborrheic dermatitis with typical nasolabial fold lesions.

4.2.1.4 Infra-auricular Fissures

Infra-auricular fissures are very common at the region where the earlobe starts, which can sometimes be superinfected. It might be interesting how dressing habits—e.g., the rapid pulling of a T-shirt over the head of the child—can contribute to these infra-auricular fissures (Fig. 4.10).

4.2.1.5 Retro-auricular Intertrigo

Similarly, signs of oozing intertrigo can be found behind the ear (Fig. 4.11).

4.2.1.6 Excoriations in the Scalp

Sometimes extremely itching skin lesions with nodules and crusts and excoriated areas can be found in the scalp as a single manifestation of atopic eczema; severe cases sometimes have been called "neurotic excoriation."

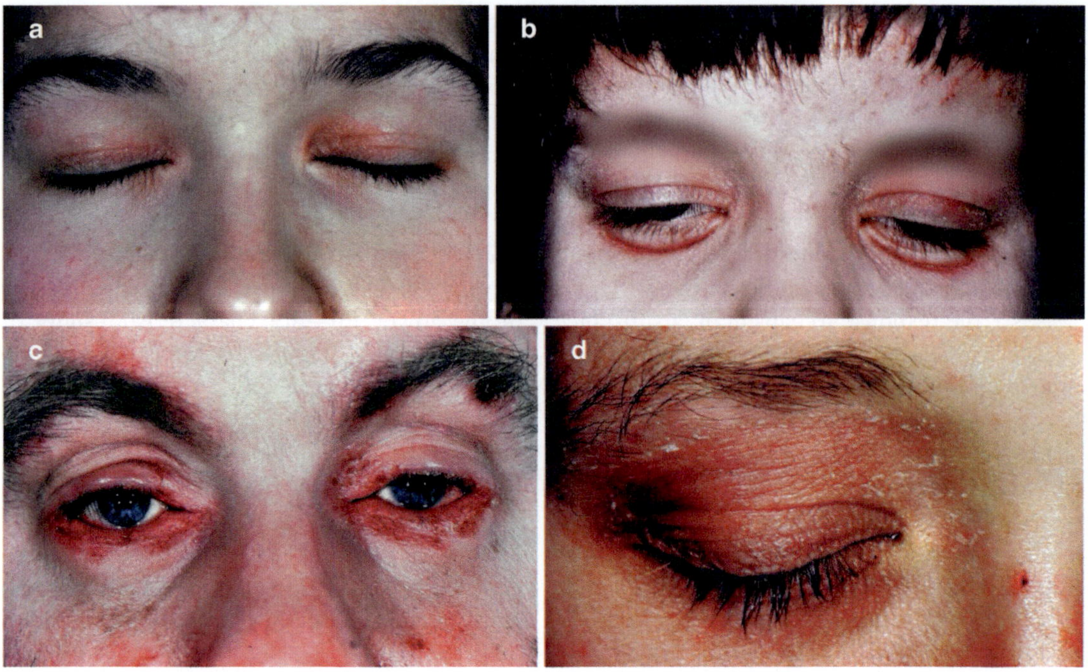

Fig. 4.7 Lid eczema in atopic dermatitis. (**a**) Upper lid eczema. (**b**) Lid eczema with edematous swelling. (**c**) Massive lid eczema of the lower lids. (**d**) Massive upper lid eczema

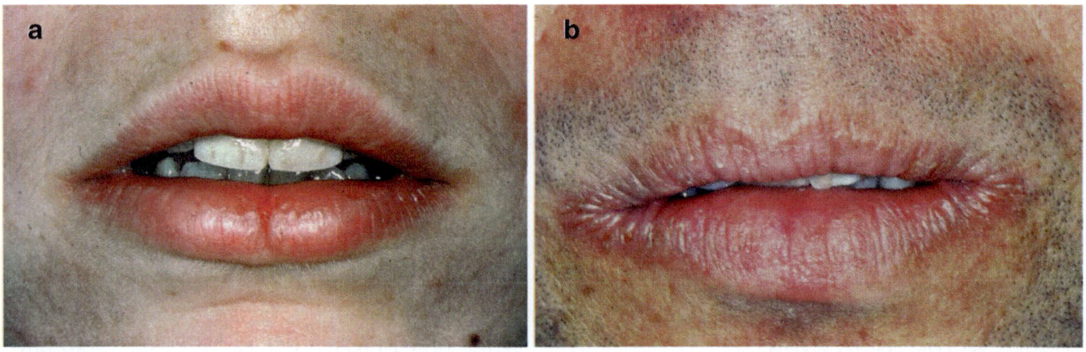

Fig. 4.8 Dry lips. (**a**) Cheilitis sicca with median lower lip fissure. (**b**) Cheilitis sicca in an adult patient with atopic dermatitis

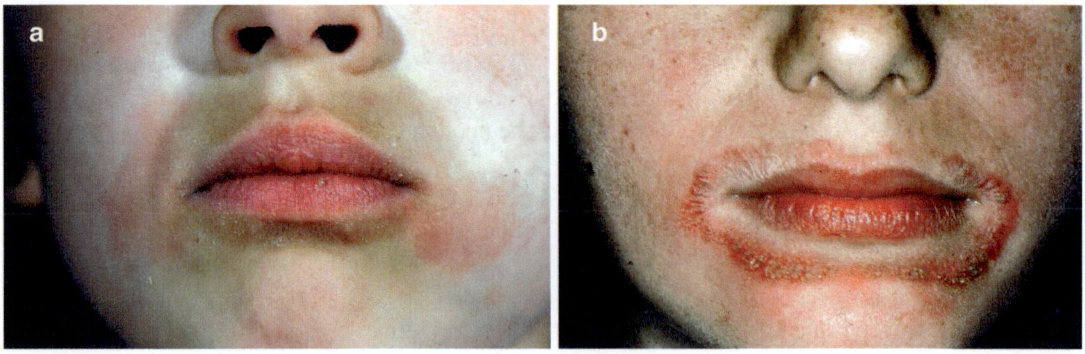

Fig. 4.9 Lip-sucking eczema. (**a**) Lip sucking eczema with hyperpigmentation. (**b**) sharply marginated perioral lip eczema and cheilitis sicca

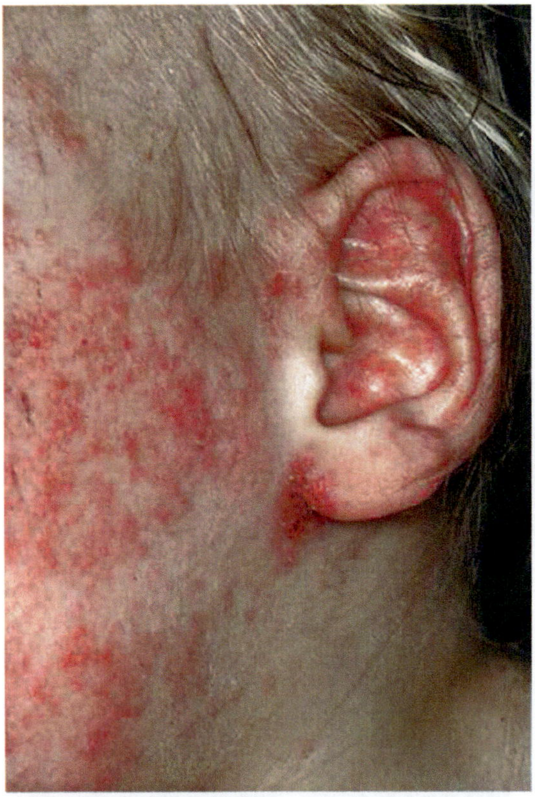

Fig. 4.10 Infra-auricular fissure in atopic dermatitis

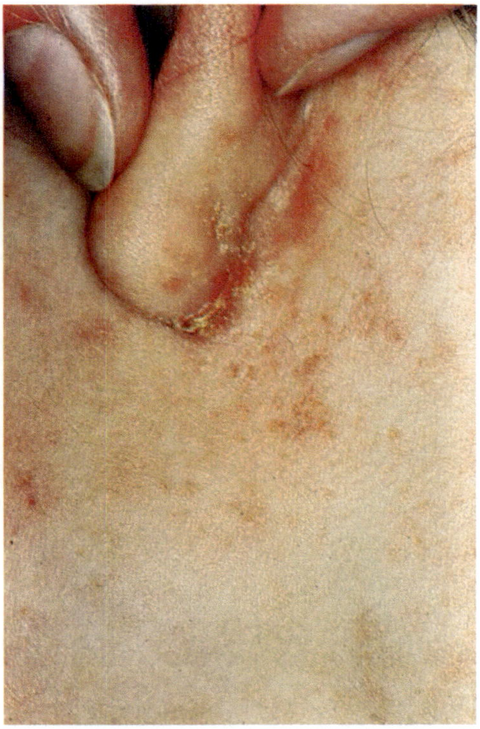

Fig. 4.11 Retro-auricular fissure in atopic dermatitis

4.2.2 Minimal Manifestations on the Trunk and Extremities

4.2.2.1 Finger and Toe Eczema

Dry finger and toe changes (pulpitis sicca) can be observed especially in winter and in small children which have been described by Möller as "atopic winter feet" [518], and sometimes were misdiagnosed as fungal infection. These changes also can look similar to dyshidrosis lamellosa sicca (Fig. 4.12).

4.2.2.2 Involvement of Nails

Strong eczematous changes on the fingers and toes can affect nail growth by matrix involvement with the development of horizontal lines (Fig. 4.13a). Sometimes also paronychia develops in atopic eczema with or without superinfection (Fig. 4.13b).

Atopic dermatitis manifestations also can affect the eponychium, leading to spontaneous loss of eponychium as "epionychitis sicca" [644].

Inspection of nails can reveal much about scratching habits (e.g., subungual crusts or shiny nails when the skin is rubbed) (Fig. 4.14).

4.2.2.3 Juvenile Plantar Dermatosis

A painful variant of atopic dermatitis can be observed on soles and lateral parts of the feet with erythema, hyperkeratosis, and fissures which is not due to contact allergy against shoe or textile material [478, 786].

4.2.2.4 Eczema of the Nipple (Mamilla)

Mamillar eczema in atopics is a very chronic and localized variant (Fig. 4.15). It has to be evaluated in differential diagnosis in order to be distinguished from M. Paget or scabies.

4.2.2.5 Localized Genital Eczema

Similarly, there are cases with exclusive affection of the genital regions as vulvar or scrotal eczema with severely lichenified variants in adults and strong psychosomatic involvement (Fig. 4.16a, b).

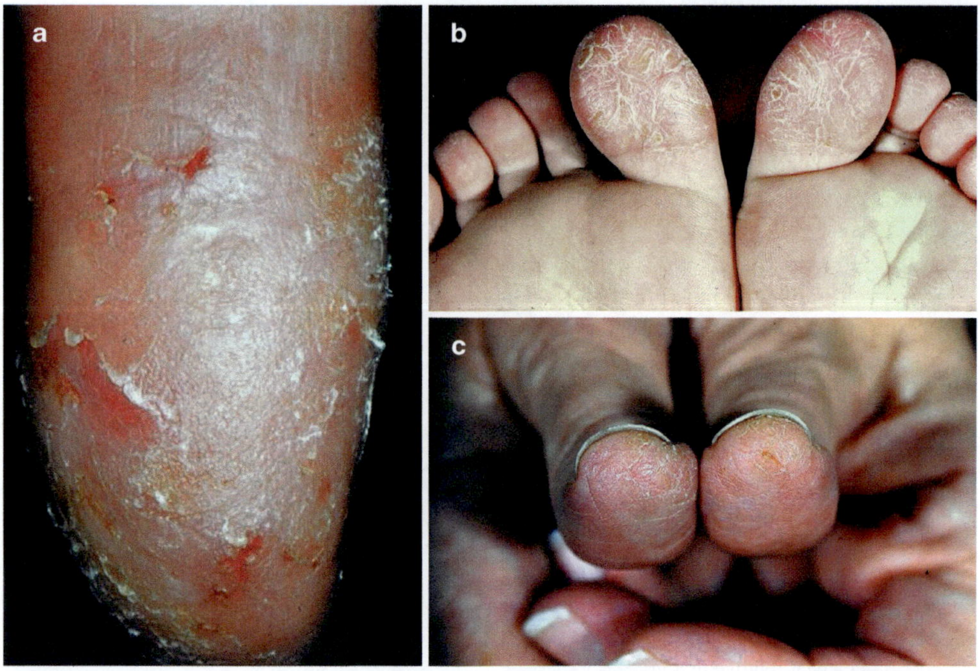

Fig. 4.12 Finger and toe eczema. (**a**) Dry fingertip eczema. (**b**) Pulpitis sicca in atopic foot dermatitis ("atopic winter feet"). (**c**) Painful eczema of the thumbs

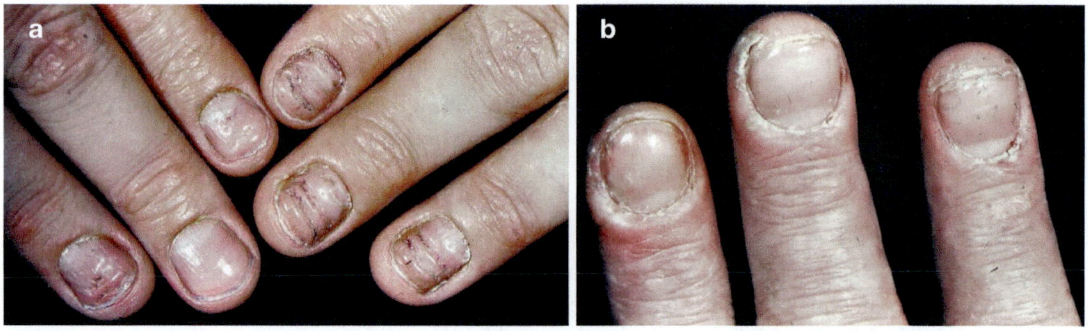

Fig. 4.13 Nail involvement in atopic dermatitis. (**a**) Eczema nails with strong horizontal grooves representing disturbance of nail growth in the matrix. (**b**) Paronychia in atopic dermatitis

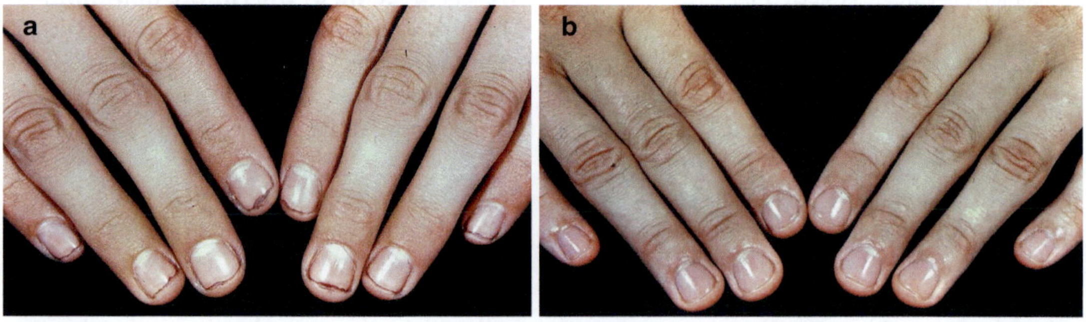

Fig. 4.14 Inspection of the nails allows information on the type of scratching. (**a**) Blood under the nail means heavy excoriation. (**b**) Shimmering nails can be derived from superficial abrasion

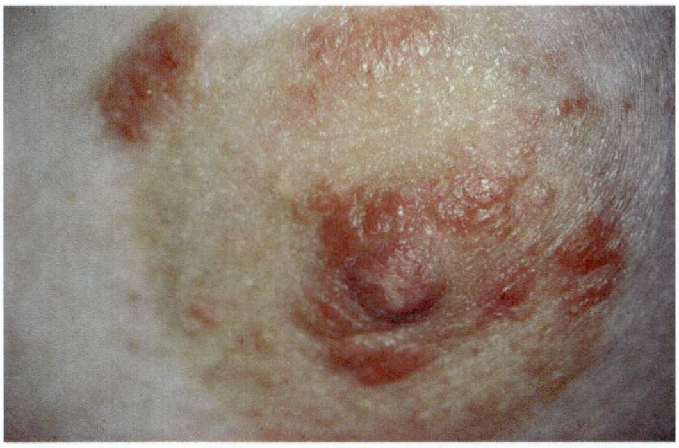

Fig. 4.15 Mamillar eczema in atopic dermatitis (when it is one-sided, scabies or Morbus Paget always have to be considered)

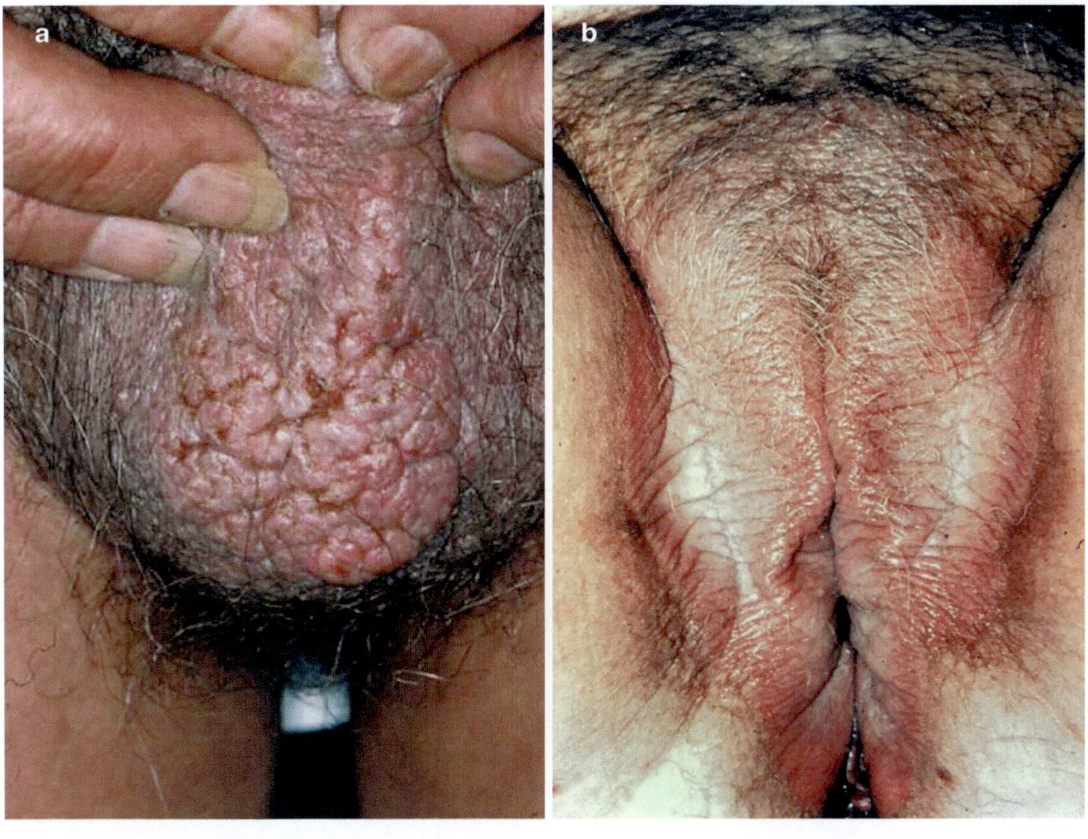

Fig. 4.16 Atopic dermatitis in the genital area. (**a**) Chronic scrotal eczema. (**b**) Chronic vulvar eczema

Fig. 4.17 Pityriasis alba in atopic dermatitis

4.2.2.6 Pityriasis Alba

The occurrence of whitish mildly scaling and relatively marked patches, especially in light-exposed skin areas during summertime is called pityriasis alba and leads to suffering in many patients, especially in colored skin (Mazenga, personal communication). Most likely it is due to minimal inflammation with superficial whitish scaling (Fig. 4.17).

4.2.3 Variants and Special Forms

4.2.3.1 Dermatitis Papulosa Juvenilis

This special variant of atopic eczema goes along with the development of fine papular skin changes, sometimes hypopigmented and often at the extensor sides of extremities in childhood [86, 239]. This manifestation can be found under different names (summertime pityriasis of the elbow and knee, dermatite du Tobogan, sandbox dermatitis, frictional lichenoid eruption, recurrent papillar eruption of childhood). Often the skin changes occur predominantly in spring and summer and are associated with pollen exposure. Also, mechanic components like friction and sensitivity to UV light have been discussed in the pathophysiology.

This manifestation seems to be more common in colored skin.

4.2.3.2 Follicular Variant of Atopic Dermatitis (Patchy Pityriasiform Lichenoid Eczema)

Kitamura, Takahashi, and Sasagawa described a skin condition in Japan as plaque-type lichenoid squamous dry skin changes in children with follicular involvement and occurring predominantly on the extensor sides, sometimes similar to "goose pimples." This variant also seems to occur more often in winter and shows improvement in summer.

In the differential diagnosis, follicular dermatoses like lichen nitidus, Gianotti-Crosti syndrome, or follicular hyperkeratosis in certain forms of ichthyosis have to be considered.

The African type of atopic dermatitis characteristically shows more often this variant with predilection of extensor sides of extremities and follicular accentuation [702].

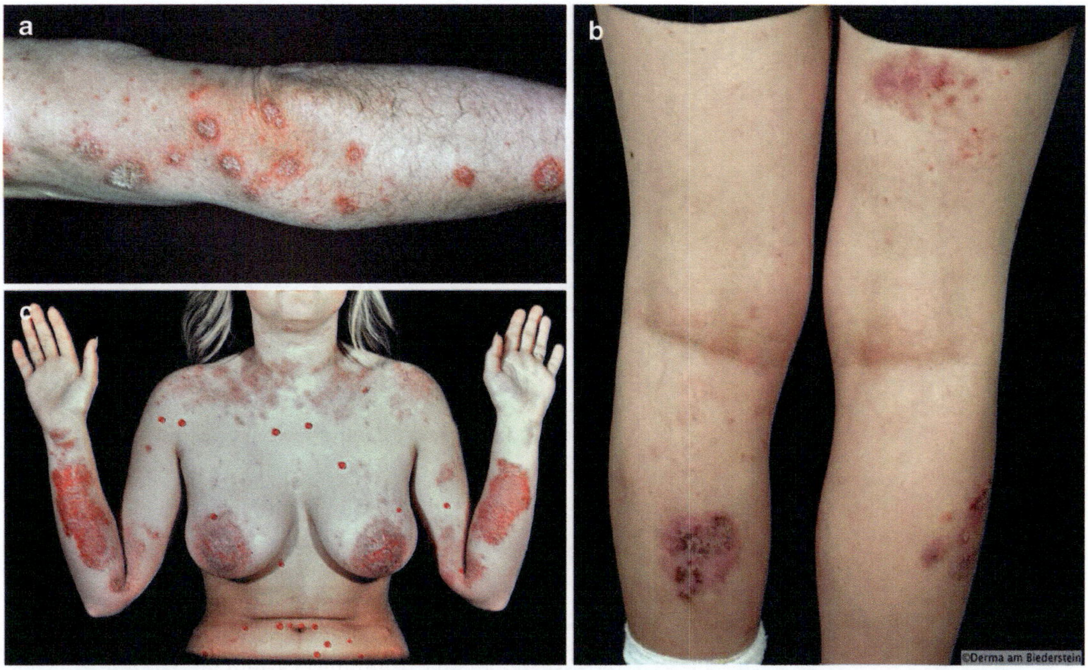

Fig. 4.18 Nummular variant of atopic dermatitis. (**a**) Scaling nummular lesions in atopic eczema. (**b**) Nummular eczema of the legs in atopic dermatitis. (**c**) Sharply marginated massive atopic eczema with nummular distribution

4.2.3.3 Nummular Variant of Atopic Eczema

Nummular eczema can occur with sharply demarcated nummular erythematous skin changes with scaling and excoriation and oozing aspect in childhood or in elderly people (Fig. 4.18). Especially lower extremities, but also arms and trunk can be involved. Our own studies of nummular eczema indicate that this entity is a variant of AD with a Th17 signature in addition to the Th2 immunity. This is why a considerable amount of biopsies showed infiltrate of neutrophil granulocytes and pronounced acanthosis in addition to the hallmarks of eczema, namely spongiosis and eosinophils. Interestingly, nummular eczema responds very well to AD therapies such as Dupilumab, but only moderately to psoriasis therapies such as Apremilast.

4.2.3.4 Special Considerations in Infants

Atopic eczema most commonly develops during or at the end of the first trimenon and then occurs in the face and extensor surfaces; commonly the so-called cradle cap is the first manifestation (Fig. 4.19). In the diaper area, there are various differential diagnoses to atopic eczema. Interestingly, the diaper area itself is often uninvolved ("diaper sign") (see Sect. 2.4 "Differential Diagnosis").

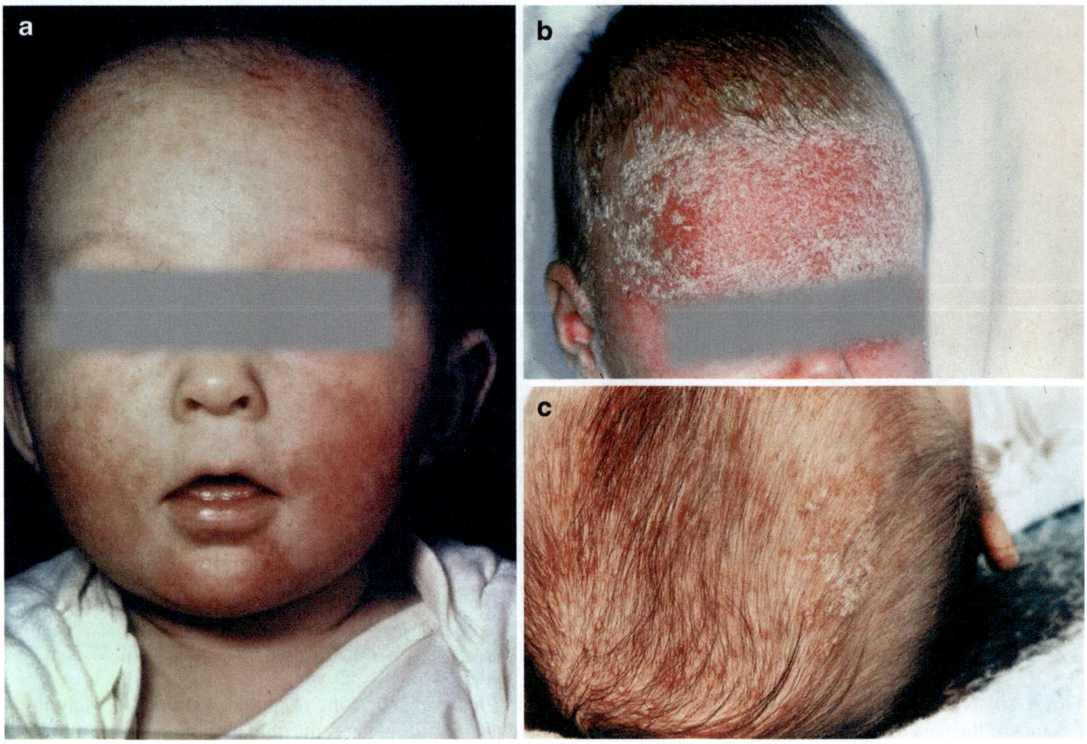

Fig. 4.19 Atopic dermatitis in infants. (**a**) Facial eczema in infants. (**b**) Cradle cap ("Crusta lactea" reminding of crusted milk in a pan). (**c**) Cradle cap on the scalp

4.2.4 Special Localizations

4.2.4.1 Face

In many patients, atopic dermatitis only affects the face (Fig. 4.20) (see above minimal manifestations).

4.2.4.2 Neck

Apart from the face, also the neck region is affected in many patients which can be regarded as a "big flexure" (Fig. 4.21). In chronic eczema, the clinical manifestation of a "dirty neck" develops as a post-inflammatory hyperpigmentation, sometimes without real symptoms [144] (Fig. 4.22).

4.2.4.3 Hand Eczema

Often hands and feet show the main manifestation of atopic eczema, with or without concomitant contact allergy. Here scaling eczematous skin changes and dry chronic skin lesions with lichenification, but also, when the palms and soles are involved, dyshidrosis and erosive crusty skin changes can be observed, leading to hyperkeratotic fissuring manifestations (Fig. 4.23). Often nails are also affected (Fig. 4.24).

Hand eczema represents a special problem as one of the most common occupational skin diseases and is pathogenetically classified between irritant, contact allergic, and atopic dermatitis [24]. Furthermore, sometimes the differential diagnosis to psoriasis of palms and soles may be difficult. In a retrospective study, the most frequent subdiagnoses of chronic hand eczema were allergic contact dermatitis, allergic plus irritative contact dermatitis, irritant contact dermatitis, atopic hand eczema, atopic plus irritant hand eczema, vesicular hand eczema (dyshidrotic = pompholyx), and hyperkeratotic eczema [183].

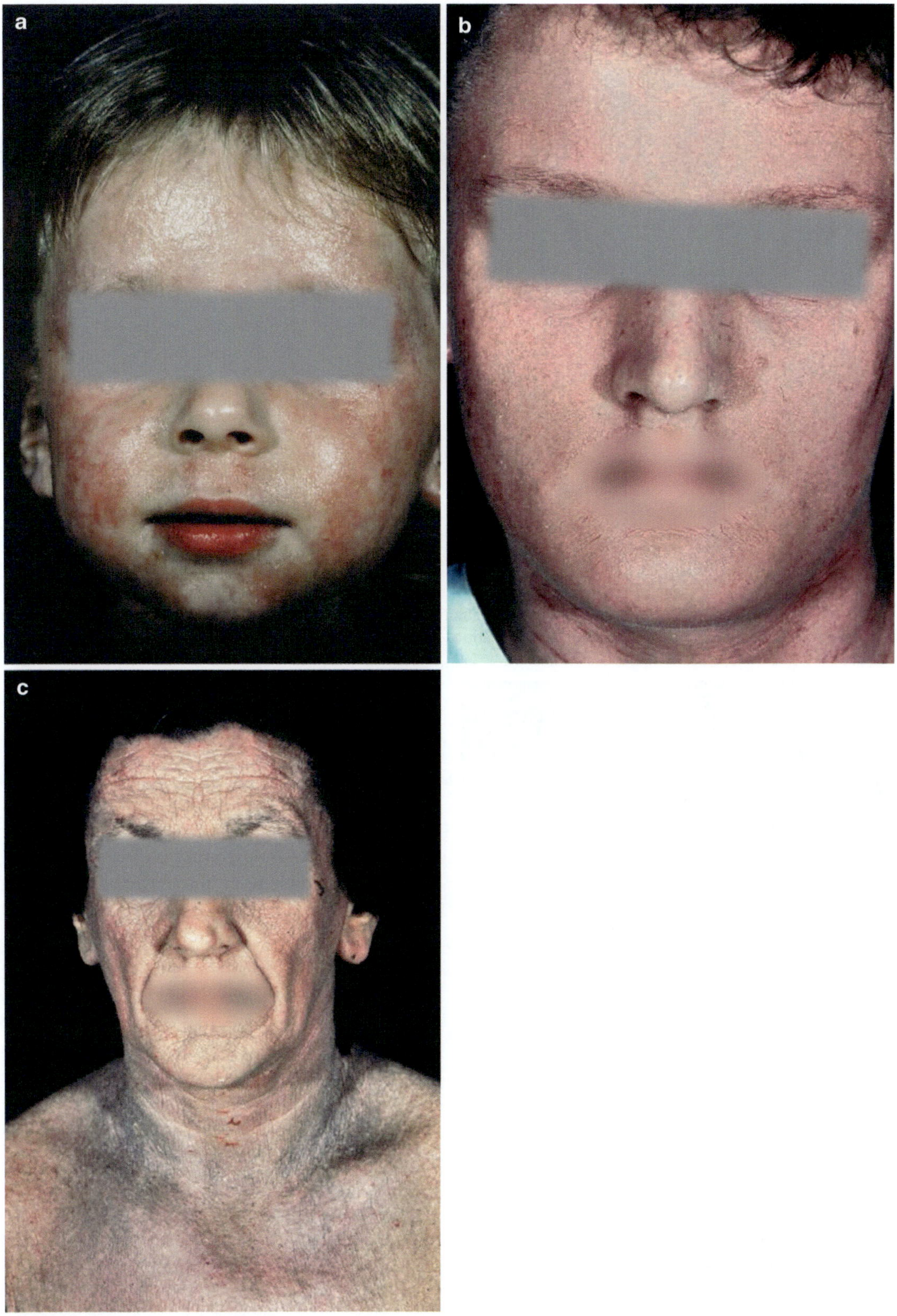

Fig. 4.20 Atopic dermatitis in the face. (**a**) in childhood. (**b**) in adulthood. (**c**) massive atopic dermatitis of the face with lichenification

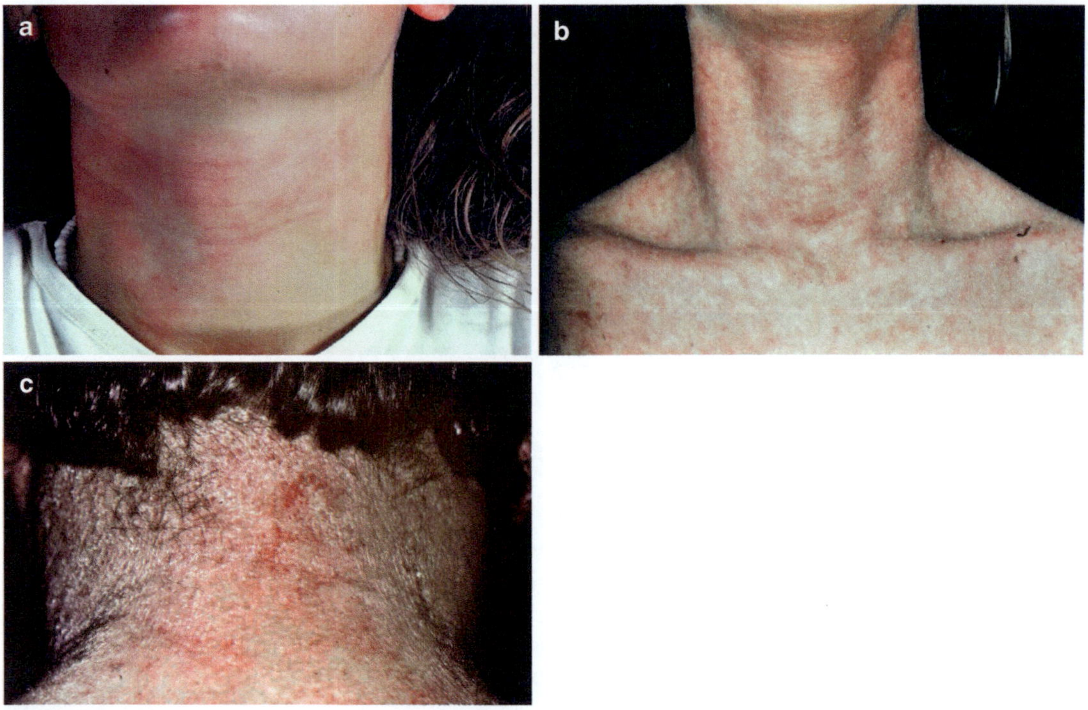

Fig. 4.21 Atopic dermatitis of the neck. (**a**) Atopic dermatitis of the neck region. (**b**) Scaling atopic dermatitis of the neck. (**c**) Atopic dermatitis of the neck with lichenification

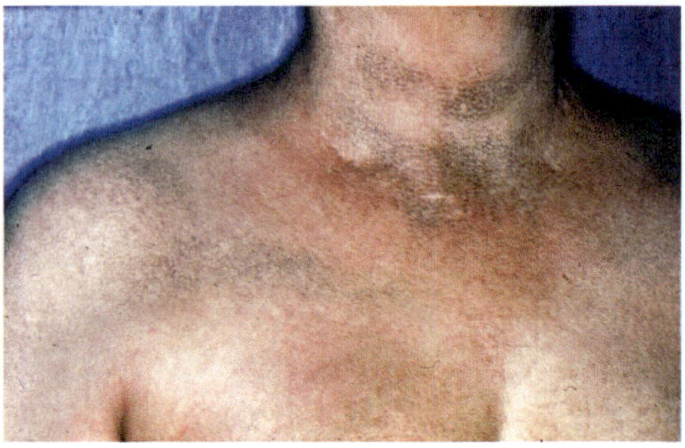

Fig. 4.22 "Dirty neck" following post-inflammatory hyperpigmentation in atopic dermatitis

4.2.4.4 Erythroderma

Atopic dermatitis also can manifest as erythroderma with involvement of the whole integument in the sense of an exfoliative dermatitis with redness and scaling. Erythroderma by definition is a clinical condition which often cannot be attributed to a single disease at first glance. Several diseases can lead to erythroderma:

- Allergic contact dermatitis.
- Atopic dermatitis.
- Psoriasis.
- Pityriasis rubra pylaris.
- Cutaneous T cell lymphoma (Sézary syndrome).
- Exanthematous drug eruption.
- Idiopathic melano-erythrodermia cachectica.

In how far this latter condition may correspond to a severe manifestation of atopic eczema at the end of the life remains to be discussed.

4.2.5 Summary

Contrary to other dermatoses, atopic dermatitis does not show a clear-cut morphology. Several variants with "infiltrated erosive erythema," "chronic lichenification," or "prurigo-type" of atopic dermatitis can be observed. Exsudative eczematous skin changes can be found predomi-

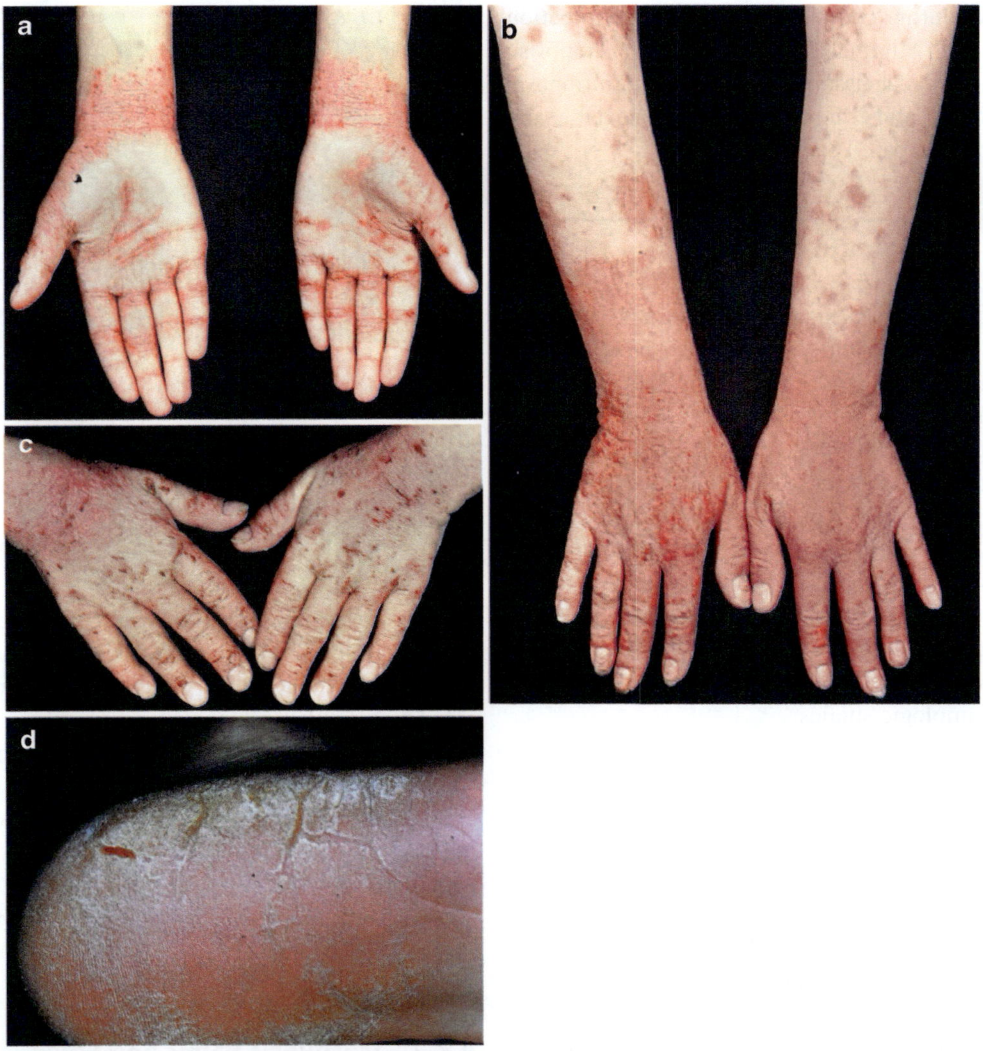

Fig. 4.23 Hand and foot eczema in atopic dermatitis. (**a**) Hand eczema with palmar involvement. (**b**) Dorsum of the hands with strong excoriations. (**c**) Dry atopic dermatitis of the dorsum of the hands. (**d**) Foot eczema with deep fissures

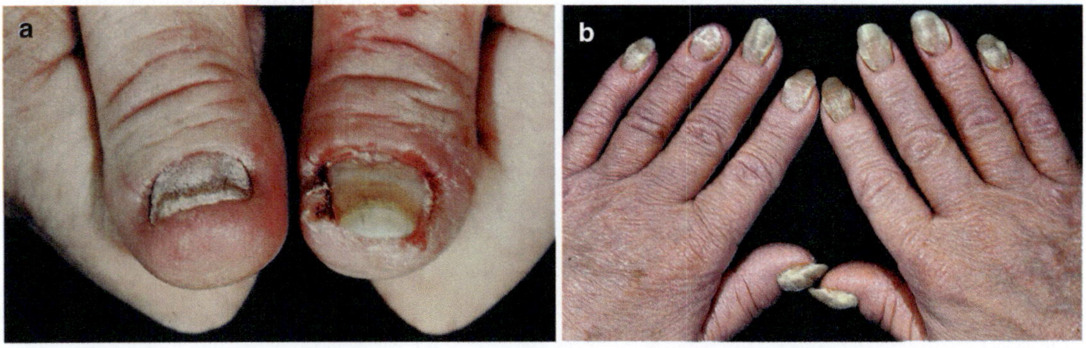

Fig. 4.24 Nail changes in hand eczema. (**a**) Eczema nails. (**b**) Nail dystrophy in eczema

nantly during childhood or when superinfection occurs. Minimal manifestations comprise infra-auricular fissures, cheilitis sicca, infranasal erosion, eyelid eczema, finger or toe eczema, and pityriasis alba.

4.3 Stigmata of Atopy

Contrary to actual signs and symptoms of disease and minimal manifestations, the so-called stigmata represent characteristics of the organ skin, not necessarily going along with feeling sick nor being sequels of the disease. Rather they can be regarded as constitutional signs of an "atopic diathesis"; thus, they can give the experienced physician valuable information without additional laboratory diagnostics or history analysis with regard to the existence of atopy in the individual.

Table 4.1 shows the most common stigmata which also have been quantitatively evaluated in epidemiologic studies.

4.3.1 Dry Skin (Xerosis, Sebostasis)

Dry skin is a major characteristic of atopic dermatitis, also called sebostasis or xerosis; it is visible as rough skin, sometimes slightly scaling (Fig. 4.25). The term "dry" skin can be questioned pathophysiologically since, in investigations with regard to the percentage of water in the skin, no real decrease has been found, but an increased transepidermal water loss (TEWL) due to disturbed skin barrier function. Furthermore, mild signs of inflammation have been found in "dry skin of atopic dermatitis" in uninvolved areas [810].

Table 4.1 Stigmata of atopic dermatitis/eczema

Dry skin (sebostasis, xerosis)
Hyperlinearity of palms and soles ("ichthyosis hands or feet")
Linear grooves of fingertips
Atopy fold of the eyelid (Dennie-Morgan)
Scattering of lateral eyebrow (Hertoghe)
Low temporal hairline
Facial pallor with periorbital halo
White dermographism
Delayed blanch reaction after acetylcholine

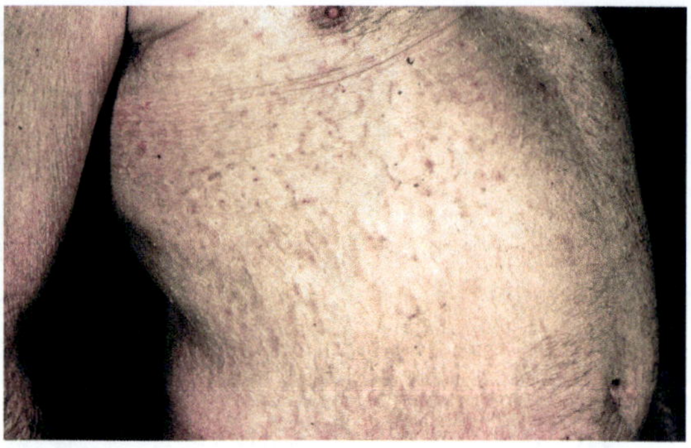

Fig. 4.25 Dry skin, eczema craquelée

The term sebostasis indicates a diminished serum secretion which is controversial. The lipid content of the epidermis has been investigated by several groups and found to be altered especially with regard to different patterns of ceramides (see Chap. 5 "Pathophysiology").

Finally, a major characteristic is roughness which can be recognized by patient and physician and feels like "dryness." It is not clear whether this "dry" aspect actually corresponds to the deficiency of the epidermal protein filaggrin (see Chap. 5 "Pathophysiology") found in many patients with atopic eczema.

4.3.2 Ichthyosis Palms and Soles (Hyperlinearity of Palms and Soles)

This stigma is well-known in patients with the autosomal dominant disease ichthyosis vulgaris. Marked linear furs or lines can be seen, partly in a bizarre or linear configuration mostly on the palms in both vertical and horizontal direction, but in infants commonly also on the soles (Fig. 4.26). This sign can be used to get information on the role of skin barrier disturbance in an individual patient [467].

This sign, first described by Leutgeb et al., was regarded for a long time as proof of concom-

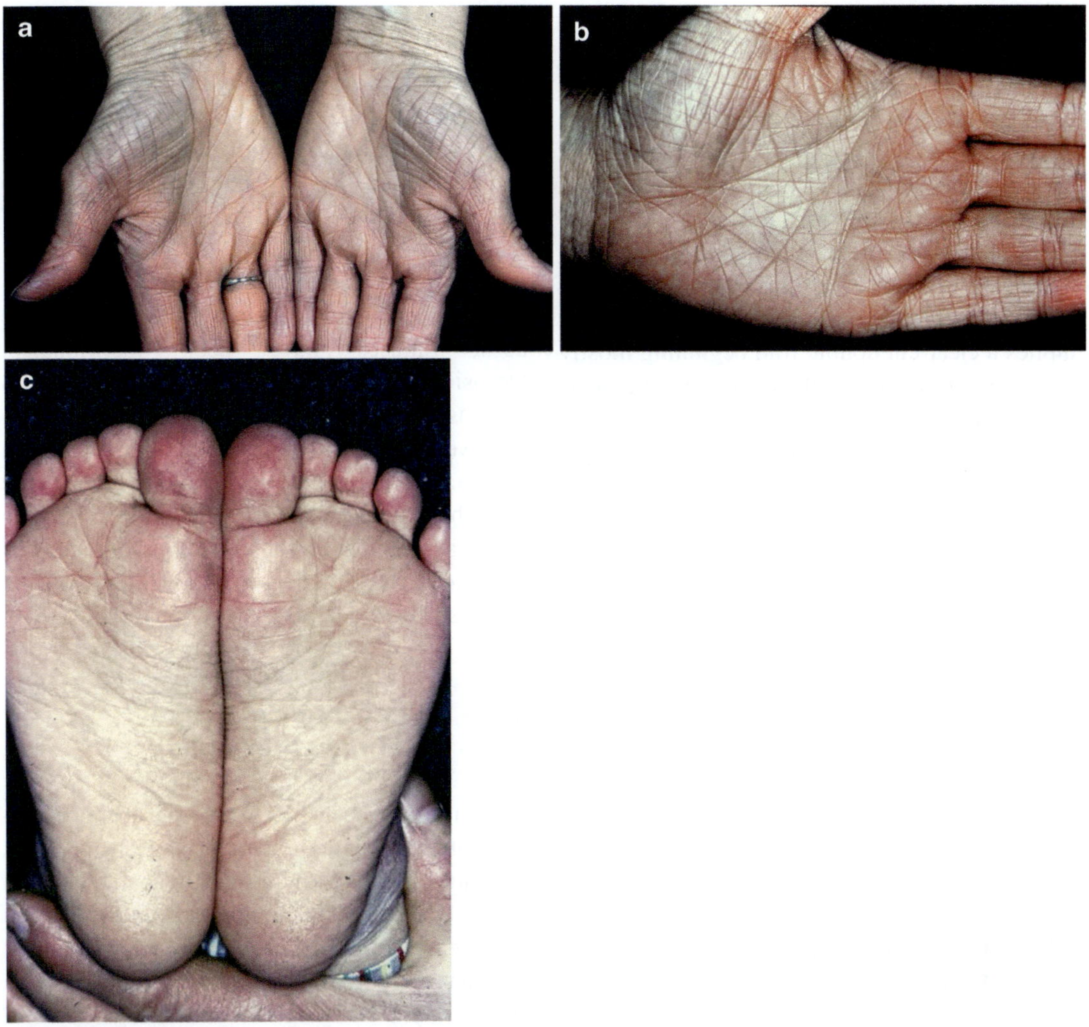

Fig. 4.26 Hyperlinearity of palms and soles (ichthyotic hands/feet). (**a**) Massive skin changes in the palms. (**b**) Hyperlinearity of hand. (**c**) Ichthyosis feet

itantly occurring ichthyosis vulgaris and can now better be explained by the filaggrin deficiency in heterozygous states in many atopic dermatitis patients. Only in a small part of eczema patients the typical signs of ichthyosis vulgaris can be seen in histopathology or by electron microscopy, namely abnormal keratohyalin granules [680].

A subgroup of ichthyosis hands or feet can be seen in linear grooves often horizontal to the papillary lines on the fingertips (Fig. 4.27).

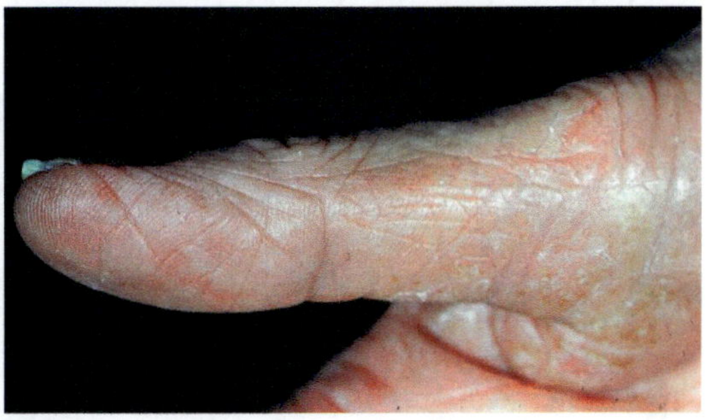

Fig. 4.27 Linear grooves on the fingertips

4.3.3 Infraorbital Fold (Atopy Fold, Dennie-Morgan)

This sign has first been described in a letter by Dr. Morgan as "definite wrinkle just beneath the margin of the lower lid of both eyes," who mentioned it to Dr. Dennie [521] as a sign of atopy. The fold can be single or double. Mostly it is present on both lower eyelids, sometimes however only unilaterally. The exact definition implies a clear-cut double fold beginning mostly at the inner (medial) canthus and reaching laterally at least beyond the center of the pupil. The atopy fold must not be confounded with the physiological sulcus palpebralis inferior [606] (Fig. 4.28). Many authors regard the Dennie-Morgan fold as a sequel of lid eczema due to increased rubbing and scratching. However, clear-cut clinical observations have shown that this stigma can be present many years before the first occurrence of atopic dermatitis, mostly starting in other body areas like elbows or knee joints and without lid eczema.

The atopy fold is also present in respiratory atopic diseases. In Asian patients, the infraorbital fold seems to be a less suitable marker.

4.3.4 Periorbital Halo and Facial Pallor

This sign, also called halo eyes (Fig. 4.29), can be observed in atopic ezema, but also in respiratory atopy as allergic rhinoconjunctivitis and has been called "allergic shiners"; the manifestation is a dark grey, brownish discoloration of the periorbital areas, sometimes associated with mild edema. The patients give an impression of sleeplessness ("bleary-eyed"). Some of our coworkers call them "disco shadows." Once an actress came to me (JR) as a patient just because of this skin change, for the director would not give her a role in a play anymore, since she looked "worn out" ("kaputt").

Pathophysiologically swellings and congestion of postcapillary venules in the area of the nasal sinuses have been incriminated. Occasionally a secondary hyperpigmentation on the basis of existing chronic eczema has been observed; this however does not correspond to a stigma. Together with the common pallor of the face, this stigma can be regarded as an imbalance of the autonomic nervous system with increased alpha-adrenergic and cholinergic impulses and decreased beta-adrenergic reactions.

4.3.5 Rarefication of Lateral Eyebrows (Hertoghe)

This sign has been first described at the beginning of the twentieth century by Hertoghe in a patient with hypothyreosis. In patients with atopic eczema, some authors see an association to increased rubbing of eyebrows, when eyebrow eczema can be diagnosed at the same time (Fig. 4.30). For a long time it was regarded as a classic stigma of altered skin independent of immune reactivity. Saurat observed a regrowth of lateral eyebrow hair after successful bone marrow transplantation in patients with Wiskott-Aldrich syndrome with massive atopic eczema

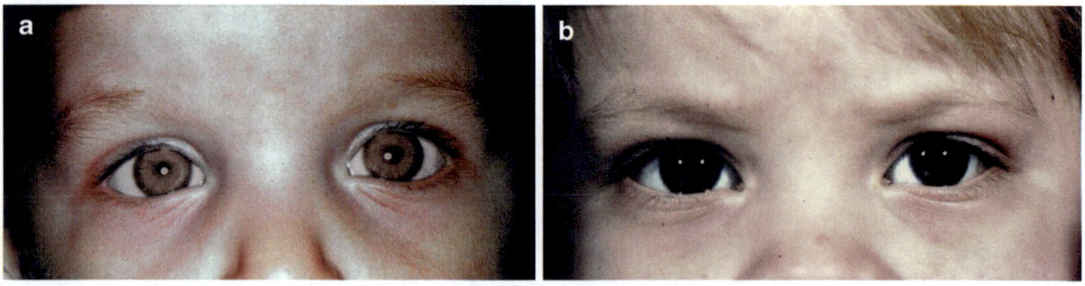

Fig. 4.28 Dennie-Morgan fold (atopy fold). (**a**) Double fold starting on the inner cantus reaching over the middle of the pupil. (**b**) Atopy fold in a child with atopic dermatitis

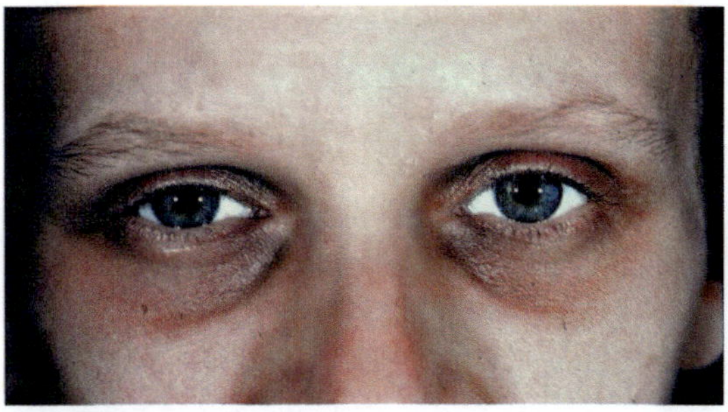

Fig. 4.29 Periorbital shadowing ("halo eyes," "disco eyes")

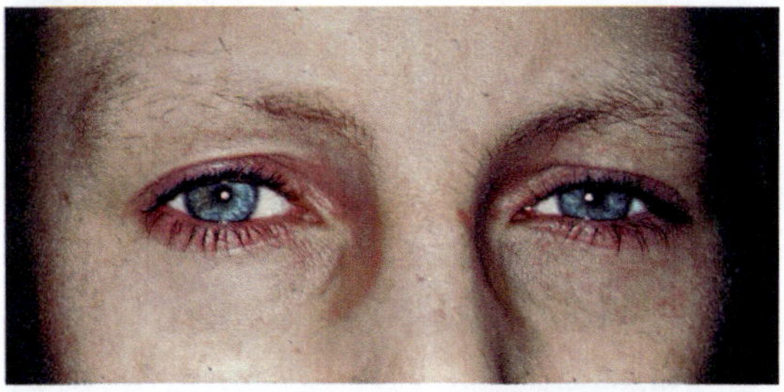

Fig. 4.30 Lateral part of eyebrows with sparse hair ("Hertoghe sign")

and atopic stigmata [683]. It is obvious that artificial manipulations (plucking of eyebrows) (pseudo-Hertoghe) have to be differentiated from the true stigma.

4.3.6 Low Temporal Hairline, "Fur Cap Hair Growth"

This stigma describes a decreased distance between the temporal hairline and the end of the lateral eyebrows; sometimes there is no distance in between (Fig. 4.31). Quantitatively the distance between temporal hairline and eyebrow should be more than 3 cm. The stigma can be observed in almost 90% of patients with atopic dermatitis [606].

A positive Hertoghe phenomenon does not exclude a low temporal hairline sign.

4.3.7 White Dermographism

The white dermographism is one of the best-known stigmata of atopy. While in healthy individuals tangential pressure (e.g., with a spatula) leads to a redness of the skin within 30–60 s (red dermographism), in atopic individuals sometimes the skin turns white (Fig. 4.32); sometimes there is a contrasting whitening next to a central red part (red dermographism with a white edge). Pathophysiologically most likely an increased local vasoconstriction is the basis of white dermographism [888].

4.3.8 Delayed Blanch

After injection of acetylcholine (intradermal), some patients with atopic eczema develop a long-lasting white discoloration in the injection area called delayed blanch reaction or delayed white reaction [304].

White dermographism and delayed blanch can be regarded as signs of autonomic dysregulation in atopics. They are not specific for atopic dermatitis but also can be seen in respiratory atopy.

It is important not to elicit white dermographism in an involved or inflamed skin area. On inflamed skin, white dermographism can be elicited also in other skin conditions.

4.3.9 Role of Stigmata in Diagnosis

Many studies have investigated the prevalence of atopy stigmata in patients with atopic eczema and other atopic diseases as well as in healthy control persons. In an intense and quantitative measurement in patients with various atopic diseases and healthy controls, we found that all of the above-mentioned stigmata were significantly more prevalent in atopics compared to non-atopic controls [606]. The strongest association with atopic eczema (and significantly higher than in respiratory atopy) were

- Dry skin,
- Ichthyosis palms and soles,
- White dermographism,
- Hertoghe phenomenon.

Similar to the parameter "increased tendency to IgE production" which sometimes only is detectable as elevated serum IgE (see Chapter

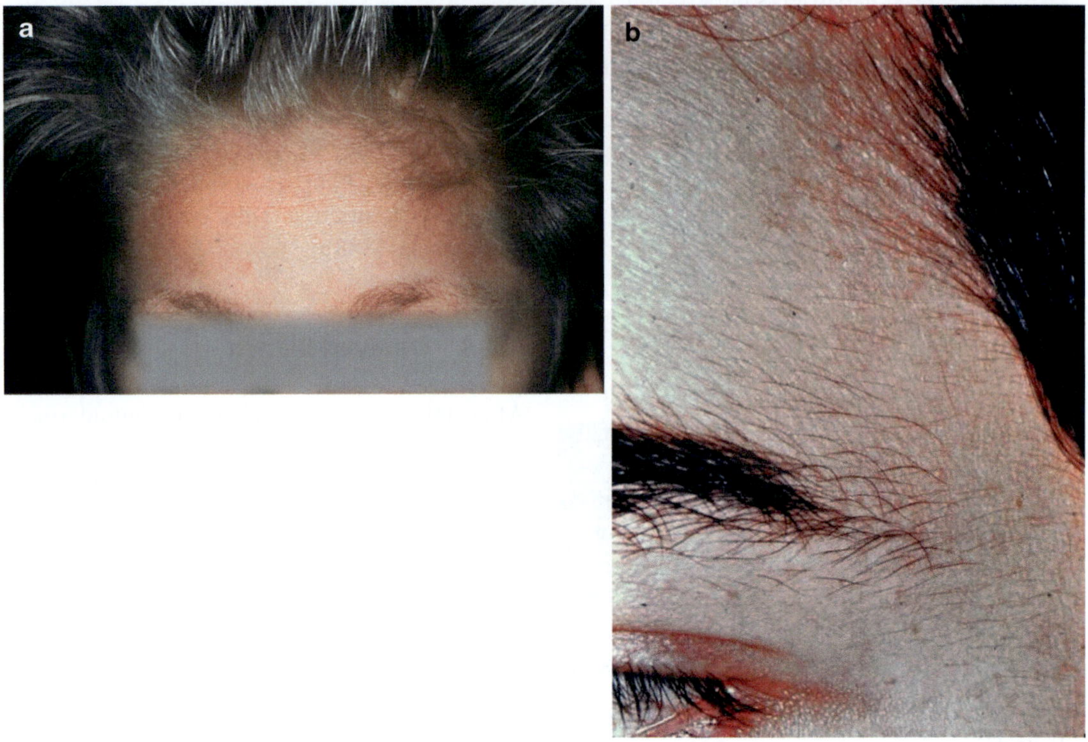

Fig. 4.31 Low temporal hairline ("fur cap"). (**a**) Reduction of the distance between temporal and hair and end of lateral eyebrows. (**b**) Low temporal hairline

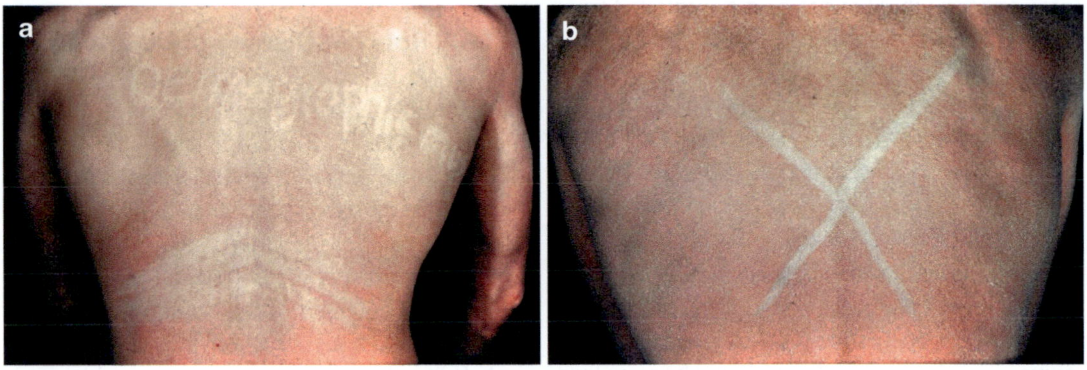

Fig. 4.32 White dermographism. (**a**) After tangential pressure, the skin turns white instead of red. (**b**) Massive whitening within 30–60 s

Terminology, Chap. 1) there also may be a gradual intensity of skin manifestation of atopy with "minimal" or "latent atopic eczema" which only becomes visible as stigma without ever turning into actual clinical eczema.

4.3.10 Summary

Stigmata have to be distinguished from actual symptoms of disease. They are signs of the organ skin not necessarily connected with feeling ill which give hints to the existence of an "atopic diathesis." They comprise dry skin (xerosis, sebostasis), hyperlinearity of palms and soles (ichthyosis "palms" or "soles"), increased infraorbital fold (atopy fold Dennie-Morgan), facial pallor with periorbital halo, rarefication of lateral eyebrows (Hertoghe), fur cap hair growth with low temporal hairline as well as white dermographism and delayed blanch.

4.4 Differential Diagnoses

Even if the diagnosis of atopic dermatitis is not difficult for an experienced dermatologist or allergist, a variety of differential diagnoses have to be considered (Table 4.2), partly depending on the age group (see also [242, 613, 658]).

Table 4.2 Differential diagnoses of atopic dermatitis

Chronic inflammatory skin diseases
• Seborrheic dermatitis
• Psoriasis
• Lichen simplex chronicus
• Allergic contact dermatitis
• Irritative toxic contact dermatitis
Infectious skin diseases
• Impetigo contagiosa
• Candidiasis
• Tinea
• Scabies
• Ictus insectorum (strophulus)
Immunodeficiency syndromes
• Ataxia teleangiectasia
• Wiskott-Aldrich syndrome
• Hyper-IgE syndrome
• Severe combined immunodeficiency (SCID)
Autoimmune diseases
• Bullous pemphigoid
• Pemphigus foliaceus
Dermatitis herpetiformis
• Dermatomyositis
• Graft-versus-host disease
Genodermatoses
• Netherton syndrome
• Dubowitz syndrome
• Erythrokeratodermia variabilis
Metabolic diseases
• Phenylketonuria
• Tyrosinemia
• Zinc deficiency
Side effects of drugs
• e.g., eczema exacerbation after anti-TNF therapy

4.4.1 Differential Diagnosis in Infants

In the first months of life, it is mainly seborrheic dermatitis or diaper dermatitis which have to be considered (Fig. 4.33). Often there is no clear-cut diagnosis in the first months of life, then the term "eczema infantum" (infantile eczema) is helpful Edgren [200] (Table 4.3).

There is a valuable rule: bipolar occurrence (especially head and scalp and genital area involved) allures seborrheic dermatitis (Fig. 4.34). Skin changes in head and trunk with uninvolved diaper area are typical for atopic eczema. This commonly observed "diaper sign" is poorly investigated scientifically. One can speculate whether the diaper offers protection against rubbing or scratching or the contents act like a wet wrap. It is surprising that in severely affected infants with atopic eczema often only the diaper area is totally uninvolved (Fig. 4.35).

Another sign visible to everybody but not often recognized is the absence of eczema on the tip of the nose (Yamamoto sign, personal communication via Kristian Thestrup-Pedersen).

Differential diagnoses in adults are enlisted in Table 4.4.

4.4.2 Chronic Inflammatory Skin Diseases

In infants, but also in small children, psoriasis can be a difficult differential diagnosis, especially in cases of so-called figurate eczema or when there is a coincidence of both diseases. Thirty years ago this was no problem; eczema and psoriasis seemed to exclude each other. Only by the epidemiological studies by Henseler and Christophers [320] it became clear that psoriasis and atopic eczema can occur in one and the same

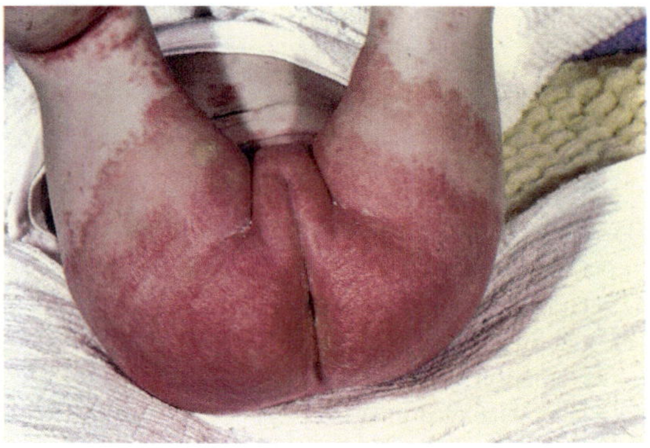

Fig. 4.33 Diaper dermatitis with marked erythema in the diaper area

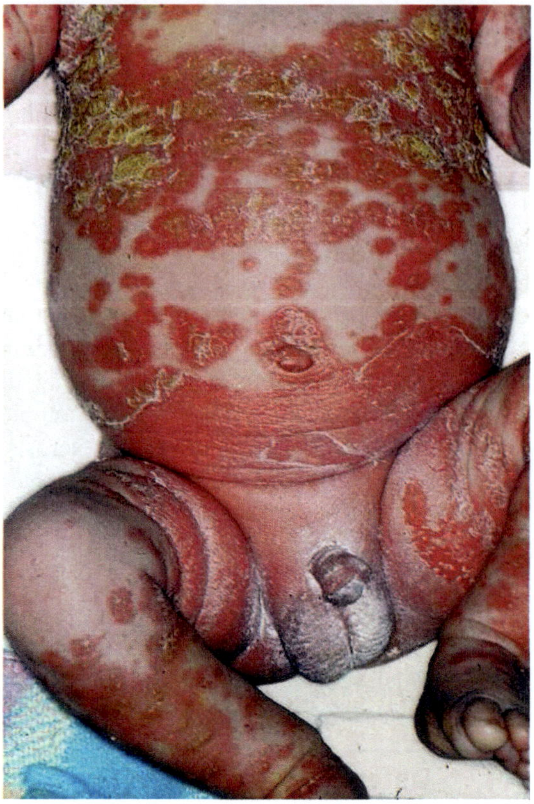

Fig. 4.34 Yellowish crusts in seborrheic dermatitis in an infant

Table 4.3 Differential diagnoses of atopic eczema in infancy (according to [242])

	Atopic dermatitis	Seborrheic dermatitis	Scabies
Onset	2–3 months	First days of life	All ages
Gender	M = F	M = F	M = F
Prevalence	Common	Common	Variable
Genetic mutation	Filaggrin +	0	0
IgE	Increased	Normal	Normal/increased
Eosinophilia	Common	Rare	Common
Morphology	Typically age-dependent	Diaper area, axillae, capillitium	Interdigital areas, genital area
Itch	Strong	Almost absent	Strong
Dermographism	White	Red	Red
S. aureus infection	Common	Rare	Rare
Other infections	Rare	Malassezia furfur	Rare
Concomitant respiratory atopy	Common	Rare	Rare
Food allergy	Common	Rare	Rare

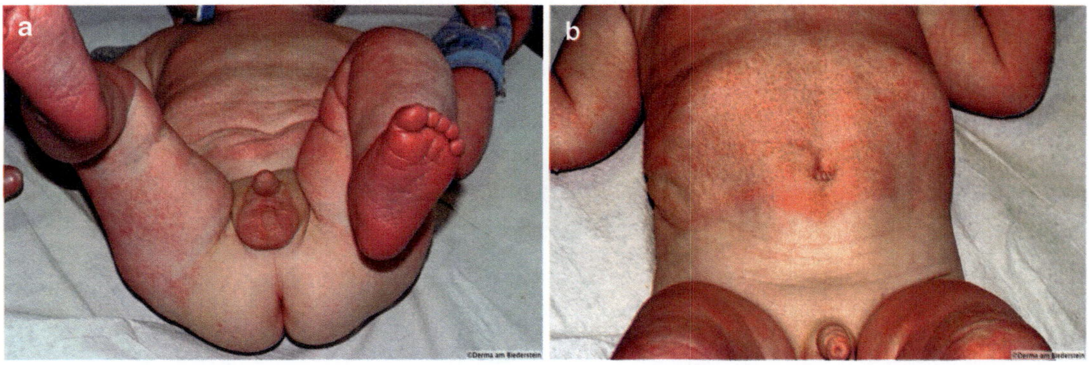

Fig. 4.35 "Diaper sign" in atopic dermatitis: the diaper area is surprisingly often uninvolved. (**a**) Uninvolved diaper area. (**b**) Uninvolved diaper area with strong general skin involvement

Table 4.4 Differential diagnosis of atopic eczema in adulthood

	Atopic dermatitis	Seborrheic dermatitis	Scabies	T cell lymphoma	Allergic contact dermatitis
Onset	Early childhood	All ages	All ages	50–60 years	Adults
IgE	High	Normal	Normal	High	Normal
Eosinophilia	Common	Rare	Common	Rare	Rare
Morphology	Large flexures	Seborrheic areas	Wrists, interdigital, and genital area	Persistent patches	Often localized
Itch	Strong	Mild	Strong	Mild	Strong
Dermographism	White	Normal	Normal	Normal	Normal
Concomitant respiratory allergy	Common	Rare	Rare	Rare	Rare
Food allergy	Common	Rare	Rare	Rare	Rare
Others			Other family members affected	T cell receptor rearrangement	Positive patch test

individual, although rarely. Due to the increase in eczema prevalence, this subgroup of patients may be seen more often.

Yet there seems to be a mutual antagonism between psoriasis and atopic eczema in the pathophysiology [224] (see Chap. 5).

Furthermore, existing eczema may trigger latent psoriasis via scratching and mechanical traumatization in the sense of a Koebner phenomenon.

A difficult differential diagnosis can be the localized involvement of palms and soles together with dyshidrosis (pompholyx). This type of hand eczema can occur in atopic eczema, but also in allergic contact dermatitis, but also in patients with tinea. According to some authors, dyshidrotic hand or foot eczema always corresponds to atopic dermatitis and should be called atopic palmoplantar eczema [725]. In the localization of the palms and soles, the differential diagnosis of eczema versus psoriasis is unclear in more than 50% of cases [413].

The cooccurrence or absence of other inflammatory diseases in atopic dermatitis is an interesting phenomenon and gives rise to new pathophysiological concepts (see Chap. 5).

Other allergic skin diseases, especially allergic contact dermatitis, have to be differentiated;

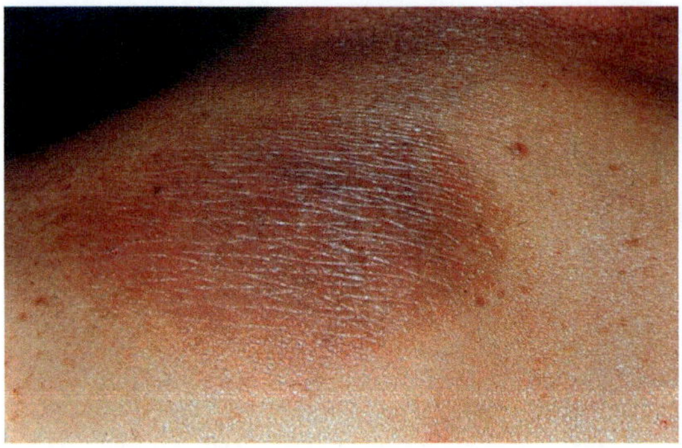

Fig. 4.36 Lichen simplex chronicus Vidal

allergic contact dermatitis also can occur in childhood, which is not mentioned in many textbooks (see Chap. 6, "Diagnosis"). Especially when the dorsum of the feet is involved, contact allergy against shoe constituents should be considered.

In adult life, lichen simplex chronicus is a differential diagnosis in chronically lichenified areas (Fig. 4.36) or may represent a subtype of atopic dermatitis in a localized variant. Similarly irritative reactions, due to strong mechanic traumatization and individual susceptibility, have to be considered as a differential diagnosis of atopic dermatitis.

Also, systemic allergic contact dermatitis (hematogenous contact eczema) may sometimes be difficult to distinguish from a generalized flare of atopic eczema. Pathophysiologically, reactivated T cells induce keratinocyte apoptosis and thereby induce generalized or symmetric eczematous skin lesions after parenteral or oral allergen application [400, 727, 781]; however, also Th2 immunity is relevant in allergic contact dermatitis, and biologics inhibiting type 2 immunity are effective [274, 470].

4.4.3 Inflammatory Tumor Responses

An interesting variant of eczematous skin disease is an inflammatory phenomenon occurring around congenital pigmentary naevi with a mostly transitory character. This inflammatorily altered nevus is called Meyerson's nevus.

4.4.4 Infectious Skin Diseases

Scabies may be overlooked by the inexperienced and diagnosed as atopic eczema, since it also goes along with extreme itch. The typical mite furrows on the wrist or in the interdigital areas together with typical papules in the genital area (penile papules) are characteristic. Using the dermatoscope, the detection of scabies mites has become much more easy (typical scabies "kite").

Regarding the existing cross-reactivities between scabies mite (Sarcoptes scabiei) and house dust mite (Dermatophagoides pteronyssinus or farinae) as well as storage mites (Lepidoglyphus destructor), one can speculate about a primitive evolutionary defense reaction against mites via IgE antibodies in the development of atopic dermatitis.

Other infectious diseases which have to be considered include staphylococcal infection (impetigo), herpes simplex, which can give rise to the serious complication of eczema herpeticum (see Chapter Complications) as well as tinea.

4.4.5 Metabolic Diseases, Immunodeficiencies or Immunopathies

A variety of metabolic diseases can become manifest in eczematous skin changes: when the orificia (perioral and perianal) are involved in infants, one has to think of zinc deficiency and acrodermatitis enteropathica.

In several congenital or acquired immune deficiencies, atopic eczema seems to be more prevalent than in the normal population [683] (see also Associated Diseases).

Immunopathies may be considered in the differential diagnosis with regard to early stages of bullous pemphigoid in the elderly or other blistering diseases like dermatitis herpetiformis Duhring or pemphigus foliaceus.

Graft-versus-host disease can show eczema-like skin changes with itch and dysesthesia and follicular papules.

Skin changes in dermatomyositis in childhood are characteristic, but can be confounded in the initial phase with facial involvement, erythema, and swelling with eczema. Sometimes lid eczema is diagnosed, although only swelling (without epidermal involvement) of the eyelids is present.

4.4.6 Malignant Diseases

Atopic dermatitis has to be differentiated from a variety of malignant skin diseases, especially T cell lymphoma of the skin and Langerhans cell histiocytosis (histiocytosis X). In infants, Langerhans cell histiocytosis can occur preferably in the diaper area or in the neck-shoulder region and looks similar to atopic eczema with crusted papules and seborrheic squamous areas. In these cases, dermatopathology is crucial.

In adults, unexplained and not clearly attributable eczematous skin changes should give rise to the differential diagnosis of lymphoproliferative disease of the skin, the most common being mycosis fungoides as a variant of cutaneous T cell lymphoma as well as Sezary syndrome [614].

Especially in the maximal variant of erythroderma which can occur in atopic eczema, the differential diagnosis of T cell lymphoma is crucial.

A hint for malignant T cell proliferation can be seen in the poor response to anti-inflammatory treatment of the eczematous skin changes. The simple question as to "whether this patch has been there in the same spot all the time or has disappeared and reoccurred at another skin area" is one of the most important questions in this differential diagnosis. There are—few—patients in which a severe form of atopic eczema finally transforms into cutaneous T cell lymphoma.

The differential diagnosis between atopic dermatitis and cutaneous T cell lymphoma, especially of an erythrodermic variant, also may be difficult. Total serum IgE or measurement of certain chemokines do not really differentiate; however, absence of specific IgE, extremely high CD4/CD8 ratio, CCR10 positivity in the skin and Sézary cells in peripheral blood and detection of Tcell receptor rearrangement may be a strong indication for cutaneous T cell lymphoma [514].

4.4.7 Summary

The most important differential diagnostic aspects of atopic dermatitis in infant and adult age are enlisted in Tables 4.3 and 4.4 and comprise chronic inflammatory skin diseases, infectious skin diseases, immunopathologies, hereditary skin diseases, metabolic disorders, malignant skin diseases, drug reactions as well as all other forms of dermatitis or eczema.

4.5 Associated Diseases

4.5.1 Hereditary Dermatoses

Some hereditary skin diseases can either directly be accompanied by atopic dermatitis or be associated with similar skin changes (Table 4.5).

In 50% of the cases with phenylketonuria, eczematous skin lesions can be observed which in early childhood can be mixed with atopic eczema, but which clear under the correct diet with avoidance of phenylalanine.

Some hereditary dermatoses have a more intense relation to atopic eczema.

4.5.1.1 Ichthyosis Vulgaris

The autosomal dominant and most common form of ichthyosis is closely associated to atopic dermatitis [613]. The basic defect is a homozygous deficiency of the epidermal protein filaggrin which, when in heterozygous manifestation, gives rise to an increased risk of atopic eczema [580] (see Chap. 5). In ichthyosis vulgaris, the second important aspect of pathophysiology in atopic dermatitis, namely the immunodeviation

Table 4.5 Hereditary dermatoses with association to atopic dermatitis

Ichthyosis vulgaris
Netherton syndrome
Dubowitz syndrome
Wiskott-Aldrich syndrome
Hyper-IgE syndrome
Anhidrotic ectodermal dysphasia
Ommen syndrome
Di George syndrome
Phenylketonuria

toward Th2 and IgE, is missing. Ichthyosis patients only suffer from extremely dry skin.

4.5.1.2 Netherton Syndrome

The triade comprises the Netherton syndrome:

- Congenital ichthyosis in linear configuration (ichthyosis linearis circumflexa),
- Atopic diathesis with increased IgE and hypereosinophilia,
- Hair growth disturbance (trichorrhexis invaginata or "bamboo hair").

Pathophysiologically the underlying defect is a deficiency of the gene for SPINK5 on chromosome 5q32 which encodes for the serine protease inhibitor LEKTI (lymphoepithelial Kazal type-related inhibitor) and plays a role in skin barrier function [151, 296].

4.5.1.3 Dubowitz Syndrome

Another autosomal recessive dermatosis going along with eczematous skin changes is the Dubowitz syndrome, which is characterized by dysmorphia of the face together with psychomotor irritations [193].

4.5.1.4 Wiskott-Aldrich Syndrome

The Wiskott-Aldrich syndrome develops through an X-chromosomal recessive defect on chromosome XpL 22 and occurs almost exclusively in boys. It goes along with eczema, thrombocytopenia, and purpura with abnormal megakaryocytes and increased susceptibility to infections. Eczematous skin changes with increased blue patches in male infants should make think of Wiskott-Aldrich syndrome.

Genetically a mutation of the WASP (Wiskott-Aldrich syndrome protein) has been found which plays a role in the actin formation of the cytoskeleton [93]. A decrease in IgM concentrations has been described in the Wiskott-Aldrich syndrome. Bone marrow transplantation is the life-saving therapy [683].

4.5.1.5 Hyper-IgE Syndrome

An extreme elevation of serum IgE levels together with skin changes often occurring in the first years of life together with severe deep tissue infections (Staphylococci, Candida) are typical for the hyper-IgE syndrome [112, 654]. In the pathology, mutations in the STAT3 gene are likely to be responsible [277, 278, 620].

A characteristic clinical sign is a delayed dentition with concomitant existence of both primary and secondary teeth.

For a long time, the differential diagnosis between severe atopic dermatitis with impetiginized and superinfected skin lesions from hyper-IgE syndrome (HIES) (Job's syndrome) was difficult. Through molecular analysis and better characterization of phenotypes, it has become clear that a papulopustular eruption especially on face and scalp in the first 8 weeks of life seems to be typical of a hyper-IgE syndrome and can be distinguished from other neonatal skin lesions. Furthermore, clinical signs of nail infection and chronic candidiasis of the oral mucosa are more often seen in HIES, where the STAT3 mutation is autosomal dominant [82].

Also, anti-IgE has been found to be helpful in occasional cases with hyper-IgE syndrome [42].

There is a subtype of hyper-IgE syndrome characterized by mutations in the DOCK8 gene (ca. 5% of hyper-IgE syndrome patients, show more severe infections) [759].

Some other severe immunodeficiency syndromes (thymic hypoplasia DiGeorge), as well as severe combined immunodeficiency (SCID), can go along with eczematous skin changes.

4.5.1.6 Keratosis Follicularis (Pilaris)

There is an endless controversy about whether keratosis follicularis should be regarded as a stigma or a minimal manifestation of atopic dermatitis which until now is not clear. According to our experiences, it is sometimes associated with atopic eczema, but is not significantly more prevalent in atopic individuals generally.

When the face is involved, so-called ulerythema ophryogenes can be a differential diagnosis to atopic eczema with involvement of eyebrows and redness of the cheeks together with keratotic papules.

Classically keratosis follicularis involves the lateral side of the upper arms and responds well to mild keratolytic treatment.

4.5.1.7 Anhidrotic Congenital Ectodermal Dysplasia

This severe skin disease can also go along with an increased prevalence of atopic diseases [819].

4.5.2 Hair Diseases

Some forms of hair disease seem to be associated with an increased prevalence of atopic dermatitis such as the syndrome of incombable hair (cheveux incoiffables) [97].

There is an association of atopic eczema and alopecia areata [23, 255].

In a study from Japan, 10–52% of patients suffering from alopecia areata have been found to be atopic [586], this association was particularly apparent in childhood.

4.5.3 Atopic Respiratory Diseases and Other Allergic Reactions

Per definition, atopic dermatitis is associated to a high degree with atopic respiratory diseases such as rhinoconjunctivitis and bronchial asthma, but also with other allergic, especially IgE-mediated reactions [56, 559, 658, 715].

4.5.3.1 Bronchial Asthma and Rhinoconjunctivitis

The occurrence of atopic respiratory diseases in atopic dermatitis is common, especially in children and adolescents. Over 50% of atopic eczema patients suffer from respiratory symptoms. The risk of allergic bronchial asthma for infants with atopic eczema is 3–4 times increased compared to the normal population; there is a clear-cut dependence on the severity of the skin disease [61]. Approximately 80% of children with atopic eczema suffer from asthma or allergic rhinoconjunctivitis. Salob et al. found in 90% of children an existing bronchial hyperreactivity which was unknown to patients and parents [678].

In the classic Venn diagram, the overlap of asthma, rhinoconjunctivitis, and eczema show a focus on eczema in childhood, while rhinoconjunctivitis is more prominent in adults (Fig. 2.6) [1].

Children with atopic dermatitis without known asthma often show bronchial hyperreactivity [147] or increased concentrations of exhalable nitric oxide (FeNO) [350].

4.5.3.2 Anaphylaxis, Food Allergy, and Gastrointestinal Diseases

IgE-mediated reactions, such as contact urticaria or protein contact dermatitis, are more frequent in atopics. IgE-associated food allergies, especially food anaphylaxis, seem to be more common in atopic eczema patients than in normals [208, 605, 913].

Apart from gastrointestinal symptoms of IgE-mediated food allergy, other gastrointestinal problems like gluten-sensitive enteropathy, eosinophilic gastroenteritis, eosinophilic esophagitis, or other inflammatory bowel diseases may be more common in atopy. Common genetic markers for M. Crohn, psoriasis, and atopic eczema have been found [145, 711].

Food Allergy and Food Anaphylaxis

In discussing the role of food hypersensitivity in atopic dermatitis, one has to consider different aspects:

Food allergens can elicit exacerbations of existing eczema lesions and contribute to the continuous maintenance of atopic dermatitis.

Food allergens—sometimes the same, but sometimes other or different allergens—can elicit life-threatening symptoms of anaphylaxis in eczema patients, independent of eczema or oral allergy syndrome with swelling of lips and tongue; this preferably occurs with pollen-associated food allergens in patients also suffering from hay fever.

Finally, non-IgE-associated food hypersensitivities may also occur in eczema patients and may contribute to eczema flares, especially after application of preservatives, e.g., sulfites or other food additives [642, 658].

Drug-Induced or Insect Venom-Induced Anaphylaxis

IgE-mediated anaphylactic reaction against drugs or insect venoms can occur in patients with atopic eczema, but they do not seem to be more prevalent than in other populations [252]. Maybe the special hyperreactivity of the mucosal surfaces in the allergen contact is a prerequisite for increased occurrence in atopic individuals.

Anaphylaxis to Seminal Plasma

This rare, but life-threatening condition affects females developing anaphylactic shock after unprotected coitus, and almost exclusively occurs in atopic females, especially in patients with severe atopic dermatitis and concomitant food allergy. The eliciting allergen could be identified as prostate-specific antigen (PSA) [847].

4.5.4 Ocular Diseases

Many different clinical and pathogenetic conditions can occur in the eye, sometimes difficult to diagnose. The major allergic diseases in the eye include

- Seasonal or perennial allergic conjunctivitis,
- Vernal keratoconjunctivitis which may be IgE-, but also non-IgE-associated,
- Giant papillary conjunctivitis with no allergy history,
- Superficial punctate keratitis,
- Atopic keratoconjunctivitis (more prevalent in atopic dermatitis),
- Classical allergic contact dermatitis (involving the eyelid and the conjunctivas as blepharoconjunctivitis) [451, 644].

In a review of the literature, it was found that atopic dermatitis alone seems to be a risk factor to develop both anterior and posterior subcapsular cataracts, the latter often being associated with systemic glucocorticosteroid use. The authors speculate about the role of oxidative stress during an inflammatory reaction as a causal factor [38].

Not only allergic rhinoconjunctivitis is more often associated with atopic dermatitis, but also a variety of other ocular complications such as atopic keratoconjunctivitis, atopic cataract, and keratoconus [417].

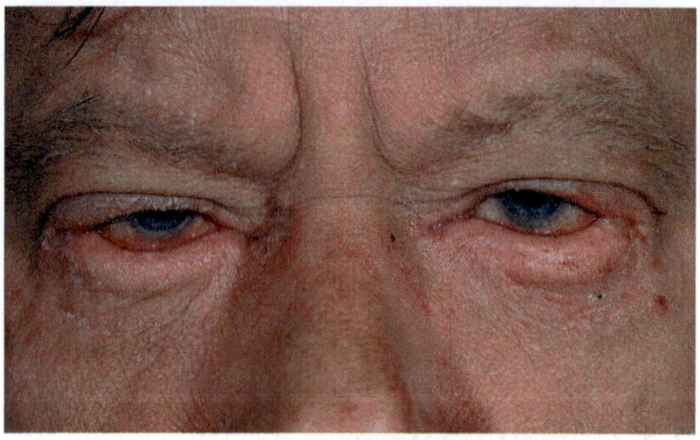

Fig. 4.37 Marked ocular changes in severe atopic dermatitis in an adult with keratoconjunctivitis and blepharitis

The association of cataract and atopic eczema is well referred to in the textbooks but may have been overestimated in earlier times with studies showing prevalences between 0.4 and 33% (!) [658]. In our own experiences this occurs much rarer. In the split lamp examination, one has to differentiate between anterior and posterior subcapsular cataracts; the latter ones usually are a sequel of long-term glucocorticosteroid use and thus can be more common in eczema patients.

It may be interesting to speculate whether common pathophysiologic mechanisms in the skin and the eye lens could play a role in the development of atopic cataract [811].

Severe eye changes usually can be seen in patients with the otherwise very severe clinical course of atopic eczema (Fig. 4.37).

In adult patients with lid eczema, of course, contact allergy to ophthalmic preparations in eye drops has to be considered.

With the development of new biologics for treatment, e.g., the interleukin 4 R antagonist dupilumab, conjunctivitis has been observed as a rather common and often unpleasant side-effect.

4.5.5 Nephrotic Syndrome

In some patients with atopic diseases, a steroid-sensitive nephrotic syndrome can occur with proteinuria, edema, and clear-cut deterioration after allergen contact (pollen, house dust mite or food allergens).

4.5.6 Vitiligo

There is an opinion in the literature that, in patients with severe atopic eczema, concomitant vitiligo has a poorer prognosis [122]. Whether there is a clear association between vitiligo and atopic dermatitis is not established [802].

4.5.7 Photosensitivity

While UV treatment and heliotherapy are benefitting many patients, ca. 10% report about deterioration or exacerbation of skin symptoms after UV exposure.

The most common—in common parlance called sun allergy—photohypersensitivity reaction is polymorphous light dermatosis (polymorphous light eruption) (PLE) which occurs characteristically in spring after the first heavy sun exposure and ameliorates during summer. This condition seems to be more prevalent among atopics compared to the general population [604]. The eliciting agent in this type of photohypersensitivity is unknown. The skin lesions clearly can be differentiated from eczematous skin lesions and are polymorphous in nature with regard to the manifestation in a group of various patients, but monomorphous in the individual patient with either urticarial or papular eruptions with a rather little itch. This is a major differential diagnostic criterion in distinguishing PLE from sun-induced atopic eczema.

4.5.8 Ear Disease

Relapsing inflammations of the middle ear (otitis media) are more common in patients with atopic diseases, especially in patients with respiratory atopy. There has been abundant literature with regard to swelling of the Eustachian tubes and also increased staphylococcal colonization and inflammation of the external auditory canal. Rarely, an association of deafness with atopic eczema has been described.

4.5.9 Inflammatory Bowel Disease

Roberts et al. found a two times higher prevalence of atopy and atopic eczema in patients with ulcerative colitis [661]. Also, Pugh et al. found a higher prevalence of eczema in ulcerative colitis and Crohn's disease [110, 607].

There was no association between atopic eczema and ulcerative colitis or M. Crohn in two studies [501, 803].

In Japan, in a large study in 47,862 adult atopic eczema patients between 18 and 62 years, Niwa found no association to Crohn's disease (OR 1.0, CE 0.45–2.2), but a clear association to ulcerative colitis with an OR of 6.5 (CE 5.1–7.3) [550].

4.5.10 Neuro-Psychiatric Diseases

4.5.10.1 Attention Deficit Hyperactivity Syndrome (ADHS)

There is a long discussion and controversy as to whether atopic dermatitis children have an increased risk for ADHS or whether symptoms of ADHS are due to allergic reactions. In a birth cohort study followed over 10 years, it was found that indeed there was an association between ADHS and atopic dermatitis which however appeared to be partly explained by sleeping problems in early childhood thus giving rise to ADHS [705].

In the survey of KiGGS (children and adolescent health survey), there was a significantly increased risk for ADHS in patients with atopic eczema (OR 1.54, CE 1.24–1.93), while there was no association to allergic rhinitis or asthma in a multivariate analysis adjusted for age, sex, SES, maternal smoking, perinatal health problems, breastfeeding, number of siblings, and family history of atopy [665]. However, in a stratified analysis taking into account sleep loss, it was found that the high association was mainly due to sleep problems since atopic eczema without sleep disturbance was no longer showing significant associations.

So there seems to be an association between atopic eczema and ADHS, whereby atopic eczema seems to temporarily precede the occurrence of ADHS. Most likely sleep problems in early childhood due to the intense itch in atopic eczema may be causal for the later development of ADHS in these patients [665].

4.5.10.2 Depression

Depression—as a psychiatric disease—is not a typical feature of atopic dermatitis.

However, the often intense individual suffering can lead to reactive depression and psychosomatic problems [268].

At the same time, psychologic stress can induce eczema exacerbations (see above).

4.5.10.3 Münchhausen by Proxy

Artificial dermatoses occur as a result of psychiatric disorders, often in the sense of delusional disease. Sometimes prurigo type of atopic dermatitis may be a differential diagnosis. Rarely also the phenomenon of "Muenchhausen by proxy" can affect AD children, when the mother (care-taker) too aggressively treats or mistreats the skin inducing irritant dermatitis. These cases are not easy to diagnose and need close observation and the help of experienced nurses.

4.5.10.4 Autism

A systematic review from Taiwan found a significant association of autism spectrum disorder with atopic eczema [804], they speculate about shared genetic and immunological determinants.

4.5.11 Summary

A variety of diseases show associations with atopic dermatitis, some of them genetic in origin—especially with defects in skin barrier or abnormalities in immune response. Also, some hair, ear, or ocular diseases as well as pigmentary disturbance can go along with atopic dermatitis. Classically and by definition the other atopic diseases of the airway like allergic rhinoconjunctivitis or asthma belong to the "atopic syndrome," but also some other IgE-mediated conditions like food allergy or anaphylaxis.

4.6 Complications of Atopic Eczema

The most common complications of atopic dermatitis regard infectious skin diseases which can give rise to very severe, partly life-threatening conditions.

4.6.1 Bacterial Infections

The skin of patients with atopic dermatitis is heavily colonized with Staphylococcus aureus (over 90%) in nonlesional skin, in the nose and under the nails. The cutaneous microbiome has been studied in atopic dermatitis and found to be characterized by a tendency to S aureus, but on nonlesional skin and during remission there is a marked diversity in species, which rapidly changes toward almost exclusive growth of *S. aureus* during exacerbation [415].

Regarding the itch-scratch processes this colonization can lead to germ transfer and impetiginization of eczematous skin changes [66, 172, 438, 452] (Fig. 4.38).

Impetiginized atopic eczema lesions are not only infected with staphylococci but also with streptococci and other microbes [5, 18, 250].

In a population-based cross-sectional study in over 1000 children between 0 and 6 years in Japan, it was found that the lifetime prevalence of impetigo contagiosa was significantly higher in atopic dermatitis than in control children, mollusca contagiosa were more pronounced in boys, while there was no difference in the prevalence of herpes simplex infection [317].

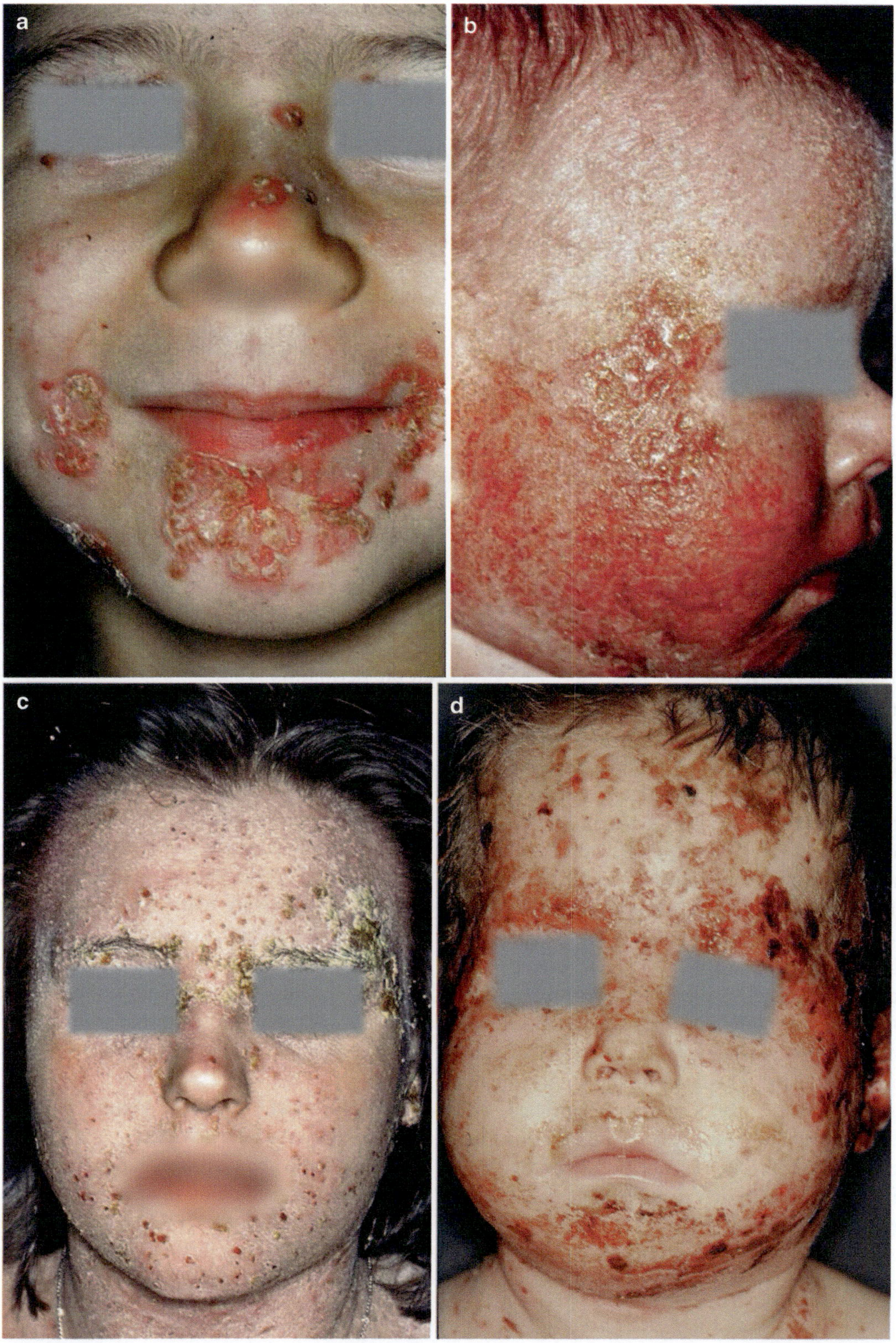

Fig. 4.38 Bacterial superinfection in atopic dermatitis. (**a**) Impetiginized eczema in the face. (**b**) Impetiginized infantile eczema. (**c**) Impetiginized atopic dermatitis with crusts and oozing. (**d**) Massive superinfected atopic dermatitis (*S. aureus*)

4.6.2 Fungal Infections

Patients with atopic eczema show an increased susceptibility to fungal infections, especially Trichophyton rubrum and Candida albicans. Some authors have found immediate-type reactions against Trichophyton rubrum antigens [372, 373], the pathophysiological relevance is unclear.

Malassezia furfur as saprophyte and inducer of pityriasis versicolor also is common in patients with atopic dermatitis and can be found especially when scalp and neck areas are involved ("head and neck dermatitis") [330]. IgE-mediated reactions against Malassezia have been detected as well as positive atopy patch test reactions with this fungus [39, 341, 552], these features seem to be less prominent in African phenotype of atopic eczema [439].

4.6.3 Viral Infections

4.6.3.1 Herpes Simplex: Eczema Herpeticum

One of the most severe complications of atopic eczema is the so-called eczema herpeticum (Kaposi's varicelliform eruption), which presents as disseminated form of infection with herpes simplex virus HSV type 1 or 2 on the basis of atopic dermatitis. It goes along with high fever and possible development of central nervous inflammation [381]. Often the diagnosis is made too late since doctors think of a mere exacerbation of atopic dermatitis. The infection occurs frequently through skin contact with affected persons (kissing, mother and child, etc.) [875, 887]. The diagnosis is made by detection of HSV antigen in the lesion together with the clinical manifestation and the acute occurrence of vesiculopustular, commonly eroded point-like skin changes (Fig. 4.39). Recurrent eczema herpeticum is observed especially in patients with severe skin disease [732].

The prognosis has been improved by the introduction of intravenous antiviral therapy with acyclovir or, for acyclovir-resistant infections, foscarnet, or ganciclovir.

4.6.3.2 Smallpox (Variola Vera): Eczema Vaccinatum

When smallpox infection (Variola vera) still was a threat to mankind and vaccination programs were common, this was a major complication of vaccination. Eczema vaccinatum occurred in patients with atopic dermatitis and corresponded clinically to eczema herpeticum with severe general disease, fever, lymph node swelling, and malaise (Fig.4.40).

Because of this complication, atopic dermatitis was regarded as a contraindication for smallpox vaccination. In those days, these individuals were not allowed to travel to the USA. By the development of a prevaccination with a modified smallpox vaccine (modified virus Ankara) (MVA) applied subcutaneously it was possible to reduce these complications [496] (see above). This vaccine also is tolerated in patients with atopic airway disease and atopic dermatitis [163].

4.6.3.3 Other Pox Virus Infections, e.g., Molluscum Contagiosum: Eczema Molluscatum

This typical infection with the epidermotropic DNA virus of the pox group is very common in childhood and occurs in especially intense manifestation in patients with atopic dermatitis; H. Wolf spoke of "eczema molluscatum" (Wolf, personal communication) (Fig. 4.41) [886].

Also, severe clinical manifestations of orf (ecthyma contagiosum) have been described in atopic eczema [197].

4.6.3.4 Human Papilloma Virus (HPV): Eczema Verrucatum

Infections with human papillomavirus (HPV) seem to be more common in atopics and show a more intense severity, especially with regard to common warts (verruca vulgaris). In some patients with severe manifestations in the hand

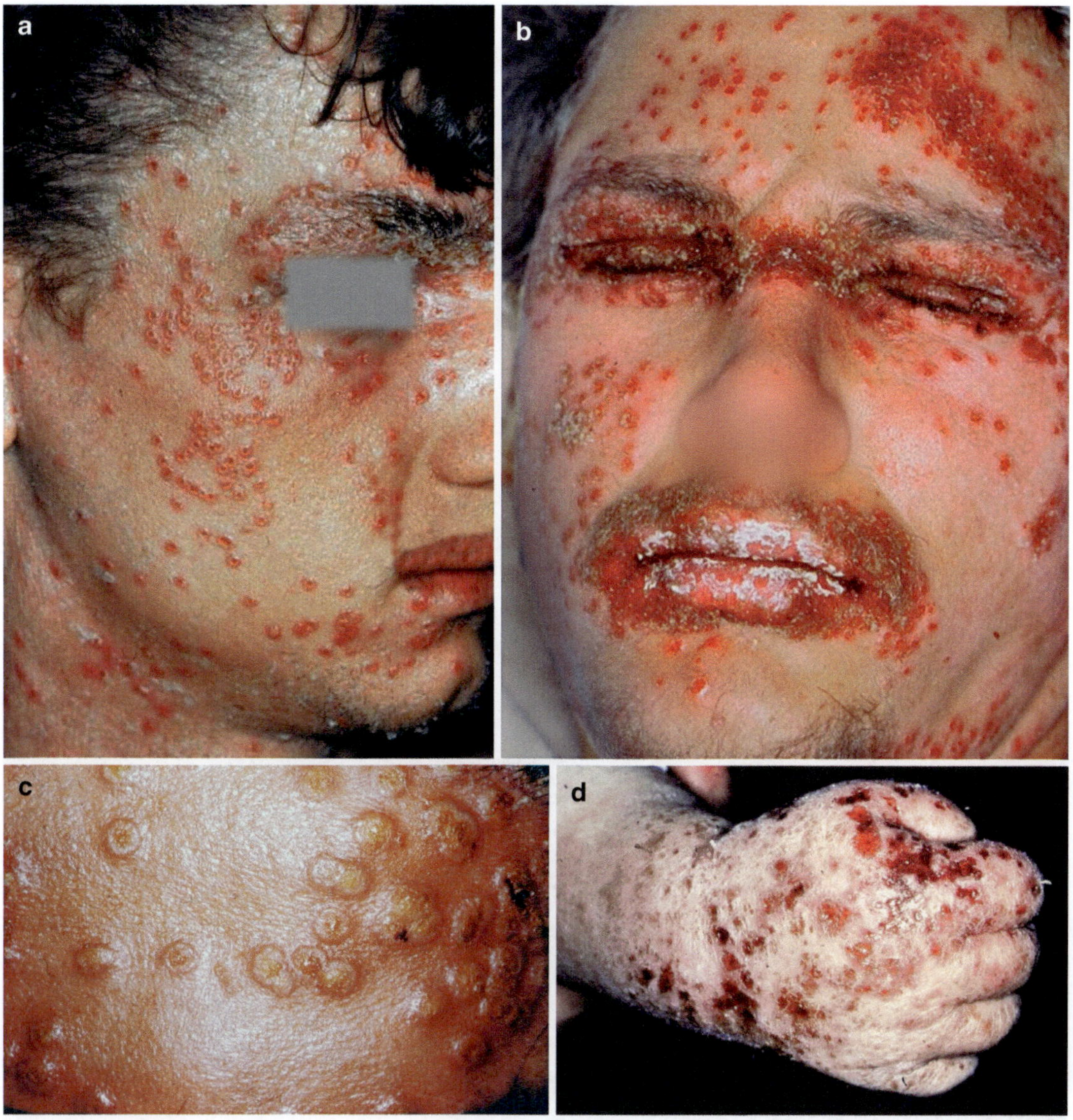

Fig. 4.39 Eczema herpeticum, a severe complication of atopic dermatitis. (**a**) Vesicular pustular skin changes. (**b**) Disseminated erosive punctate skin changes. (**c**) In the magnifying perspective the vesicular pustular character resembles varicella. (**d**) Eczema herpeticium of the hand with large erosions

and around the nails, the term "eczema verrucatum" could be used (Fig. 4.42).

4.6.3.5 HIV Infection

The association of HIV infection and IgE-mediated diseases is controversially discussed; in the initial phase of HIV infection, atopic diseases and immunoglobulin E do not seem to play a role; however, in manifested AIDS, severe exacerbations of atopic eczema together with superinfection can be observed.

4.6.3.6 Other Viral Diseases

An increased prevalence of extracutaneous viral infections has been discussed with regard to the pathophysiological immunodeficiency of Th1 reactions. Compared to the normal population,

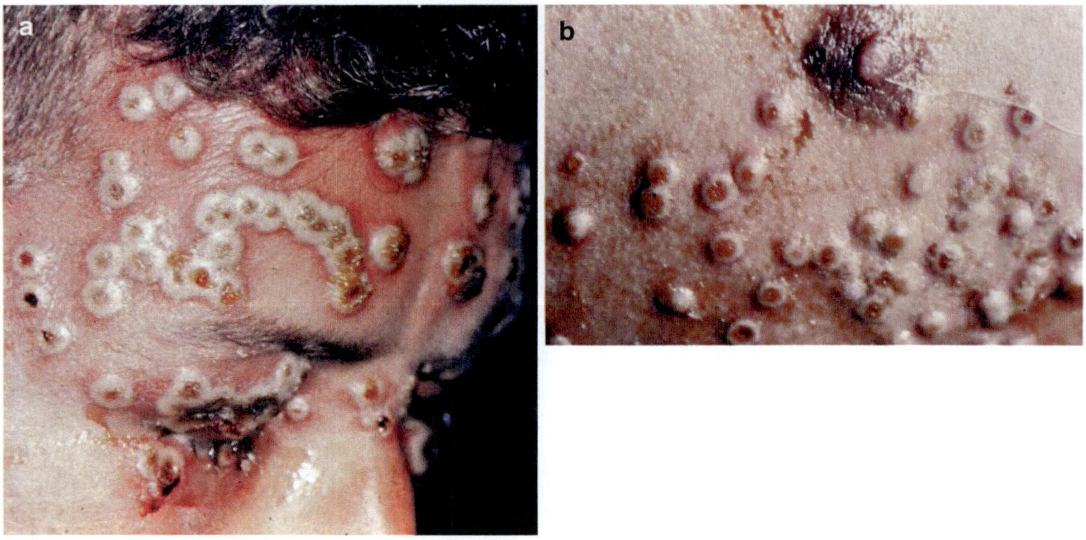

Fig. 4.40 Eczema vaccinatum. (**a**) Severe complication of smallpox vaccination in a person with atopic dermatitis. (**b**) Detail

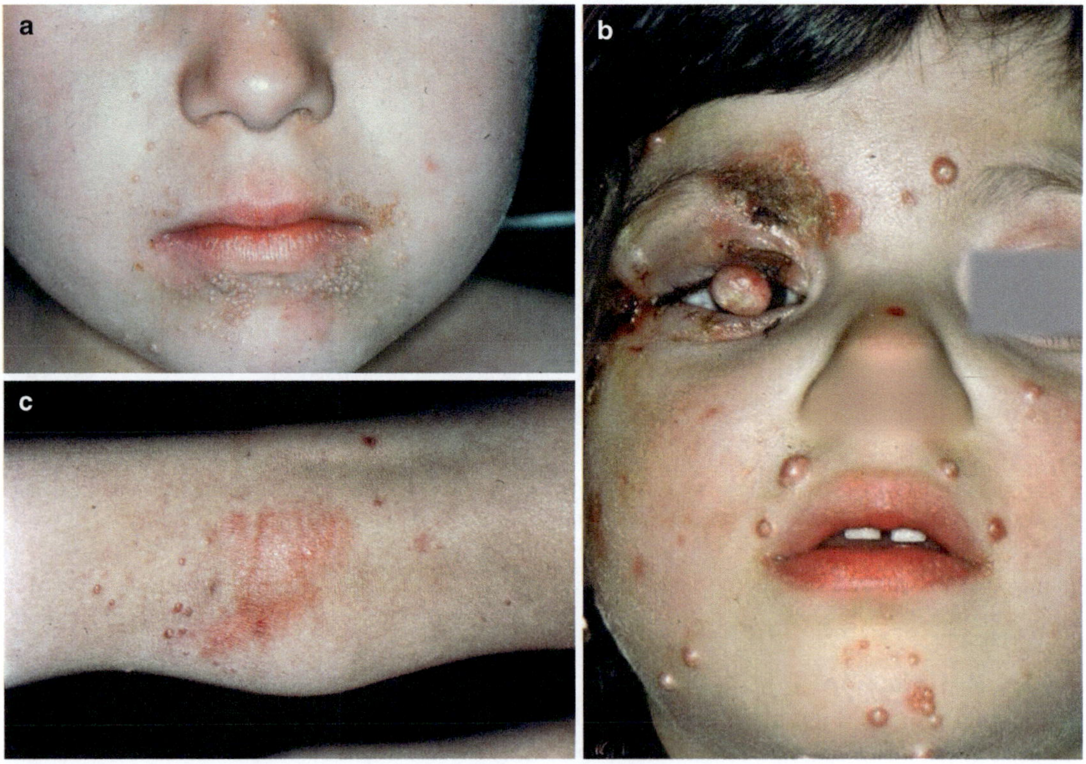

Fig. 4.41 Mollusca contagiosa. (**a**) Intensive appearance of Mollusca contagiosa in the perioral region with cheilitis sicca. (**b**) Massive Mollusca contagiosa in a child with atopic dermatitis. (**c**) Mollusca contagiosa immediately next to flexural eczema

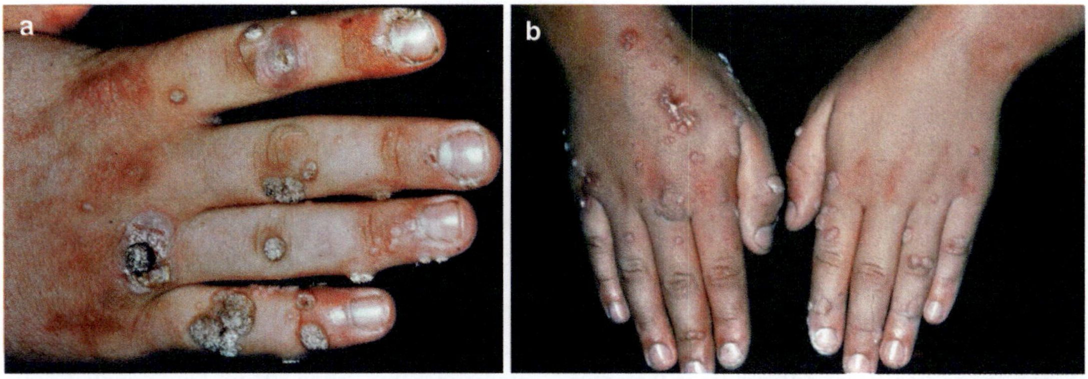

Fig. 4.42 Eczema verrucatum. (**a**) Intensive warts on the hands, especially periungual, in atopic dermatitis. (**b**) Massive appearance of warts on both hands

viral infections of the upper respiratory tract seem to be increased in prevalence in atopic dermatitis.

Infections with Epstein-Barr Virus (EBV) also seem to be more frequent in atopics (both respiratory atopy and atopic eczema).

Activation of a subclinically existing cytomegalovirus infection (CMV) in patients with severe eczema has been observed.

Also, cases with severe Coxsackievirus infection have been observed in atopic dermatitis (see 2.5.8).

With regard to COVID-19, there does not seem to be an increased risk for patients with atopic eczema. Also, standard treatment regimens including immunomodulatory medications can be used according to position statements of scientific societies (see above). Some authors recommend not to start biological and systemic immunosuppressive therapy during active COVID-19 disease [797].

4.6.4 Summary

Complications of atopic eczema comprise especially infectious skin diseases, either viral (eczema herpeticum), bacterial (Staphylococcus aureus, streptococci), or fungal (Pityriasis versicolor) in origin.

Some viral infections—especially of the herpes and pox virus group—can spread intensively in patients with atopic eczema leading to severe generalized conditions. Care should be taken to prevent these infections in patients seriously affected.

4.7 Diseases Rarely Associated with Atopic Eczema

While the literature is abundant regarding atopy-associated diseases and complications, only a few epidemiological trials study the occurrence of certain diseases which, according to general experience, are less prominent in atopic individuals compared to the normal population. On the basis of the pathophysiological concept of Th1 and Th2 [224], this may be apparent [571] for the following diseases:

4.7.1 Diabetes Mellitus

Juvenile diabetes mellitus (type 1) occurs by an autoimmune Th1 reaction against the beta cells in the pancreas. It therefore was of interest whether diabetes type 1 is more common in atopics.

A study from the Netherlands found a lower prevalence of atopic diseases in 7–12-year-old children with insulin-dependent diabetes mellitus (IDDM) Meerwaldt et al. [502]. Another study reported an increased prevalence of atopic diseases, especially asthma, in IDDM with controversial results regarding atopic eczema (EURODIAB).

A Danish study in 3–15-year-old children with IDDM found a significantly lower incidence of atopic eczema in diabetes patients in comparison to the normal population (OR 0.49, CT 0.39–0.63). When diabetes mellitus was manifest, there were no significant differences in the prevalence of atopic eczema in diabetics compared to normal persons [571].

The increased prevalence of type 2 diabetes in middle-aged adults was also investigated: Again lower prevalence rates of atopy were found in diabetes patients [789].

4.7.2 Rheumatoid Arthritis

A similar situation seems to be found in rheumatoid arthritis with data showing an inverse association between atopic diseases and rheumatoid arthritis [820].

There was a significantly lower incidence of atopy among rheumatoid arthritis patients compared to healthy controls (OR 0.39, CE 0.19–0.81) [328]. On the other hand, there was a significantly lower incidence of eczema among rheumatoid arthritis (2.9% compared to healthy controls 4.9%) [300].

4.7.3 Psoriasis

The association of atopic eczema and psoriasis has been discussed and is controversial, although with regard to the Th1/Th2 hypothesis lower prevalences of atopy in psoriasis and vice versa should be expected and represent a general experience. In selected cases with concomitant simultaneous occurrence of clear-cut psoriasis and atopic eczema, interesting immunological findings could be observed with interleukin-4-producing T cell clones only to be isolated from eczema, or atopy patch test lesions and interferon gamma-, interleukin 17- or TNF-secreting T cell clones from psoriasis lesions [224] (see Chap. 5 "Pathophysiology").

4.7.4 Melanocytic Nevi

Many doctors have seen however few have realized the specific phenomenon that patients with atopic eczema often show fewer melanocytic nevi than normal persons. The inspection and registration of the eczematous skin lesions are in the focus. Sometimes nevi are registered as side finding, sometimes they give rise to further investigations because of atypia. There are few scientific investigations with regard to the incidence and prevalence of melanocytic nevi in atopy or atopic dermatitis.

In a Swedish study, Broberg et al. found in a group of patients with severe atopic eczema significantly decreased numbers of melanocytic nevi compared to non-atopic controls. They found a significant negative association between the level of serum IgE and the number of melanocytic nevi in atopic eczema [102].

In a larger Danish study, 2030 adult patients with atopic eczema were examined and compared with the General Cancer Registry in Denmark. Thereby, no single case of malignant melanoma was found in the group of patients with atopic eczema, although 2.4 cases should have been expected theoretically [368].

There are other studies showing similar findings.

However, it seems too early to generally speculate whether atopic individuals or atopic dermatitis patients have a really decreased risk to develop malignant melanoma.

4.7.5 Atopic Eczema and Cancer

There is abundant literature with regard to the incidence of cancer and allergy; however, the literature is controversial [110].

Some studies have found decreased prevalences in neurological or brain tumors (glioblastoma) [726].

In a recent large review investigating 23 publications from 1985 to 2004, Wang et al. found that atopic eczema may be associated with a decreased risk of pancreatic cancer, brain tumor, and childhood leukemia (the latter not significant) with no consistent findings with regard to skin cancer or non-Hodgkin lymphoma [836].

In 575 children with brain tumors from the UK childhood cancer study, atopic children (asthma and/or atopic eczema) showed a reduced risk for CNS tumors while there was no significant inverse correlation for atopic eczema alone [311].

On the contrary, in a study involving 2030 adult patients with atopic eczema, compared to the Danish Cancer Registry from 1977–1996, an increased risk of cancer was observed overall (OR 1.5, CE 1.2–1.9), whereby half the excess cases of cancer were non-melanoma skin cancer diagnosed within the first 9 years of the follow-up. Others conclude that this increased rate may be due to the carcinogenic potential of therapies used for severe atopic dermatitis [368].

In a study of 550 children 8–9 years old, those with active eczema had fewer melanocytic naevi than children without atopic disease with a median of 4 (mean 7.4) versus a median of 9 (mean 11.2) in controls [779] (see above).

When the same authors studied the incidence of malignant melanoma in 6280 patients with atopic dermatitis and a mean follow-up of 36.7 years, they found 6 cases with malignant melanoma representing an OR of 0.49 (CE 0.27–1.35) which was not significant [779].

A large study from UK and Denmark showed no increased risk for cancer in atopic eczema, except for lymphoma [485].

Another study found decreased rates of allergic disorders in patients with breast cancer raising the question of whether atopy might be able to protect from cancer [92].

4.7.6 Contact Allergy

For a long time, it was postulated that contact allergy would be rarer in atopic dermatitis [488], also under the light of the Th1/Th2 paradigm, this seemed to be logical. However, intense studies examining the prevalence of contact allergy in atopic dermatitis find similar rates; in an own study, we found a prevalence of positive patch tests in 41% of atopic eczema patients compared to 40% in the whole group of other diagnoses tested [215] (see Chap. 4 "Diagnostics"). Atopic eczema patients also can suffer from contact allergies, especially to metal salts like nickel.

4.7.7 Debates on Association of Common Diseases with Atopy

4.7.7.1 Cardiovascular Diseases, Metabolic Syndrome

There are opinions that cardiovascular disease and metabolic syndrome may occur rarer in atopy patients. The clinical impression of many dermatologists treating eczema patients describes more leptosome instead pyknic individuals with rather low blood pressure and not so many obese or with hypertension. Some epidemiological studies found associations, others did not. The debate is ongoing. Clear analytical studies are missing [110].

4.7.8 Summary

While some diseases are associated significantly more often with atopic eczema as especially respiratory atopic diseases, asthma, allergic rhinoconjunctivitis, food anaphylaxis, there are other diseases which probably occur less often in eczema patients like type I diabetes mellitus, rheumatoid arthritis, psoriasis, but also melanocytic naevi. This area needs further research. The concomitant occurrence of psoriasis and atopic eczema seems to be possible but rare and gives rise to interesting studies regarding the mechanisms and therapeutic effects of new strategies.

For a long time, the prevalence of contact allergy was regarded to be decreased in atopic dermatitis; however, allergic contact dermatitis also occurs in atopic eczema and also in childhood. Therefore, a patch test belongs to the diagnostic standard in atopic dermatitis also in childhood.

Complications of atopic eczema comprise especially infectious skin diseases, both viral (eczema herpeticum) and bacterial (Staphylococcus aureus, streptococci) in origin.

4.8 Atopic Eczema: Diagnostic Criteria and Severity Scoring

Many factors contribute via various mechanisms to the development and chronification of this disease, which is partly reflected in the colorful terminology. The diffuse and variable morphology with the lack of a true primary lesion and variable clinical course over lifetime can make diagnosis sometimes difficult.

4.8.1 Diagnostic Criteria

4.8.1.1 Diagnostic Criteria According to Hanifin and Rajka

Therefore, it can be regarded as a breakthrough that two dermatologists, Jon Hanifin from Portland, Oregon, and Georg Rajka from Oslo, developed an internationally accepted list of diagnostic criteria based on clinical and anamnestic findings [305] (Table 4.6). In most scientific studies, these criteria are the gold standard for the diagnosis of atopic dermatitis. The diagnosis of atopic dermatitis can be made when a minimum of three major and additional three minor criteria are fulfilled.

In an analysis by Diepgen et al., [184] in 110 patients with atopic eczema and healthy controls, the following five criteria were the most common:

Table 4.6 Diagnostic criteria for atopic dermatitis according to Hanifin and Rajka [305]

A minimum of three major criteria	+3 or more "minor" criteria
Itch	Dry skin
Typical morphology and distribution: • Big flexures and linearity in adults	Ichthyosis (palmar/ hyperlinearity, keratosis pilaris)
• Facial and extensor sites in infants and children	Skin test reactivity of the immediate-type (type I)
• Chronically relapsing dermatitis	Increased serum IgE
Personal or family history of atopy (asthma, allergic rhinitis, atopic dermatitis)	Onset in early life
	Tendency to skin infections (especially *S. aureus* and herpes simplex/decreased cell-mediated immunity)
	Itch when sweating
	Incompatibility of wool and solvents
	Perifollicular accentuation
	Food hypersensitivity
	Influenced by environment or emotional factors
	White dermographism/delayed blanch

- Itch when sweating.
- Wool incompatibility.
- Dry skin.
- White dermographism.
- Hertoghe phenomenon.

The multitude of criteria is sometimes difficult to define in signs and symptoms. The mixture of the actual clinical findings and data from history and laboratory make the application of Hanifin and Rajka's criteria in daily practice difficult.

4.8.1.2 Diagnostic Criteria of the UK Working Party

With regard to epidemiological trials, an English working group around H. Williams came up with the UK Working Party's diagnostic criteria in 1994 which were based on clinical examination and validation of dermatological criteria, whereby sensitivity and specificity were around 90% [868, 869] (Table 4.7).

According to this definition, the diagnosis "atopic dermatitis" can be made when there is an itchy skin rash together with three or more criteria from Table 4.7.

4.8.1.3 Criteria According to Ring

In 1982, JR published a list of diagnostic criteria for atopic eczema [637] (Table 4.8) which in daily practice allows the diagnosis in a simpler way, namely when four of the six criteria are fulfilled.

4.8.1.4 Other Criteria

There are a number of further criteria in the last 30 years [380], the millennium criteria [89], the ISAAC questionnaire [30], and recently also from Asia for children and adults [138].

Table 4.7 Diagnostic criteria for atopic dermatitis according to the UK Working Party (1994)

The diagnosis of atopic dermatitis can be made when there is an itchy skin rash together with three or more of the following criteria:
• History of flexural involvement (elbow, anterior foot, neck, in childhood also cheeks)
• History of asthma or hay fever in patients with one atopic disease in a near relative first grade (mother, father, brother, sister) in children under 4 years
• History of general skin dryness in the last year
• Actually existing flexural eczema (or eczema of cheeks, forehead, or extensor sides of extremities in children under 4 years)
• Onset during the first years of life (not relevant for children under 4 years)

Table 4.8 Diagnostic criteria for atopic eczema according to Ring [637–639]

The diagnosis of atopic dermatitis can be made when at least four of the following six criteria are fulfilled:
• Age-specific morphology
• Itch
• Age-specific distribution of skin lesions
• Stigmata of atopic eczema (typus neurodermitis or atopic diathesis)
• Personal or family history of atopy
• Detection of IgE-mediated sensitization (in vitro or in skin test)

Some of these diagnostic criteria have been studied in a systematic review for their specificity and sensitivity with overall satisfying results [98].

4.8.2 Evaluation of Severity of Eczema

When the diagnostic criteria had been established, the problem of variable severity of the disease in different patients became apparent. It is obvious that there are mild and very severe courses which are not exactly defined beforehand. Several attempts were made to quantify the severity [135, 213, 610]. Therefore, a task force of the European Society for Pediatric Dermatology (European Task Force on Atopic Dermatitis (ETFAD) developed a scoring system for atopic dermatitis (SCORAD) at the beginning of the 90s [436].

4.8.3 Objective Signs and Subjective Symptoms

The SCORAD consists of an objective score which quantifies both the extent of the body surface involved and the intensity of the qualitatively different skin lesions together with a subjective evaluation of the intensity of suffering. The latter is measured as the intensity of itch and sleep loss on a visual analog scale. The various qualitatively different skin lesions registered in the SCORAD are

- Erythema.
- Edema/papules.
- Oozing/crusting.
- Excoriation.
- Lichenification.
- Skin dryness.

These different skin lesions are semiquantitatively evaluated from 0 (absent) to 3 (maximal). The subjective complaints are registered on a visual analog scale (VAS) from 0 to 10 by the patient (or the parents, respectively). In order to measure the SCORAD, there are standard figures and forms (Fig. 4.43). Special training sessions are offered.

SCORAD European task force for atopic dermatitis (EFTAD)

Patient: Name/First name	Birth Date	Date of Investigation

Topical steroid used

Active Substance (brand name, concentration)	Amount/Month (g)	Number of flares per month

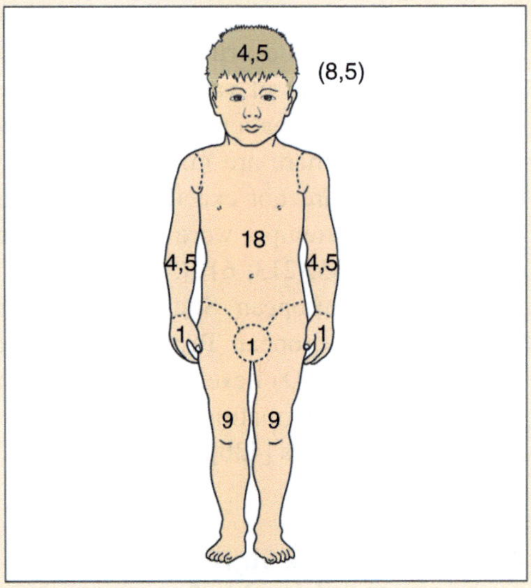

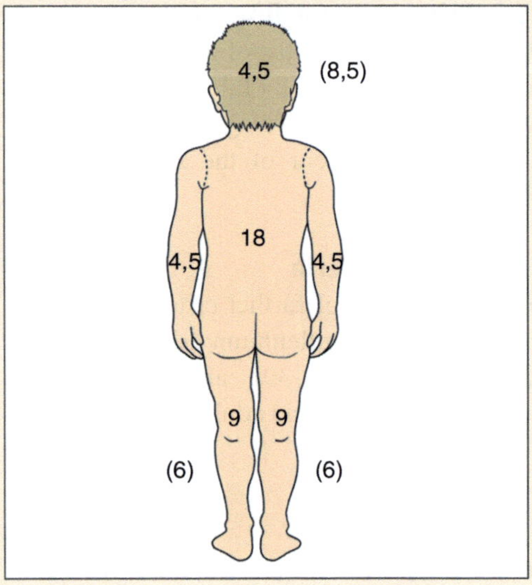

Numbers in brackets for children below 2 years

A: Extent
Please add the sum of affected skin areas

B: Intensity
Values for intensity
(on maximal affected skin location)

0 = non 1 = mild 2 = moderate 3 = Severe

Criteria	Intensity	Criteria	Intensity
Erythema		Excoriation	
Edema/Papules		Lichenification	
Oozing/Crusting		Dryness (evaluated at non-lesional skins)	

C: Subjective symptoms

Itch and loss of sleep

SCORAD A/5 + 7B/2 + C

Visual analogue scale (average the last 3 days or nights)

Pruritus (0–10) 0 1 2 3 4 5 6 7 8 9 10

Loss of sleep (0–10) 0 1 2 3 4 5 6 7 8 9 10

Treatment	Remarks

Fig. 4.43 Scoring system for atopic dermatitis (SCORAD) with objective and subjective scales

Using the SCORAD it is possible to follow the actual severity of the disease objectively and reproducibly over long time periods. Especially for clinical trials with regard to the effect of therapeutic strategies the SCORAD has been proven valuable.

It should be mentioned that various groups (partly authors of the original ETFAD group) started to develop more simple versions of SCORAD for faster analyses. However, for the experienced the examination of the SCORAD means 10 min of time. In specialized hospitals, the SCORAD belongs to the routine diagnostic procedure for every eczema patient.

The SCORAD offers the advantage that it can also be used for single parts; thus, it is possible to measure the clinical course of certain symptoms independent of the total score over time. So the effect of therapeutic treatment can be studied with regard to the effect upon morphologically different skin lesions.

The SCORAD was developed by the ETFAD and studied in several hundred patients in 11 European countries over several years before it was finally established and refined. In these studies, the statistical analysis came to a maximum of 103 points for the most severe patient. Many have not understood why one could not more simply come to 100 points as a maximum. This is due to the fact that the SCORAD was not developed only arbitrarily, but really studied in hundreds of patients and measured and evaluated in statistical analysis.

4.8.3.1 Patient-Oriented Self-Evaluation

Recently in a clinical trial, the validation of a patient-oriented (PO) SCORAD has been shown valuable so that patients themselves or parents can measure the severity of atopic eczema over time [833].

This instrument also works quite well on African skin [227].

Also, with an instrument called Patient-Oriented Eczema Measure (POEM) is it rather simple to get self-evaluated impression of actual severity of eczema in the preceding week [134].

4.8.3.2 Eczema Area and Severity Index (EASI)

In some countries, the Eczema Area and Severity Index (EASI) is more popular than SCORAD. The EASI was developed in analogy to the Psoriasis Area and Severity Index (PASI); however, it is only measuring signs but not the major symptom of atopic dermatitis which is the itch sensation. In America, the EASI is preferred by many authors, while the SCORAD has its home in Europe.

4.8.4 Quality of Life as Health Outcome Measure in Atopic Eczema

Several Quality of Life (QOL) instruments are available in dermatology, starting with the Dermatology Life Quality Index (DLQI) developed by A Finlay [234].

On the way to more specific instruments for atopic dermatitis the following tools have been developed:

Quality of Life—atopic dermatitis (QUOLIAD),
Atopic Dermatitis Burden Scale for Adults (ADBS-A)
Skindex
Atopic Eczema Score for Emotional Consequences (AESEC), the latter focussing on the individual suffering of the patients.

For children, special instruments include the following:

Infant's Dermatitis Quality of Life Index (IDQoL) [459],
Children's Dermatology Life Quality Index (CDLQI) [459],
Childhood Atopic Dermatitis Impact Scale (CADIS) in a long and a short form [129].
Infants and Toddlers Dermatology Quality of Life (InToDermQoL).

Recently, by the HOME (health outcome measures for eczema) initiative the IDQoL, the CDLQI, and the CADIS have been found suitable for clinical trials [251].

4.8.5 Summary

The diagnosis of atopic dermatitis can be made on the basis of various diagnostic criteria. Most commonly used are those of Hanifin and Rajka [305]. For daily practice in epidemiological trials, the UK Working Party's criteria [868] and those of Ring [637–639] have proven valuable.

In a task force of the European Society for Pediatric Dermatology (European Task Force on Atopic Dermatitis ETFAD) a scoring system to measure the severity of atopic dermatitis (SCORAD) has been developed which not only registered the extent of skin lesions over the body surface but also the intensity of six different morphologically apparent skin lesions together with the subjective impairment due to itch or sleep loss. The SCORAD can also be used with regard to single parameters for scientific studies or therapeutic trials.

Also often used is the Eczema Area and Severity Index (EASI) which measures only signs and not symptoms.

Instruments for patient self-evaluation are available such as the Patient-Oriented (PO)-SCORAD, as well as the Patient-Oriented Eczema Measure (POEM).

Similar tools are also available for children. The international initiative "Health Outcome Measures for Eczema" (HOME) constantly updates recommendations. Currently, the DLQI, the RECAP or ADCT, and a NRS assessing maximum itch intensity over the last 24 h is recommended [792].

5 Etiopathophysiology of Atopic Eczema

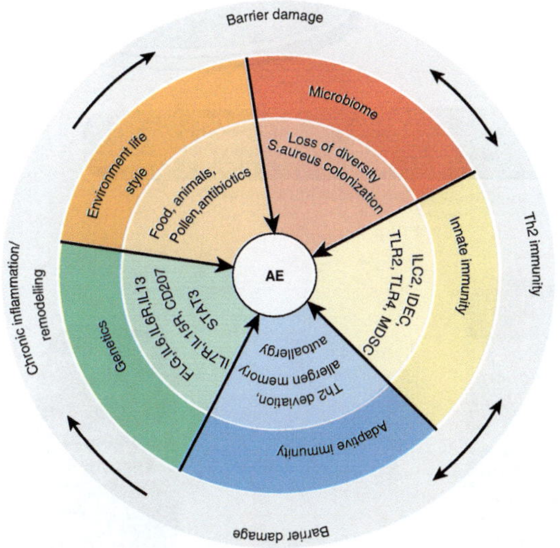

5.1 Pathophysiological Concepts

The pathogenesis of atopic dermatitis is based on complex interactions of genetic predisposition and environmental triggers that result in a triage of (1) impaired epidermal barrier, (2) altered cutaneous microbiome, and (3) type 2 immunity mediating inflammation (Fig. 5.1). All three aspects are connected and influence each other: type 2 immunity directly impacts the epidermal barrier by downregulation of genes such as filaggrin and leads to a dysfunctional local innate immune system which favors certain microbiota such as *S. aureus*; *S. aureus* decreases the epidermal barrier by inducing proteases and triggers inflammation by superantigen release; barrier dysfunction promotes cutaneous inflammation. Furthermore, type 2 immunity drives itch, the cardinal symptom of atopic dermatitis, through neuroimmune interactions. In the course of inflammation, the local microenvironment impacts the pathogenesis of atopic dermatitis. That means chronic inflammation is distinct from acute lesions. Finally, the clinical heterogeneity of atopic dermatitis is reflected by its pathogenesis—there are possibly distinct endotypes defined by age ethnicity and severity of inflammation.

K. Eyerich, J. Ring, *Atopic Dermatitis - Eczema*, https://doi.org/10.1007/978-3-031-12499-0_5

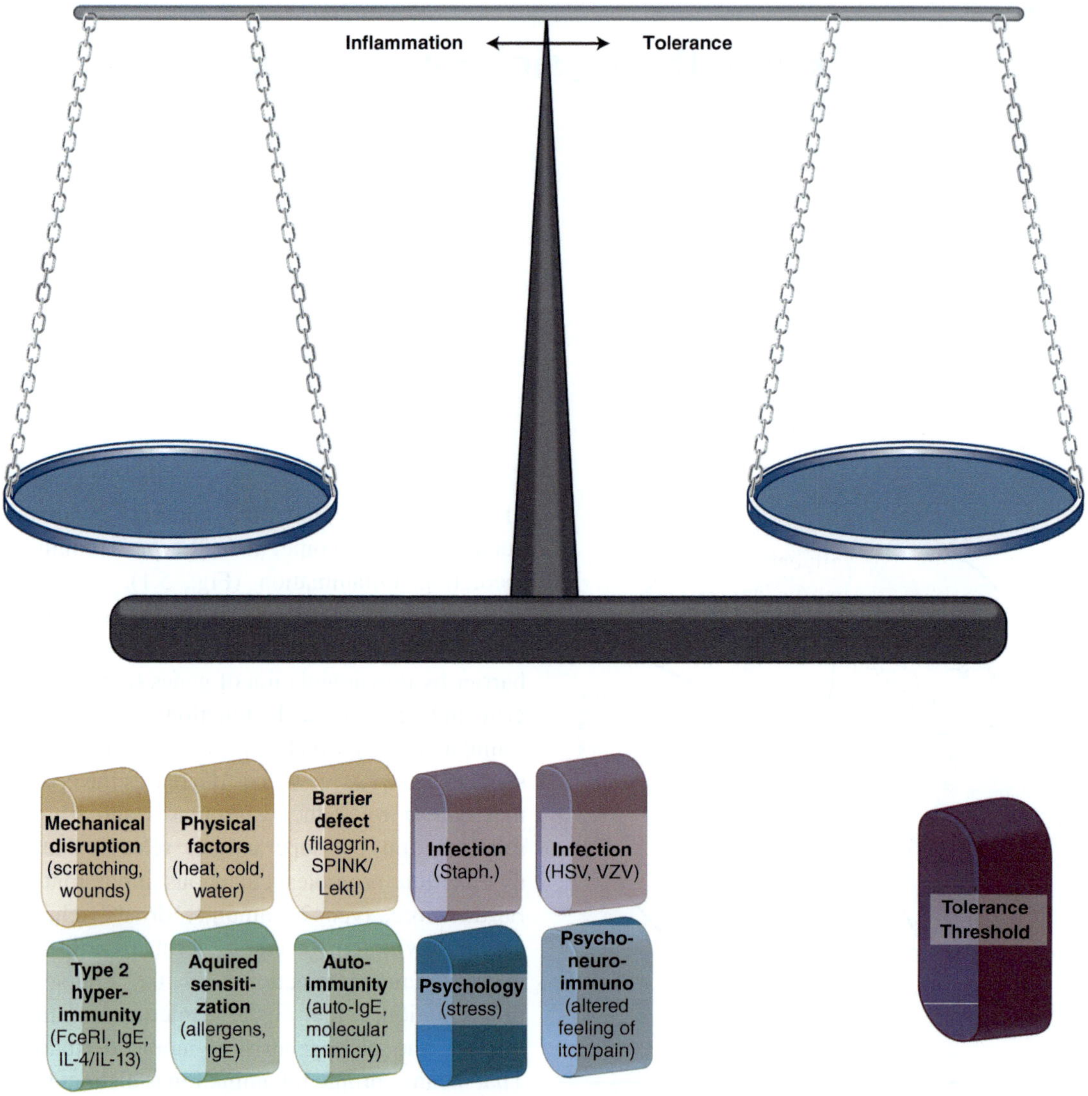

Fig. 5.1 The pathogenesis of atopic dermatitis is based on multiple mosaics such as type 2 immunity, barrier disruption, and microbial dysbalance. Modified from [649]

5.2 Genetics of Atopic Dermatitis

Atopic dermatitis is a complex disease that does not follow the simple Mendel heredity. However, epidemiological studies consistently report a positive family history of atopic dermatitis as the strongest risk factor to develop atopic dermatitis disease; it is around three times higher than in the rest of the population. This is more or less consistent in large population-based trials and older studies, with the latter tending to generally overestimate the prevalence of atopic dermatitis due to methodological weaknesses. Furthermore, a meta-analysis of twin studies suggest an approximately three times higher concordance rate in monozygotic twins (ranging from 15% to 86%) than in dizygotic twins (ranging from 5% to 41%).

5.2.1 Genome-Wide Association Studies (GWAS)

Since it became clear that atopic dermatitis as a complex disease cannot show monogeneous hereditary traits following Mendel's laws, there was the hope to define an atopy gene. In the meantime, we know that a multitude of gene loci on various chromosomes is involved in the manifestation of the many phenotypes of atopic diseases. These loci have been identified by determination of variations at single sites of the DNA in patients versus nonaffected controls, so-called Single nucleotide polymorphisms (SNP's). While historically candidate gene analyses were followed, the technical advances and cost-developments led to increasingly used hypothesis-free investigations of the whole genome of atopic dermatitis patients, so-called GWAS's (genome-wide association study). To date, more than 30 loci associated with atopic dermatitis have been identified using GWAS. While this method does not allow to attribute a function or a causative role for these loci in the pathogenesis of atopic dermatitis, the identified genomic regions contain genes that are important in epidermal barrier function, acute phase, or type 2 immunity (Table 5.1). Altogether, these loci still explain less than 20% of the heritability of AD [583], while at least another 12% are explained by rare protein-coding variation.

Table 5.1 Susceptibility loci and candidate genes associated with atopic dermatitis. Modified from [843]

Susceptibility locus	Candidate genes	Function
Epidermal differentiation		
1q21.3	FLG, FLG2, HRNR	Terminal differentiation
2q24.3	XIRP2	Cytoskeletal function
3q13.2	CCDC80	Cell adhesion
11p13	PRR5L	Cytoskeletal organization
11q13.1	OVOL1	Transcription factor regulating FLG
19p13.2	ACTL9, ADAMTS10	Cytoskeletal function
Acute phase (innate) immunity		
2q12.1	IL1RL1, IL18R1, IL18RAP	Inflammation mediated via NF-kB
2q13.3	CD207	Antigen processing and presentation
6p21.32	HLA-DRB1	
6p21.33	HLA-B	
4q27	IL2, IL21	Activation and survival of lymphocytes
5q13.2	IL7R	
10p15.1	IL15RA, IL2RA	
1q21.3	IL6R	Acute phase inflammation
7qp22.2	CARD11	
11p15.4	NLRP10	
16p13.13	CLEC16A	
17q21.2	STAT3	Inflammatory signaling
20q13.33	TNFRSF6B	
Type 2-associated immunity		
5q31.1	IL4, IL13	Type 2 cytokines
5q22.1	TSLP	Recruitment and differentiation of type 2 cells

5.2.2 Filaggrin

The strongest genetic predisposition factor of atopic dermatitis is mutations in the filaggrin (FLG) gene. While homozygous mutations in the FLG gene cause ichthyosis, heterozygous mutations predispose to atopic dermatitis with an Odd's ratio of around three. These mutations occur in around 10% of the European and Japanese populations and result in a diminished expression of filaggrin protein of about 50%. FLG is part of the epidermal differentiation complex which is a cluster of more than 60 genes that cooperatively regulate epidermal differentiation and barrier function. The FLG gene encodes for pro-filaggrin which is expressed in the upper layers of the epidermis. During terminal differentiation of the epidermis, pro-filaggrin is dephosphorylated and cleaved into filaggrin protein. This process is mediated by several endogenous proteases and is balanced by serine protease inhibitors such as LEKTI (SPINK5). Filaggrin protein is most highly expressed in the outer layers of the epidermis, the stratum corneum. Here, it is further processed and lysed. Components of filaggrin act as natural moisturizing factor, protect against UV light, regulate the pH of the skin, and have antimicrobial activity. In vitro and in animal models, loss-of-function mutations of FLG result in an impaired epidermal barrier as shown by enhanced penetration of allergens or dye. This enhanced penetration occurs from inside the body to the environment ("inside-out") and vice versa ("outside-in") thus leading to enhanced transepidermal water loss on the one hand side, and to increased irritative reactions on the other side. In summary, FLG is central to the regulation of epidermal differentiation and lipid formation—this explains why it is the strongest genetic risk factor for atopic dermatitis. However, less than 20% of AD patients carry a loss-of-function mutation of FLG and more than 50% of people carrying such a mutation do not suffer from atopic dermatitis—so neither does a mutation in FLG explain the whole phenotype of atopic dermatitis, nor is it a prerequisite to develop this disease (Fig. 5.2).

5.2.3 Protease Inhibitors

On the basis of the protease inhibitor defect in Netherton syndrome (SPINK5), which encodes an important serine protease inhibitor LEKTI, corresponding investigations have been performed in atopic dermatitis [345]. There were decreased levels of kallikrein (KLK)-dependent peptidases. In a transgenic mouse model with overexpression of KLK7 with chymotryptase activity, skin changes similar to atopic dermatitis developed. In a candidate gene analysis however no significant association of KLK7 mutations to atopic eczema was found in humans [842].

On the other hand, associations of polymorphisms of mast cell chymase have been shown with infantile atopic eczema [486].

Epidermal serine proteases act via signal transduction of protease-activated receptor (PAR)2 G-protein-coupled receptor which plays a role in innate immunity, but also in the mediation of itch sensation [768]. Activation of PAR2 leads to inhibition of "lamellar" bodies and stratum corneum formation. The change in potassium gradients with concomitant activation of PAR2 receptors leads to a rapid transformation of the external keratinocytes in the stratum granulosum to terminally differentiated corneocytes [296].

The thickness of epidermis, the thickness of stratum corneum, and the size of the corneocytes also influence barrier function. Found smaller corneocytes in atopic dermatitis compared to healthy controls (1977). The smallest corneocytes were found in the retroauricular area and on the forehead, sites commonly affected by atopic eczema.

Other studies found an association of SPINK5 gene mutations to atopic eczema [842].

In addition to the SPINK5 locus, a mutation in cysteine protease inhibitor cystatin A (CSTA and chromosome 3q21) was described which shows association to atopic dermatitis [450].

5.2.4 Genes of Innate Immunity

The innate immune system is the oldest active defense system in the evolution and protects the organism against a variety of exogenous intruders with a rather rapid reaction which somehow is able to recognize and differentiate pathogenic structures on microbes or other "danger" signals [365, 493]. Apart from the physicochemical barrier at the surface, various cellular and secretory elements are involved which are activated after stimulation of so-called pathogen-related receptors (PRR) [16]; all of them may be altered in a sense of being "defective" or "less efficient" in atopic dermatitis such as the response of the following PRRs:

- Toll-like receptors (TLRs).
- Nucleotide-binding oligomerization domain (NOD).
- Leucine-rich repeat-containing proteins (NLR) as well as the endotoxin receptor CD14.
- Some soluble PRRs [174].

Thus, major cells of the innate immune response like polymorphonuclear leukocytes, natural killer cells, and dendritic cells, especially pDC, have been found to show reduced functions [174]. Also, the production of antimicrobial peptides (AMPs) from keratinocytes is reduced as well as the secretion of CCL20/MIP-3-α or CXCL8/interleukin-8.

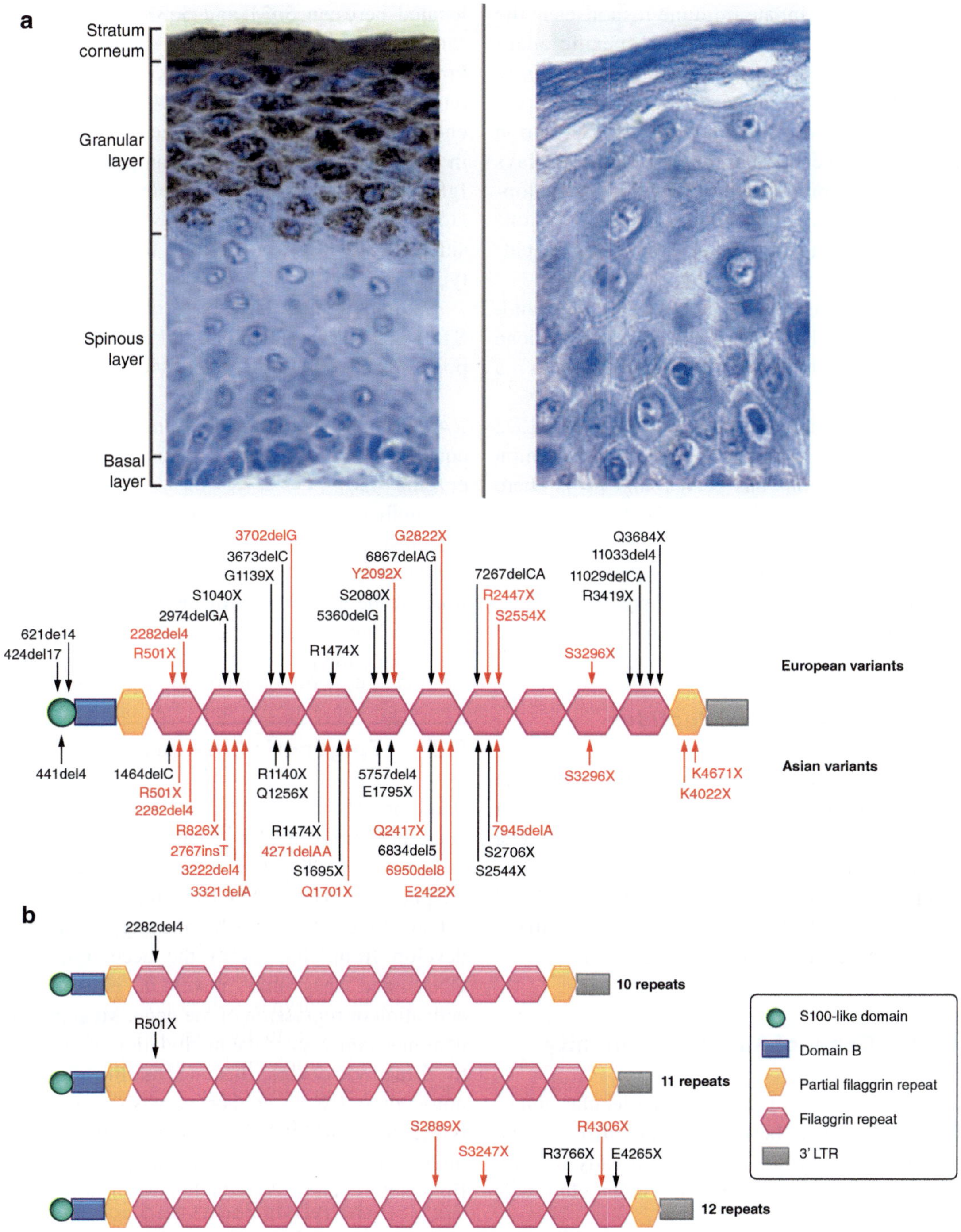

Fig. 5.2 The role of *filaggrin* in the pathogenesis of atopic dermatitis. Upper panel: Filaggrin immunohistochemistry of normal (left) and lesional atopic eczema skin (right). Middle and lower panel: described mutations in the filaggrin gene that are associated with atopic dermatitis. From [78]. (**a**) Upper panel; (**b**) Lower panel

Functioning innate immune responses is the basis of the establishment of a specific adaptive immune response. When innate immunity is weaker, dysregulation of T cell reaction patterns may occur. Toll-like receptor activation after epicutaneous allergen sensitization plays an important protective role in allergy development [295]. Impaired innate immune reactions can give rise to Th2-dominated reaction patterns [523].

These findings may lead to a new understanding of the mechanisms of the so-called hygiene hypothesis with regard to allergy and eczema development [245, 388].

An association of polymorphisms of TLR2 gene with severe atopic eczema and common bacterial infections has been found [10]. There was no association between TLR4 and TLR6 [848]; however, there was a significant association to a polymorphism in TLR9 [556] similar to the NOD1 gene, a molecule of signal transduction in innate immunity against bacteria [845].

5.2.5 Antimicrobial Peptides

An important part of innate immunity in the skin is antimicrobial peptides in the epidermis, such as defensin or cathelicidin. A study from Korea found significant polymorphisms for Defensin Beta1 (DFB1) in atopic eczema (rs5743399 and C haplotype) which are especially common in the extrinsic variant of atopic eczema [394].

5.2.6 Genes of Adaptive Immunity

At the beginning of the era of molecular genetics, associations between atopic disease and genes on chromosome 5 were already discovered, where the so-called cytokine cluster is located between 5q31 and 5q33 and encoding for a variety of candidate genes such as interleukin-4, interleukin-13, interleukin-9, and interleukin-5, but also for CD14 (receptor for endotoxin) [490, 670]. Many gene associations in this cluster were found for atopy in general, IgE, but also respiratory atopic diseases; for atopic dermatitis, they have to be specially considered and only associations for certain subtypes were found [551].

Similar findings have been observed for the STAT6 signal transduction marker (signal transport and activation in T cells) [846].

The genes encoding for the chemokine RANTES or the transcription factor GATA equally were found to be associated with atopic eczema [450].

Another interesting association between polymorphisms of the high-affinity IgE receptor FcεR1 [145] has been found. Obviously mutations in the alpha chain of the high-affinity IgE receptor have a special importance with regard to IgE production [844].

5.3 Epigenetic Changes

The complex heritability of atopic dermatitis does not only involve changes in the DNA sequences encoding for proteins, but also heritable phenotypes caused by DNA modification, so-called epigenetics. Such phenotypes usually develop from changes in the accessibility of DNA, and they may result in either over-activation or repression of the gene. Most prominent mechanisms are the methylation of cytosine to 5-methylcytosine, histone modification, or non-coding RNA's (either very short microRNA's, short siRNA's, or long non-coding RNA's) interfering with protein-coding mRNA's. Epigenetics is a well-studied phenomenon that is

Table 5.2 miRNA's associated with the pathogenesis of atopic dermatitis. (Modified from 5)

miRNA Expression Change in AD Lesions or Serum	Associated Effect
↓Let-7 a-d	↑IL-13↑CCR7
↓miR-375	↑TSLP (Thymic stromal lymphopoietin)
↓hsa-miR-26a-5a	↑HAS3 (hyaluronian 3 synthase)
↑miR-21	↓IL12
↑miR-29b	Promotion of INF-γ-induced keratinocyte apoptosis
↑miR-146a	↓STAT1 and decrease in Treg activation ↓NFκB–pro-inflammatory transcription factor
↑miR-155	↓CTLA-4 and decrease in Treg proliferation ↑Promotion of Th17 differentiation ↓Inhibition of tight junction formation
↑miR-223 in umbilical cord blood	Decrease in Treg activation
↑MiR-151a in serum	Inhibition of IL-12 signaling
Other miRNA expression changes in atopic skin: ↑ miR-17-5p, ↑ miR142-3p/5p, ↓ miR-122a, ↓miR-326, ↓miR-133b, ↓miR-125b, ↓miR375, ↓ miR193c, ↓miR365	

essential for the differentiation of cells, including immune cells. More recently, epigenetics is also studied in the context of atopic dermatitis [541]. Demethylation of promoter regions of genes associated to atopic dermatitis has been reported, in particular for type 2 immunity-associated genes such as TSLP and the high-affinity IgE receptor gene FCER1G but also for genes involved in epidermal differentiation including FLG. Furthermore, several miRNA's have been reported to be relevant for the pathogenesis of atopic dermatitis (Table 5.2) (Fig. 5.3).

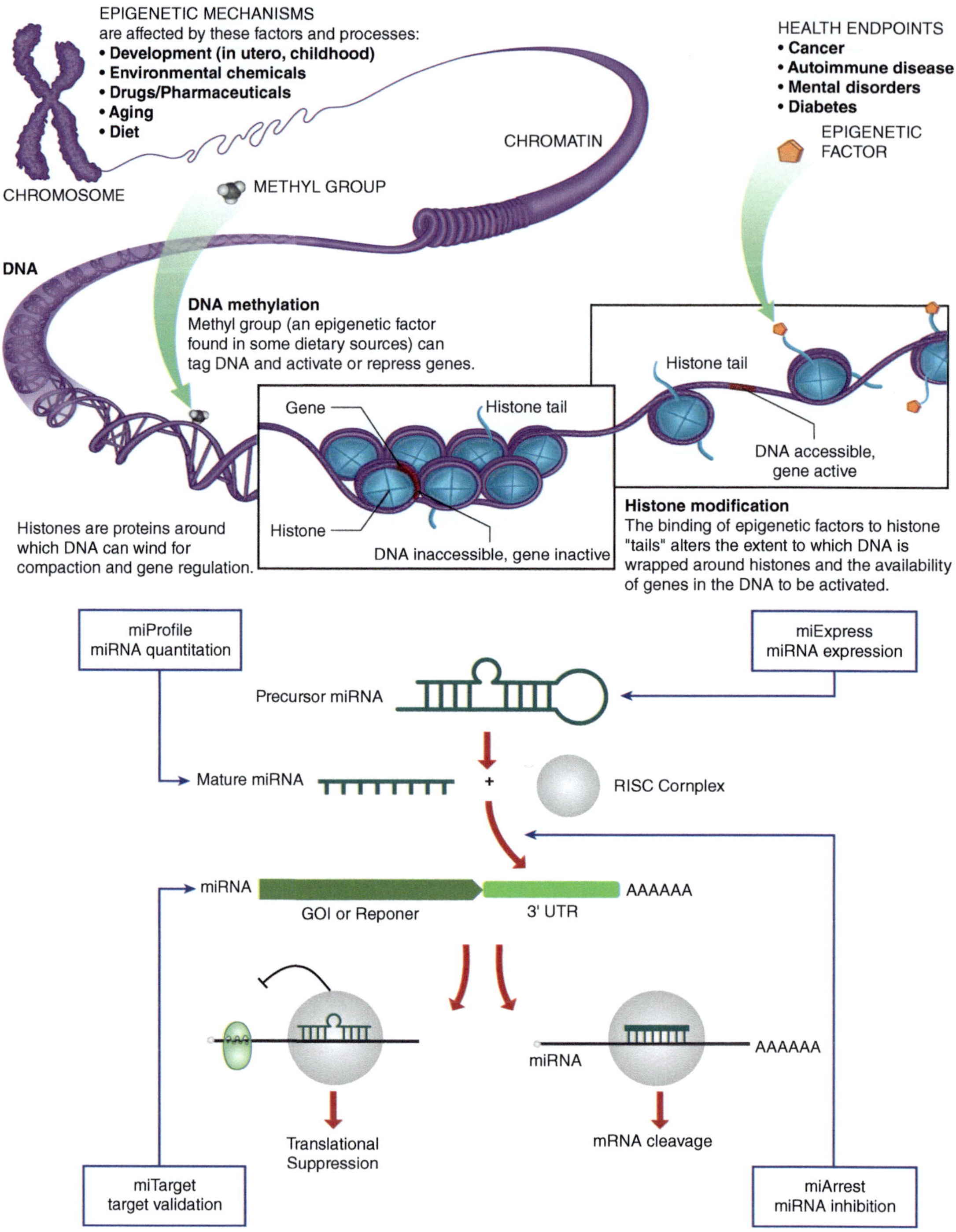

Fig. 5.3 Mechanisms of epigenetics: DANN methylation and chromatin formation (upper panel) and the principle of action of miRNA (lower panel). Zhang L et al. Epigenetics in health and disease. Adv Exp Med Biol. 2020; 1253:3–55. https://doi.org/10.1007/978-981-15-3449-2_1. PMID: 32445090

5.4 Skin Barrier

The skin was historically seen as an inert physical barrier to prevent from external harm (outside-in) and maintain body integrity (inside-out). In the last decades, numerous studies began to draw a very different picture, namely that of the skin as an active organ that is critically involved in homeostasis of our body with its environment. In particular, the skin barrier is built by four carefully orchestrated functional units—the microbial, the chemical, the physical, and the immune barrier (Fig. 5.4) [222].

5.4.1 The Skin in Evolution

When the species Homo sapiens is regarded with respect to the particularly advantageous development of certain organs over the millions of years of evolution, normally the research focuses on the nervous system and the development of the brain. Few studies take the development of the human skin with regard to evolution into account. Therefore, a short reflection on this aspect will be given. The earliest correlate of a "skin" can be found in the Metazoa (e.g., Porifera [sponges]) which have not yet really separated their internal body from the external aqueous environment densely. A structure called pinacoderm represents a very thin one-cell layer which is often disrupted to allow water flow. The Coelenterata (e.g., hydra) already show real epithelium closing the internal part of the body with a one-layered ectodermis overlaying an endodermis.

Further specialization with the development of mesoderm or endomesoderm between the two other layers can be found in helminths. Arthropods have an important feature, namely, an exoskeleton consisting of chitin and proteins as cuticula connected to the underlying epidermis via hemidesmosomes. This cuticula becomes even more pronounced in Echinodermata (e.g., sea urchin).

Fish also produce an exoskeleton with a multilayered epithelium and the development of scales in the upper dermis (placoid scales). The major change occurred in Amphibia when they as the first animals conquered the land and had to cope with a dry environment. Here cornification of the most upper layers of the epidermis occurs; the secretory glands migrate down to the dermis. Cornification is more pronounced in Reptilia with a dry epidermis which periodically is shaded off sometimes within minutes as in the gecko species.

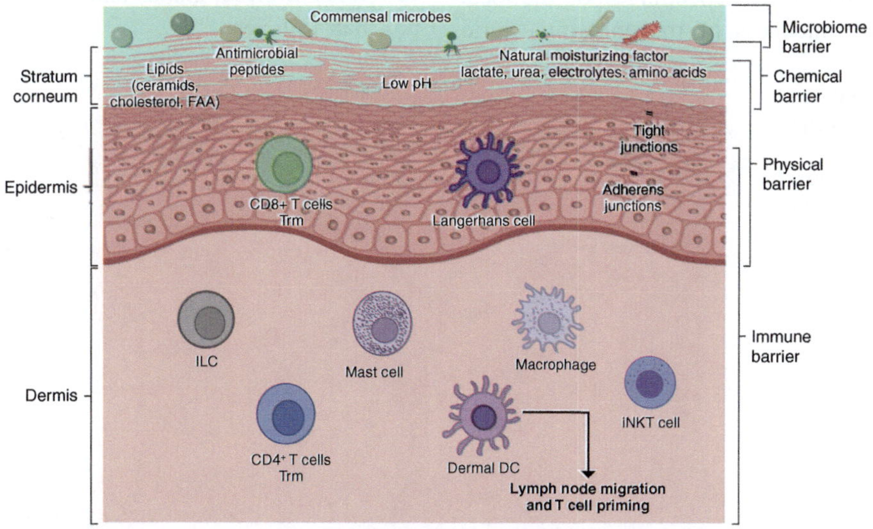

Fig. 5.4 The skin barrier consists of four interdependent layers. Modified from

In birds, the skin developed feathers important for temperature equilibrium and for movement in the air. The avian epidermis only consists of two layers: the stratum germinativum and the stratum corneum. There are no sweat or sebaceous glands. Feathers develop from a protrusion of epidermis with a central dermal pulpa. Finally, they consist completely of keratin, only showing connective tissue rests in the papilla.

Mammalians finally have a wide variability from reptile-like corneal scales via dense furs to the relatively thin and reduced skin of humans. Homo sapiens, among all members, has the most reduced type of skin with regard to thickness, scales, or adnexal tissues, except for innervation which is rather well represented with many sensory cells and free nerve endings over the whole skin surface.

This part has been taken from the excellent reviews of Jablonski [360] and Schempp et al. [698].

5.4.2 Anatomical Structure of the Skin

Anatomically, one can classify the skin from outside to inside into epidermis, dermis or corium, and subcutis (Fig. 5.5).

The epidermis is not of the same thickness on all sites of the body. Depending upon the localization, the thickness of the epidermis varies between 0.014 and 1.5 mm. The epidermis is formed from inside to outside in four layers:

- Stratum basale or stratum germinativum (basal layer).
- Stratum spinosum (spinal layer).
- Stratum granulosum (granular layer).
- Stratum corneum (corneal layer).

Within the epidermis, fine dendritic cells can be found (Langerhans cells) which represent the most external sentinels of the immune system. They act as antigen-presenting cells together with dendritic cells in the dermis which take up foreign substances and present them after migrating to lymphocytes in lymph nodes.

The multitude of cells in the epidermis are formed in the basal layer as keratinocytes producing the most important protein of the epidermis, keratin, but also other proteins (see below). Also, keratinocytes are immunologically active and able to produce important cytokines such as interleukin-1 and -6 as well as defensins and other antimicrobial peptides.

The corium, or dermis, consists of connective tissue with collagen and an extracellular matrix produced by fibroblasts. Here also lymphocytes, nerves, and blood vessels are embedded. In the corium reaching into the subcutis are the adnexal structures of sweat glands and sebaceous glands plus hair follicles.

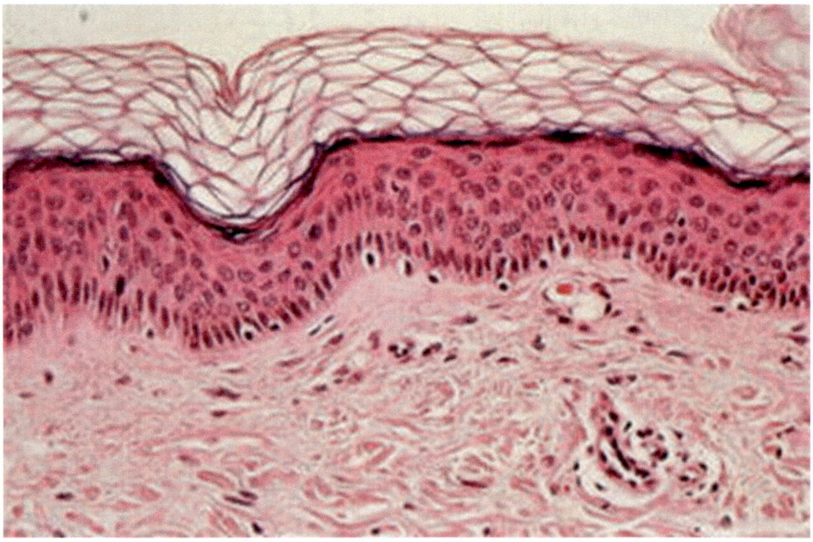

Fig. 5.5 Histological structure of normal skin with dermis and epidermis (hematoxylin-eosin staining) (With friendly permission from Volker Steinkraus)

The adipose tissue forms the mass of the subcutis above the fascia of the muscle.

5.4.3 Microbial Barrier

As a barrier organ, the skin is constantly colonized by a multitude of microorganisms such as bacteria, viruses, or fungi that collectively form the skin microbiome. During evolution, a symbiotic coexistence was established with diverse microbial communities that form a characteristic microenvironment. This microenvironment is fairly stable over time and is reestablished after disturbances. It is very different depending on the body site, as anatomical differences such as the density of glands and hair follicles, thickness of the skin, and exposure to air differ over the body thus creating different microbial niches. There are 19 different phyla with in total more than 1000 different bacterial species reported to colonize the skin. In general, the skin microbiome is dominated by the species *Staphylococcus* and *Cutibacterium* (formerly known as *Propionibacterium*) in sebaceous areas such as the face and intertrigines and by *Staphylococcus* and *Corynebacterium* species in dry areas. Interactions of the skin microbiome with the host immune system are critical to maintain a mutual coexistence of microbiota and our organism. Commensal bacteria are critically involved in protection against potentially harmful pathogens. This is achieved either by stimulating the human immune system to secrete antimicrobial peptides or by secretion of antimicrobial peptides derived from the commensal itself. Prominent examples of induction of the innate immune system are induction of the innate immune system and secretion of antimicrobial peptides by *S. epidermidis* or *C. acnes*. S. epidermidis also directly releases antimicrobial peptides such as the serine protease Esp that destroys *S. aureus* biofilms and reduces *S. aureus* colonization. Of note, overgrowth with *S. aureus* is critically involved in the pathogenesis of atopic dermatitis ([416], discussed in Sect. 5.5), and this overgrowth is associated with reduced antimicrobial activity of *S. epidermidis*. Taken together, the skin microbiome barrier is an active part of the skin that prevents pathogen encounter not only by sophisticated host immune interactions but also by influencing the chemical barrier that is described below.

5.4.4 Chemical Barrier

The second layer of the epidermal barrier is the so-called chemical barrier. It regulates the skin pH and hydration as well as desquamation of corneocytes and epidermal plasticity. The chemical layer consists of hygroscopic amino acids, mostly derivates of urocanic acid or pyrrolidone carboxylic acid together with specific salts and electrolytes. Collectively, these low molecular hygroscopic products of the stratum corneum are named the natural moisturizing factor (NMF). Many of the components of the NMF are filaggrin degradation products. In line with this, filaggrin mutations as the strongest genetic risk factor of atopic dermatitis (see Sect. 5.2.2) lead to reduction of the NMF, and a reduced NMF correlates with the severity of atopic dermatitis. The NMF can be measured in the epidermis using Raman spectroscopy. This measurement is suggested as a biomarker of atopic dermatitis.

Besides control of the hydration, regulation of the skin pH is a hallmark of the NMF. The skin is covered by a so-called acid mantle, a tightly regulated pH gradient in the stratum corneum with values of around 5,5 in the upper layers. This gradient is involved in the physical barrier formation, as several enzymes regulating desquamation and lamellar arrangement of ceramides and other lipids in the "brick and mortar" model (see Sect. 5.4.5) are pH-dependent. The skin pH is influenced by multiple factors such as age, anatomic site, ethnicity, genetic predisposition, or sweat, but also by exogeneous factors including emollients, cosmetics, and topical antiseptics. Mechanistically, urocanic acid and derivates as well as lactate and potassium ions are central NMF components regulating skin pH. Of note, skin pH in atopic dermatitis is frequently higher than in healthy volunteers. Furthermore, a higher skin pH correlates with severity and burden of itch in atopic dermatitis patients.

The NMF is critical for protection against microbial pathogens: corneocytes containing low NMF show nanoscale villus protrusions, and these seem to be important for adhesion of *S. aureus* to the stratum corneum.

In summary, the chemical barrier controls skin hydration and barrier formation in the stratum corneum through a carefully orchestrated process of skin pH-dependent degradation of hygroscopic amino acids. The microbial and chemical barrier are tightly connected, and so are the chemical and the physical barrier (see Sect. 5.4.5).

5.4.5 Physical Barrier

The barrier function of the skin is important to form a frontier between the organism and the environment. Physiologically it protects the body from pathogenic noxes and is anatomically realized mostly in the stratum corneum. This barrier is not totally impermeable but has permeability to a degree to allow transport between the internal milieu of the organism and the outside. The corneal layer is not "dead skin" but is the end product of a highly differentiated epidermal process where skin cells transform into corneocytes from inside to outside with increasing numbers of keratin filaments which, together with lipids, form the stratum corneum according to the model of "bricks and mortar" [209].

The structural integrity of the stratum corneum is guaranteed by so-called modified desmosomes (corneodesmosomes) which bind corneocytes together and thus build a defense against tangential forces and mechanical trauma. In the model of Peter Elias, corneocytes can be compared to bricks, while the lipid lamellar layers can be compared to mortar. Corneal desmosomes could be regarded as iron rods [148] which supply resistance against mechanical stress [603].

5.4.6 Corneocytes

Corneocytes are flat cells in the terminal differentiation of epidermal keratinocytes which takes place in the stratum granulosum. Here the cells lose their nuclei as well as intracytoplasmic organelles and are connected densely with keratin fibrils. The human stratum corneum consists of approximately 20 layers of corneocytes, each 30 μm in diameter. The keratinocytes of the stratum granulosum release the contents of the keratohyalin granules which then together with keratin filaments form the lipid lamellar matrix of the mortar. The lipid layer consists of cholesterol, ceramides, fatty acids, and cholesterol esters which represent as a coherent lamellar layer in the stratum corneum. In the terminal differentiation of keratinocytes, the cell membrane changes into an insoluble protein matrix, called cornified envelope, to which the lipid layer binds. The cornified envelope consists mainly of structural proteins such as loricrin, involucrin, filaggrin, and smaller proline-rich proteins which are bound together by transglutaminases.

5.4.7 Corneodesmosomes

The corneodesmosomes are part of corneocyte envelopes and consist mainly of proteins of the cadherin family, a group of extracellular transmembrane glycoproteins. Corneodesmosin is a 52 kD protein especially expressed in cornifying epithelia, which, after its secretion in the extracellular space between stratum granulosum and stratum corneum, is integrated into the desmosomes in a way that corneodesmosomes develop.

A very rare disturbance of cornification and skin barrier function has been described as "peeling skin disease" which shares some features with Netherton syndrome, but without "bamboo hair" and SPINK5 mutation. In a family with this rare autosomal recessive ichthyosiform erythroderma, a defect in corneodesmosin has been found to be relevant and another very important factor for epidermal barrier integrity [567].

5.4.8 Desquamation

A natural decay of superficial corneocytes leads to a continuous process of desquamation in an equilibrium between keratinocyte proliferation in the stratum basale and desquamation on the surface. The process of desquamation depends upon a network of active proteases and protease inhibitors which degrade extracellular corneodesmosomal structures and thus allow the desquamation of superficial corneocytes. In this process, kallikrein-associated peptidases such as stratum corneum chymotryptic enzyme (SCCE) KLK7 as well as stratum corneum tryptic enzyme (SCTE) KLK5 are involved [202]. Apart from serine proteases, also cysteine proteases like cathepsin L2 (SC thiol protease) and aspartate protease cathepsin D with a pH optimum in the acid range are active. KLK-related serine proteases have their activity optimum in the mild alkaline pH.

All the activities of these proteases are regulated by a mixture of protease inhibitors such as serine leukoprotease inhibitors, but also cystatin protease inhibitors. Cystatin A is formed in sweat and forms a protective film against exogenic proteases from microbes or parasites (*S. aureus* or house dust mite) on the skin surface. The lymphoepithelial Kazal-type 5 protease inhibitor (LEKTI), which is encoded via the serine protease inhibitor Kazal-type 5 gene (SPINK5), is a special pH-dependent regulator of desquamation. LEKTI is formed in the stratum granulosum and secreted into the intracellular space between stratum granulosum and stratum corneum (lamellar bodies) where it is found colocalized with the abovementioned kallikrein peptidases in the neutral pH. The more acid the pH to the outside, the weaker the inhibitory potential of LEKTI thus allowing a normal desquamation in the most superficial layers.

5.4.9 Summary

Genetic alterations are a central component of the atopic dermatitis pathogenesis. Twin studies and large genetic association trials give clear evidence for this. However, AD follows a complex genetic trait, and to date only a minority of cases can be explained by mutations in the genome. The most important factor driving the susceptibility to AD is filaggrin, a central gene of the epidermal barrier complex, but also other genes regulating the epidermal structure, innate or adaptive immunity are identified. Less is known about permanent or long-term modifications of the readability of genes, so-called epigenetics. Most likely, epigenetic changes play an important role in the pathogenesis of AD.

5.5 Changes in the Microbiome

As discussed above, microbiota colonizing the skin contribute to the skin barrier formation by interacting with the chemical barrier, ensuring a regular formation of the physical barrier, and protecting against pathogens both by activating the human immune system and own production of antimicrobial peptides. In atopic dermatitis, this mutual way of coexistence is critically disturbed, and pathogenic microbiota overgrow the commensals. Of particular importance is a dysbalance of S. epidermidis, an essential commensal, versus *S. aureus*, a pro-inflammatory bacterium critically involved in several aspects of atopic dermatitis pathogenesis.

The prevalence of *S. aureus* is around 20% in healthy volunteers while it doubles in atopic dermatitis patients at non-lesional sites. Lesional atopic dermatitis skin is colonized by *S. aureus* in 30%–100%, depending on the study and method used, with a mean prevalence across 95 observational trials of 70% according to a meta-analysis. Thus, a change in the microbiome occurs during atopic dermatitis flares—that includes a reduced diversity of the genera *Streptococcus*, *Corynebacterium*, and *Cutibacterium* and an increased abundance of *Staphylococcus*, in particular of the species *S. aureus*. In fact, it is usually only a single strain of *S. aureus* that colonizes lesional skin of atopic dermatitis.

S. aureus drives the pathogenesis of atopic dermatitis in different ways. First, *S. aureus* impairs the epidermal barrier. This is mediated by at least ten *S. aureus*-derived proteases that attack both keratinocytes and cell-cell interaction molecules. Besides these endogeneous proteases, *S. aureus* triggers protease secretion of keratinocytes, in particular of kallikreins, which further impairs the epidermal barrier. Some *S. aureus* strains produce *S. aureus* a-toxin, a cytotoxin that forms pores in keratinocytes thus adding another mechanism to *S. aureus*-mediated disruption of the epidermal barrier. Of note, the effects of these proteases are enhanced in a more alkaline milieu such as observed in atopic dermatitis (see Sect. 5.4.4) and type 2 cytokines induce certain kallikreins in keratinocytes. Thus, the typical chemical and immune microenvironment of atopic dermatitis skin are ideal for *S. aureus* to bind to the epidermis and exert its pathogenic effects.

Second, *S. aureus* induces pro-inflammatory immune responses in the host that contribute to the pathogenesis of atopic dermatitis. This is mediated in part by *S. aureus*-derived factors such as superantigen A, B, or C (SEA, SEB, SEC). These superantigens enhance the binding of T cells to antigen-presenting cells and therefore cause an immune response independent of an antigen. SEA and SEB induce type 3 immunity, namely secretion of IL-17A or IL-22 by T cells in atopic dermatitis skin (see Sect. 5.7). Also other toxins such as toxic shock syndrome toxin 1 or the cell-bound protein A induce pro-inflammatory immune reactions involving the NF-kB pathway in the host. Finally, lipoproteins derived from *S. aureus* trigger Toll-like receptors such as TLR2/6 to induce TSLP secretion in keratinocytes and thus contribute to type 2 inflammation, the hallmark of atopic dermatitis.

In summary, various *S. aureus*-derived products act pro-inflammatory in the skin. It is still under debate whether these changes may be causative or an epiphenomenon of ongoing inflammation—in other words, what is the chicken and what is the egg in the complex pathogenesis of atopic dermatitis.

In contrast, other frequently observed changes in the skin microbiome of atopic dermatitis patients are usually regarded to be secondary events. This is the case for infection with certain viruses such as vaccinia virus or herpes viruses that are usually associated with a decreased epidermal barrier or type 2 immune microenvironment.

Besides *S. aureus* and secondary virus infection, a third commonly observed phenomenon in atopic dermatitis is inflammation caused by yeasts of the *Malassezia* species. Depending on the study and method used, *Malassezia* species comprise 1–22% of the total skin microbiome. Usually, they are commensals. That means Malassezia induces Th17 immune responses, but usually does not cause dysbalanced inflammation. However, *Malassezia* is the cause of pityriasis versicolor and may also be involved in the pathogenesis of atopic dermatitis. Here, *Malassezia* induces eczema-like reactions in a subgroup of patients when using the Atopy Patch Tests model. Furthermore, IgE-medited sensitization levels against Malassezia are frequently observed and correlate with the severity of atopic dermatitis.

5.5.1 Summary

For decades, colonization of lesional (and non-lesional) skin of atopic dermatitis patients with *S. aureus* is known. More granular molecular techniques have proven that there is a very close interaction between the host and specific *S. aureus* strains, and that *S. aureus* overgrows other, potentially beneficial, commensals, during a flare. The mechanistic role of how *S. aureus* contributes to further impairment of the epidermal barrier as well as to inflammation is now better understood; however, there is no direct therapeutic translation of these findings as of yet.

5.6 Excursion into a New Concept for Classification of Pathogenic Immune Reactions in Noncommunicable Inflammatory Skin Diseases

This paragraph is modified from [221]. When discussing the immunology of atopic dermatitis, an excursion into how we historically classify inflammatory skin diseases is necessary, as we have to overcome certain limitations that result from a misfit between our traditional disease ontology and molecular therapies. Disease classification in dermatology relies on precise clini-

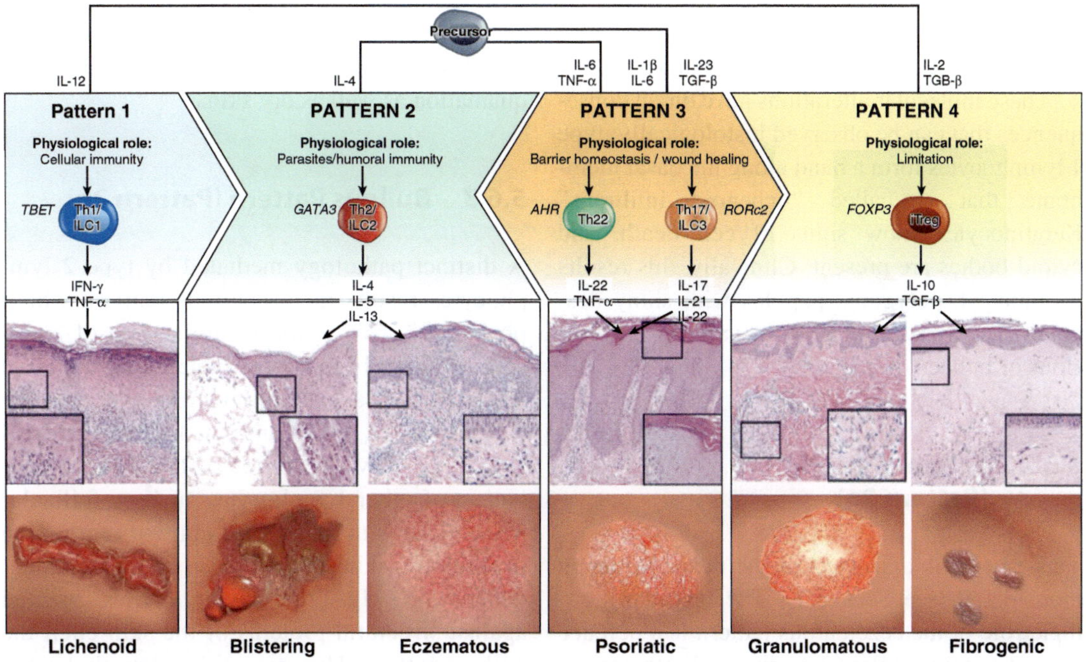

Fig. 5.6 Distinct T cells induce characteristic clinical and histological disease patterns. Modified from

cal description in combination with histological description of microscopic tissue alterations and infiltrating immune cells. This classification is complex, and at times misleading. At the same time, insights into mechanisms of how distinct lymphocyte subsets terminally orchestrate the inflammatory response and how these lymphocytes interact with resident skin cells resulted in a translational revolution leading to more and more specific therapeutics. To acknowledge these recent advances made in the design and approval of specific immune-mediating therapeutics, a classification of inflammatory skin diseases according to their immune response patterns is required (Fig. 5.1). Here follows a brief summary of what is known about immunology, histopathology, and clinical phenotype for each of the immune response patterns (Fig. 5.6).

5.6.1 Lichenoid Pattern (Pattern 1)

The major physiologic role of the lichenoid pattern is the disposal of keratinocytes that are potentially infected with intracellular microbes or are (pre-)carcinogenic due to DNA damages beyond repair. It is characterized by a cytotoxic immune response against keratinocytes of the basal layer ("interface dermatitis") that is mediated by killer T cells (Tc1), Th1 cells, ILC1, NKT, and NK cells (type 1 lymphocytes). This cytotoxic reaction is driven by the master regulator of type 1 lymphocytes, IFN-g, and cytotoxic granules such as granulysin, perforin, granzyme B, and Fas/FasL. In line with that observation, transcriptional network comparison of lesional lichen planus and lupus erythematosus with non-interface skin diseases revealed that differentially expressed genes are attributable to type 1 lymphocytes as well as to the effect of IFN-g on keratinocytes, including apoptosis and necroptosis. Furthermore, interface dermatitis is induced in murine models of xenotransplantation or adoptive transfer of keratinocyte-reactive cytotoxic T cells. In cell culture models, FasL induces the characteristic hypergranulosis while IFN-g causes keratinocyte apoptosis with cytoid body formation, and ICAM-1 expression. This is mediated via janus kinase (JAK)-dependent upregulation of class 2 HLA molecules in keratinocytes that lead to increased binding of cytotoxic T cells and subsequent killing. In line with this, JAK inhibition could be beneficial in treating interface dermatitis diseases such as lichen planus.

These molecular alterations have direct consequences that can be observed histologically: type 1 lymphocytes form a band along the basal membrane that is called "lichenoid infiltrate." Keratinocytes show signs of cell death, and cytoid bodies are present. Clinically, this results in flattened, polygonal papules with shiny desquamation; maximum clinical variants are erosions or bullae.

5.6.2 Eczematous Pattern (Pattern 2a)

This pattern is discussed in the next chapter in more detail (see Sect. 5.7). The major physiologic role of the eczematous pattern is a defence against extracellular parasites. Furthermore, recent evidence suggests a role in protection against toxins. Skin lesions are dominated by Th2 and ILC2 cells (type 2 lymphocytes) secreting IL-4, IL-5, IL-13, and IL-31. These cytokines affect the epidermis in two ways: IL-4 and IL-13 downregulate genes of the epidermal differentiation complex thus impairing the epidermal barrier and resulting in dry skin [340]. Furthermore, IL-4 and IL-13 inhibit cutaneous innate immunity which explains why most patients affected by eczematous diseases suffer from skin colonization with *S. aureus* or other microbials. Th2-derived IL-31 also impacts the epidermal barrier and is a critical mediator of itch, a leading symptom of most diseases grouped into the eczematous pattern. IL-5 is a strong activator of eosinophil and basophil granulocytes as well as mast cells. The release of a plethora of mediators from these cells leads to edema and influx of further immune cells into the skin.

The type 2 immune deviation results in histological hallmarks such as spongiosis, serum crusts, and a mixed cellular infiltrate composed of lymphocytes and eosinophil granulocytes in the acute phase and irregular acanthosis in the chronic phase characterize the eczematous pattern. Clinically, the phenotype eczema presents as epidermo-dermatitis with cooccurrence of vesicles, papules, erythema, erosions, and desquamation as well as dry skin.

5.6.3 Bullous Pattern (Pattern 2b)

A distinct pathology mediated by type 2 lymphocytes results in the bullous pattern, whose physiologic role is the neutralization of extracellular microbes. Type 2 lymphocytes instruct B cells and plasma cells to form the antibody subclasses IgE, IgG1, and IgG4 via secretion of IL-4 and IgA via secretion of IL-5. The contribution of other lymphocytes such as follicular helper T cells to pathogenic antibody formation in bullous skin diseases is currently under debate. IgG, IgA, or IgE antibodies directed against structural proteins of the skin elicit the bullous pattern. They may either directly lead to keratinocyte apoptosis and loss of cellular adhesion, a concept called apoptolysis, or bind to their target and cause secondary inflammation via opsonization .

Histological hallmark of type 2 lymphocyte-mediated auto-antibody formation is the destruction of the skin integrity as a result of acantholysis, a gap between epidermis and dermis, or dermal split. An inflammatory infiltrate composed of lymphocytes, eosinophil, or neutrophil granulocytes is always observed. Using immunofluorescence, antibody deposits of distinct patterns are disease-defining. Clinically, the primary resulting lesion is a blister with surrounding erythema; depending on the thickness of the epidermal roof and manipulation, also erosions and crusts are frequently observed. Circulating specific antibodies are typical and represent biomarkers of bullous skin diseases. Of note, diseases of the lichenoid or eczematous pattern may show a bullous clinical variant; those variants are not regarded as bullous pattern diseases, but rather as maximal variants of interface dermatitis or spongiosis, respectively, due to their distinct primary pathology.

5.6.4 Psoriatic Pattern (Pattern 3)

The psoriatic pattern is mediated by a group of lymphocytes comprised of Th17, Tc17, ILC3, and Th22 cells (type 3 lymphocytes) that share the physiologic role to warrant homeostasis at barrier organs such as the skin and mucous membranes of lung and gastrointestinal tract. The pattern is caused by increased epidermal metabolism as well as by activation of innate immune signals. IL-21 and IL-22 increase keratinocyte proliferation and migration and inhibit their differentiation thus contributing to acanthosis and parakeratosis. IL-17A and IL-17F induce keratinocyte secretion of several antimicrobial peptides as well as of CXCL8, a chemokine recruiting neutrophils to the epidermis, and VEGF that stimulates vascularization.

Collectively, this results in histological hallmarks such as regular acanthosis with hyperparakeratosis, (micro)-abscesses in the upper layers of the epidermis, dilated dermal capillaries and a lymphocytic dermal infiltrate. Clinically, a type 3 lymphocyte response is reflected by sharply demarcated plaques with thick desquamation. Sterile pustules are a further hallmark of the psoriatic pattern. IL-36 proteins and inducible nitric oxidase (NOS2) in the skin and the antimicrobial peptide HBD-2 in the serum are valid biomarkers of the psoriatic pattern.

5.6.5 Fibrogenic Pattern (Pattern 4a)

The fibrogenic pattern is a consequence of prolonged lymphocyte anti-inflammatory activity, usually a counter-regulation of a preceding inflammatory response. Lead cytokines of causative regulatory T cells (Tregs) such as iTreg, Th3, and Tr1 (type 4 lymphocytes) are IL-10 and TGF-b. The fibrogenic pattern is mediated via TGF-b that induces numerous pro-fibrotic genes in distinct tissue cells. Furthermore, it is central in endothelial-to-mesenchymal transition to pro-fibrotic myofibroblasts. The consequence is excessive extracellular matrix production, deposition, and tissue remodeling (fibrosis).

Alterations in the regulatory T cell department histologically lead to fibrosis that is observed as thickened collagen bundles and a diminished number of cells. The lymphoid infiltrate is typically mild and located in deeper skin layers. The epidermis is normal or atrophic. This is reflected by clinical hallmarks such as well-demarcated thickening of the whole skin and a shiny, atrophic epidermis that may be surrounded by erythema in active lesions.

5.6.6 Granulomatous Pattern (Pattern 4b)

Granuloma formation is a general mechanism of the immune system after identification of a potentially harmful molecule that cannot be eliminated. In the skin, such molecules may be of infectious nature or degenerated extracellular matrix. Recently, the term "Immunocompromised districts" (ICD) has been proposed for a localized immune dysbalance in the skin after trauma. Interestingly, granulomatous skin diseases occur frequently in ICD predilection sites. As compared to the other patterns, the level of evidence for a dominating role of a single lymphocyte subset is low for the granulomatous pattern. Both pro-inflammatory and regulatory T cells are involved. The balance of TNF-a and type 4 lymphocyte-derived IL-10 expression seems to be critical for granuloma development and sustainability. Interestingly, Tregs decrease after therapy with TNF-a blocking antibodies, indicating a functional link between Tregs and Th1/Th17 cells via TNF receptor 2.

The histological architecture of a granuloma is comprised of a center of epitheloid cells and histiocytes that may melt into giant cells or die and leave a cell-free mass (caseating granuloma). This center is surrounded by lymphocytes to a varying degree. In the skin, granulomas develop in the dermis, the epidermis is typically noninvolved or atrophic. Clinically, granulomatous diseases present as brownish papules of sharp demarcation with or without epidermal desquamation. Figurated or annular manifestation is regularly observed.

5.6.7 Summary

The growing possibilities to modulate specific immune pathways therapeutically is opposed by our traditional way to look at skin diseases. We know that virtually all chronic inflammatory skin diseases are either caused by (mono)genetic autoinflammation or by a complex interplay of adaptive immune cells and resident stromal cells or keratinocytes. There is a limited number of reaction, or response, patterns in the skin; each has a physiological role, but may turn into harmful inflammation if the response is inadequate. While the concept of immune response patterns is over-simplified, it helps us in making therapeutic decisions in the era of highly specific symptomatic treatments such as biologics.

5.7 Type 2 Immunity, Allergy, and Its Consequences for Atopic Dermatitis

5.7.1 Definition and Occurrence of Type 2 Immune Cells

A common denominator of all variants of atopic dermatitis is the presence of type 2 immune cells in the skin. Type 2 immune cells are a group of lymphocytes characterized by secretion of cytokines such as interleukin(IL)-4, IL-5, IL-9, IL-13, and IL-31 under the control of the master transcription factor GATA3. The group of type 2 immune cells comprises T helper (Th) 2 cells, Th9 cells, and innate lymphoid cells type 2 (ILC2). Th2 cells differentiate from naive precursor cells in the presence of IL-4. Th9 cells need additional stimulation with TGF-b. ILC2 differentiates from a multipotent precursor cell under the influence of IL-33 and potentially IL-17E (formerly called IL-25). Type 2 immune cells are dominant, especially in acute forms of atopic dermatitis. In a provocation model of early atopic dermatitis, the Atopy Patch Test (APT), early lesions can be induced by allergen challenge of sensitized individuals. In an APT to house dust mite, virtually all antigen-specific T cells had a type 2 phenotype thus confirming the causative role for this T cell subtype in atopic dermatitis.

Historically, a “switch”was proposed from acute to chronic immune reactions. This means that while early lesions are dominated by type 2 cells, more chronic lesions show an infiltrate of type 1 immune cells (Fig. 5.7). This “switch”occurred as a consequence of several immune cells being activated in the course of inflammation, e.g., inflammatory dendritic epidermal cells (IDEC) that secrete the master cytokine of the type 1 program, namely IFN-g. Subsequently, also type 3 immunity was found to be induced in ongoing inflammatory reactions in atopic dermatitis, primarily by *S. aureus*-derived substances such as superantigens (see Sect. 5.5). While the evidence that more chronic lesions show a mixed T cellular infiltrate is clear, the idea of a “switch” is now proven wrong—type 2 immunity is at all times of eczematous lesions relevant and present. Nevertheless, type 1 and type 3 immunity have a clear impact on atopic dermatitis. They account for many differences in the clinical and histological differences of acute and chronic atopic dermatitis, with the first showing a higher number of infiltrating lymphocytes and spongiosis, and the latter acanthosis that might be related to type 3 immunity and in particular IL-22.

5.7.2 Functions of Type 2 Immune Cells in the Context of Atopic Dermatitis

Type 2 immune cells drive several hallmarks of atopic dermatitis (Fig. 5.7). In the skin, cytokines released by type 2 immune cells such as IL-13 and IL-4 downregulate keratinocyte differentiation genes such as filaggrin, loricrin, and involucrin through modulation of the transcription factor STAT6. This leads to an impaired epidermal barrier function. IL-4 and IL-13 also impact the innate immune response of the skin. Namely, the secretion of antimicrobial peptides

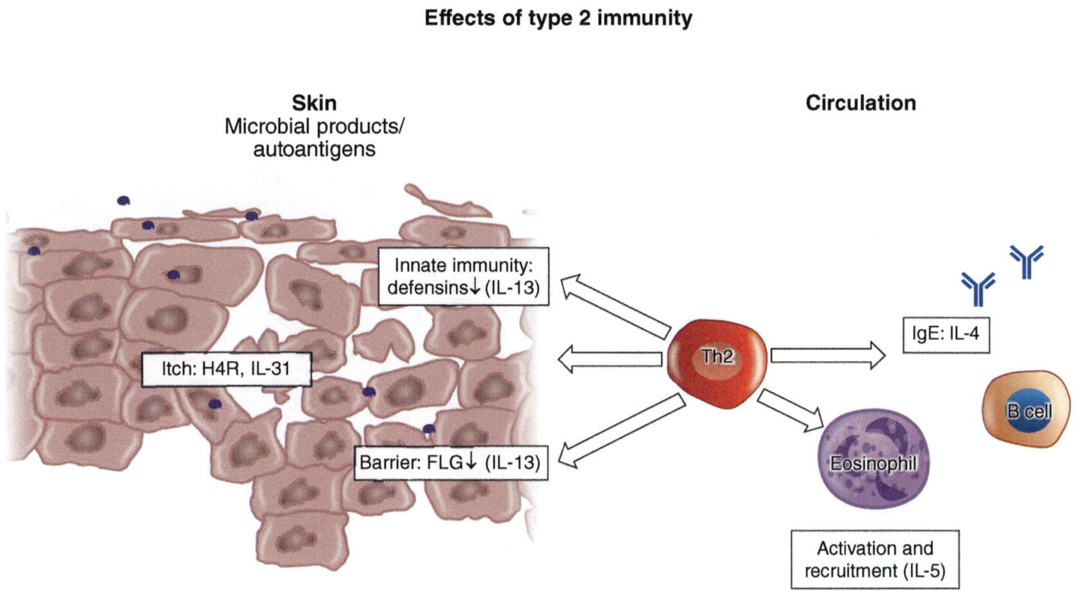

Fig. 5.7 Effects of type 2 immunity in the skin (left side) and the circulation (right side)

such as defensins by keratinocytes is controlled by type 1 (IFN-g, TNF-a) or type 3 (IL-17, IL-22, TNF-a) immunity. However, type 2 cytokines such as IL-4 or IL-13 strongly diminish this induction of antimicrobial peptides. Furthermore, IL-4 and IL-13 impair migration and activation of neutrophils into tissue. Thus, type 2 immunity partially impairs innate immunity in the skin which can be one reason for the altered microbiome frequently observed in atopic dermatitis patients (see Sect. 5.5).

A third function of type 2 immune cells in the skin is the induction of itch, the main symptom of atopic dermatitis. These effects are discussed in Sect. 5.8.

Besides its local functions in the skin and effects on myeloid immune cells, type 2 immune cells impact immunity in the circulation, lymph nodes, and bone marrow. Type 2 cytokines are essential to steer antibody production in B cells and plasma cells: IL-4 induces an isotype switch to the immunoglobulin subclasses G1 (IgG1), G4 (IgG4), and E (IgE); IL-5 instructs IgA production. Especially production of high levels of IgE is a typical phenomenon observed in the majority of atopic dermatitis patients. In a subpopulation of atopic dermatitis patients, allergen-specific IgE may be of clinical relevance. These patients show an exacerbation upon stimulation with pollen under experimental conditions. For the majority of patients however a causative role in humoral immunity is not demonstrated and the question of whether increased IgE levels are an epiphenomenon or causative is discussed controversially. However, only a small minority of atopic dermatitis patients benefit from neutralizing IgE therapeutically by treatment with omalizumab. Furthermore, up to 20% of atopic dermatitis patients do not show increased IgE levels (historically called "intrinsic"atopic dermatitis), so high IgE levels are not a *conditio* sine qua non in atopic dermatitis pathogenesis.

Type 2 lymphocytes also activate and recruit myeloid cells to the skin. In particular, IL-5 is an important survival factor for both eosinophil and basophil granulocytes, as well as mast cells. (Chemokines induced) These cell types are typically increased in both circulation and lesional skin in atopic dermatitis. They release numerous cytokines, chemokines, and other inflammatory mediators that contribute to the pathogenesis of atopic dermatitis, in particular to spongiosis and edema in lesional skin (Fig. 5.8).

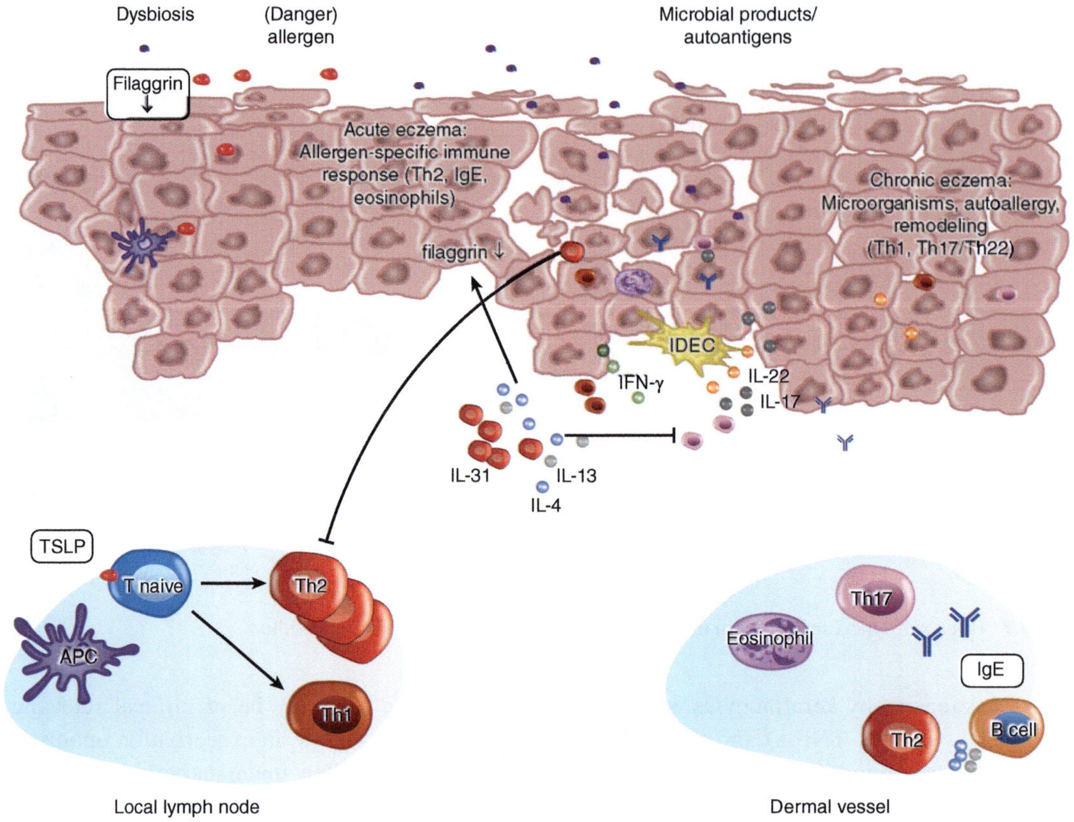

Fig. 5.8 The pathogenesis of atopic dermatitis. Filaggrin deficiency and type 2 inflammation predispose to barrier damage. Antigens are processed by antigen-presenting cells (APC) and then presented to naive T cells in the local lymph node. Both the nature of the antigen and genetic factors such as enhanced activity of TSLP lead to preferential induction of type 2 immune cells. These encounter the skin and release cytokines such as IL-13 and IL-31, which in turn impairs the epidermal barrier, induces itch, and facilitates the growth of pathogens such as *S. aureus*. *S. aureus*-derived products and activation of dendritic cells such as IDEC subsequently induce the second wave of inflammation that trigger type 1 and type 3 immune cells to enter the skin and contribute to chronic inflammation

5.8 Autoimmunity and Atopic Dermatitis

Parts of this chapter were modified from [287]. Taking an immunological perspective, autoimmune diseases are caused by T cells or antibodies specifically recognizing self-antigens, while the term inflammatory diseases is a much broader term that comprises autoimmunity and autoinflammatory responses arising from any type of, or a mix of, adaptive and innate immune responses. As discussed in Sect. 5.6, the disease ontology in dermatology is largely misleading, as some ncISD is called "inflammatory," although they might well be autoimmune—and vice versa. In that context, there are reports demonstrating both autoreactive T cells or IgE autoantibodies in atopic dermatitis, but their relevance for the pathogenesis is controversially discussed.

Antigen-specific T cells have been identified in the skin and/or periphery of patients with atopic dermatitis. The overarching question is whether these T cell antigens are the primary cause of ncISD or rather an epiphenomenon that occurs in the course of inflammation. To date, this question cannot be clearly answered, as animal models that capture the full complexity of the human disease, as well as a "standardized human"do not exist for atopic dermatitis. Thus, adequate tools are lacking to investigate the early events of these diseases. The fact that atopic dermatitis and psoriasis follow an antagonistic disease course, but may develop in close proximity to each other in the same patient, suggests that distinct adaptive immunity is the driving force at least in a subgroup of these diseases, but this leaves the question open whether the disease-driving T cells are recognizing environmental or autoantigens.

In atopic dermatitis, both CD4+ and CD8+ T cells reacting against self-antigens have been reported over decades. Best described are T cells recognizing a-NAC/Hom s 2 or the human alarmin thioredoxin (hTrx). They most likely originate from a phenomenon called molecular mimicry. This means similarities in the protein structure of potentially harmful antigens lead to cross-reactivity against human structures. It is one of the main mechanisms of how autoimmunity may develop (Fig. 5.9). hTrx cross-reacts with *Malassezia*-derived products. Thus, T cell autoreactivity is observed in patients with atopic dermatitis, but their functional role is not yet well established.

While the causative role for autoantibodies in bullous autoimmune diseases and potentially in CSU is well established, the relevance of autoantibodies observed in atopic dermatitis is still under debate (Table 5.1). In a meta-analysis of 14 studies, IgE autoantibodies were reported in 23–91% of atopic dermatitis patients, depending on the origin of the study and detection methods used. Of these 14 studies, only two report a significant correlation between the presence of autoantibodies and skin severity. Furthermore, IgE autoantibodies seem to be quite frequent in healthy children, which further questions the causative relevance of autoantibodies in atopic dermatitis (personal communication, Prof. Jan Gutermuth, Brussels). The origin of autoantibodies is still under debate, but just like autoreactive T cells, the majority seem to develop from molecular mimicry. In atopic dermatitis, causative structures seem to be derived from *Aspergillus* or *Malassezia*. There are 140 different autoantigens described so far in atopic dermatitis. The most relevant are displayed in Table 5.3.

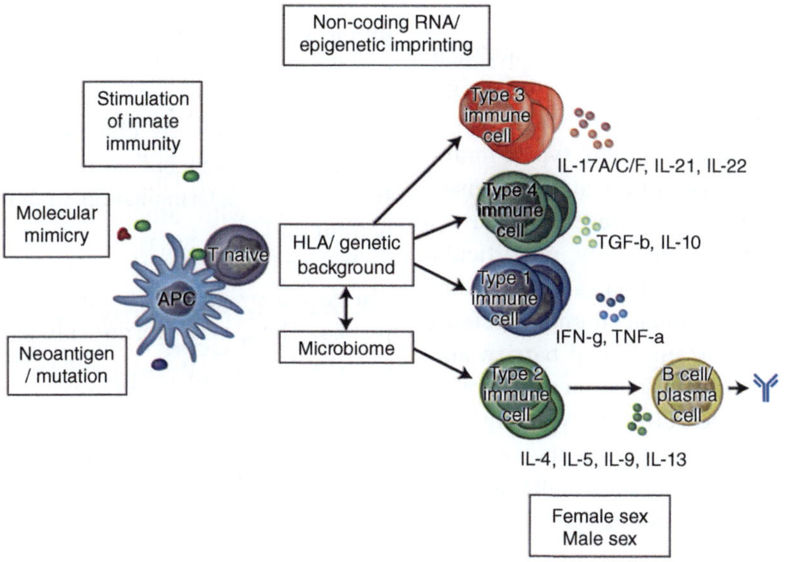

Fig. 5.9 Mechanisms of skin autoimmunity. Modified from. Inflammation due to harmless self-antigens can be due to the formation of new antigens (e.g., in cancer), structural similarities to potentially harmful pathogens (molecular mimicry, main mechanism in atopic dermatitis), inherent danger signals of antigens (such as in the house dust mite) antigen Der p 2 that stimulates Toll-like receptors, microbial dysbiosis, epigenetic modifications (see Sect. 5.3), or female sex (especially in humoral autoimmune diseases) Gudjonsson JE et al. Mechanisms of skin autoimmunity: cellular and soluble immune components of the skin. J Allergy Clin Immunol. 2020; 146:8–16. https://doi.org/10.1016/j.jaci.202005.009. PMID: 32631499

Table 5.3 Autoantigens recognized by IgE in atopic dermatitis (Modified from 5)

IgE against	Prevalence
Manganese superoxide dismutase (MnSOD, SOD2)	42%
Ribosomal protein P2 (RPLP2)	8%
Profilin 1 (PFN1)	n.a.
Thioredoxin (TXN, hTrx)	n.a.
SART-1/Hom s1	n.a.
α-NAC/Hom s2	30%
BCL7B/Hom s3	n.a.
MICU1/Hom s4	16.7%
Cytokeratin 6A/Hom s5	n.a.
Cyclophilins A, B, C (PPIA, PPIB, PPIC)	n.a.
Dense fine speckles (DFS70/LEDGF)	10–30%
Actin-α	15.5%
Tubulin-α	21.7%
eIF6	25.4%
HLA-DR-α	8.7%
RP-1	21%

5.8.1 Summary

In addition to genetic and epigenetic modifications of the epidermal barrier and to dysregulated colonization of the skin with microorganisms such as *S. aureus*, type 2 immunity is the third main axis of the atopic dermatitis pathogenesis. Type 2 immune cells have a central role in humoral immunity, in particular the production of IgE antibodies; in the skin, they downregulate the innate immune defense and further damage the epidermal barrier, and, finally, they induce itch (see next chapter). While type 2 immune cells are typically triggered by environmental allergens, such as aeroallergens or food, more chronic inflammation may be caused by autoreactive type 2 immune cells.

5.9 Itch and Neuroimmunology

5.9.1 The Itch Sensation

Itch is the dysesthesia or unpleasant sensation which induces the urge to scratch. There is no better definition for this major symptom of allergic skin disease even 300 years after the first description by Hafenreffer [294]. When itch persists over a period of more than 6 weeks, it is called "chronic pruritus" [903]. This condition occurs preferably in atopic eczema, but also in a variety of other inflammatory skin diseases like psoriasis, scabies, or lichen planus or especially among the group of so-called prurigo diseases. In these conditions, often topical therapy is not enough, but systemic treatment strategies have to be considered with neuroactive medications like gabapentin, naltrexone, or pregabalin [484] or antidepressants like sertraline or paroxetine or mirtazapine [108, 764].

Chronic pruritus is not a rare condition. A cross-sectional observational study in 11,730 persons working in 144 companies in Germany showed a point prevalence of chronic pruritus of 16.8%. There was an age dependence as this condition was more frequent in elderly patients (12.3% in young adults of 16–30 years, 20.3% in persons with 61–70 years) [765].

In some cases of chronic pruritus, disturbances in iron metabolism have been suspected. If at all, the determaination of ferritin may be helpful [62].

Itch and pain have in common that they only can be felt by the patient and not seen by other people. Thus, they are difficult to be measured objectively. While patients with pain raise feelings of compassion immediately and everywhere, patients with itchy skin diseases are not taken seriously and often encounter the flippant sentence "just stop scratching!" This recommendation shows complete ignorance about the dermatoneuropsychological mechanisms involved in pruritus.

5.9.2 Itch Research

While over many decades itch was regarded as the little brother of pain, this concept has been abandoned. Itch is mediated by a special subgroup of unmyelinated sensory C fibers and originates from the upper part of the dermis or the dermo-epidermal junction. These fibers are sensitive to temperature but insensitive to mechanical stimulation. They express the vanillin receptor (TRPV1 = transient receptor potential vanilloid type 1), which is a nonselective ion channel expressed on keratinocytes and peripheral sensory C nerve fibers. Therefore, also antagonists to this receptor, like, e.g., PAC-14028, have shown to have an antipruritic effect in an atopic dermatitis model of mice [905].

These sensory nerves then transmit the sensation to dorsal route ganglia and from there via the spinal cord to the brain.

Altered neuronal response is a hallmark of atopic dermatitis (and other atopic diseases) and goes along with pathological reflexes. One result is a white dermographism, but more importantly it is the cardinal symptom of atopic dermatitis (Sect. 4.1), namely itch that is often devastating and severely impacts the quality of life of atopic dermatitis patients. Early studies reported a higher innervation of atopic dermatitis skin, giving a first hint that the nerve system might somehow interact with the cutaneous inflammation [799].

The interaction of sensory neurons and immune cells is mutual. That means immune-mediated factors stimulate sensory neurons, and vice versa neuronal products are pro-inflammatory. As for the first, the main mediators of itch are histamine and tryptase. Histamine is released primarily by mast cells and basophil granulocytes and directly induces action potential firing in sensory neurons via one of four specific receptors (histamine 1–4 receptor [H1R]). H1R and H4R are highly expressed in the skin and are therapeutic targets to treat atopic dermatitis (see chapter therapy) [795]. Engagement of histamine with one of its receptors results in activation of central channels mediating itch, the so-called transient receptor potential (TRP) channels. Best described in atopic dermatitis are the two TRP channels TRP ankyrin 1 (TRPA1) and TRP vanilloid 1 (TRPV1) [229, 378]. They are central to many known immune triggers of itch. Besides histamine, tryptase is a central direct mediator of itch. It activates protease activated receptors (PAR), in particular PAR2, and further downstream also TRP channels [768]. The third well-known factor to directly stimulate sensory neurons is IL-31 [127, 384]. This type 2 cytokine signals via the IL-31 receptor expressed on sensory neurons, with subsequent activation of TRPA1 and TRPV1 [127]. It is also a potential target to treat atopic dermatitis [376].

Interestingly, also the main receptor transmitting IL-4 and IL-13 signals, the IL-4ra, is expressed on sensory neurons. In contrast to histamine, tryptase, and IL-31, stimulation of this receptor leads to calcium influx, but not spontaneous action potential firing in sensory neurons thus pointing toward a role for IL-4 and IL-13 to sensitize the nervous system to other pruritogenic stimuli [563]. Of note, IL-4 signaling is dependent on intracellular JAK1 signaling in sensory neurons. JAK1 inhibition is a target of several small molecules tested or approved for atopic dermatitis. A characteristic of these substances is the rapid relief from itch ([780], see chapter therapy).

Thus, immune cells activate sensory neurons in multiple ways to induce itch (Fig. 5.10). In this context, also factors derived from keratinocytes may contribute to the stimulation of sensory neurons, and evidence suggests this is even more relevant if the epidermal barrier is disturbed. In particular, Thymic stromal lymphopoietin (TSLP) and IL-33, two epithelial molecules upstream of type 2 immunity, directly stimulate sensory neurons via their cognate receptors TSLPR or IL-33R, respectively [462, 871].

Vice versa, neuronal derived products activate the immune system (Fig. 5.10). The best-explored molecule in this context is substance P (SP). It has multiple effects on diverse immune cells via the neurokinin 1 receptor (NK1R), among them degranulation of mast cells [778], survival and activation of eosinophils [611] and T cells [585]. Other neuron-derived factors such as calcitonin

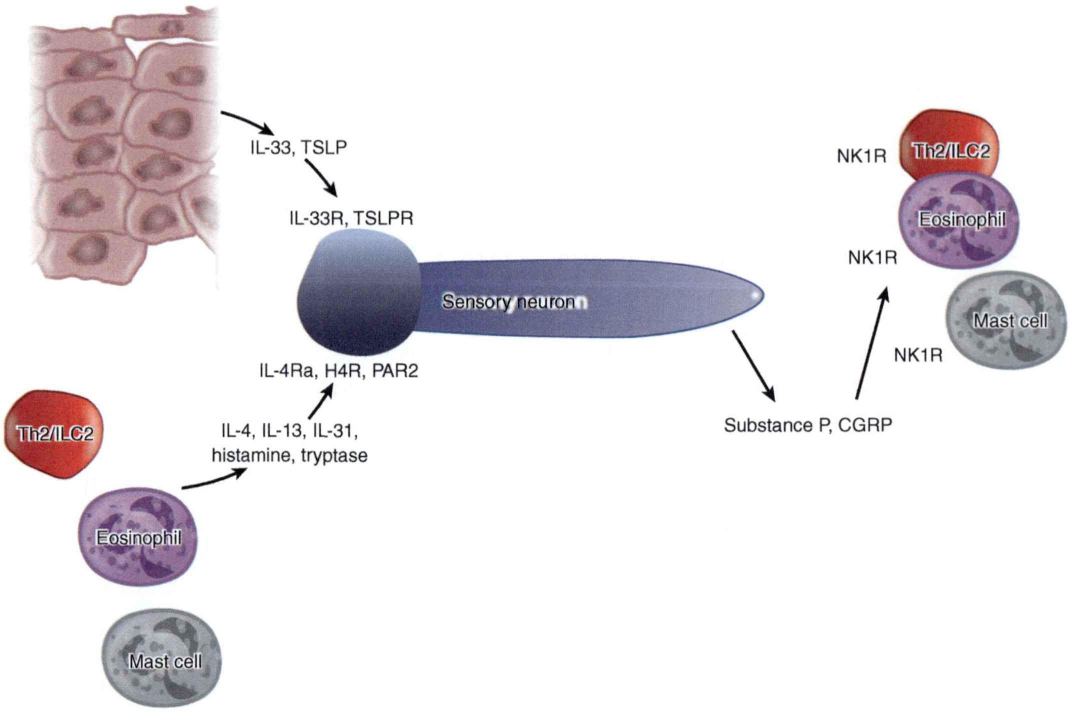

Fig. 5.10 The neuroimmunology axis of atopic dermatitis. Epithelial cells via upstream type 2 cytokines (IL-33, TSLP) and type 2 lymphocytes, eosinophils, and mast cells via IL-4, IL-13, IL-31, histamine, and tryptase release stimulate sensory neurons to axon potential firing that causes itch. In turn, sensory neurons secrete substances such as Substance P or CGRP that stimulate immune cells via the NK1 receptor

gene-related peptide (CGRP), vasoactive intestinal peptide (VIP), or neuromedin U (NMU) also impact the immune system [574]; however, their role is less well established in the context of atopic dermatitis.

Taken together, the neuroimmune axis is involved in the pathogenesis of atopic dermatitis both by mediating the central symptom itch and by shaping a type 2 inflammation, further closing the vicious circle of type 2 immunity, epidermal barrier disruption, and microbial dysbalance in atopic dermatitis.

5.9.3 Measurement of Itch

Recent imaging studies have shown that not only the thalamus is the major sensory organ, but also areas of the anterior cingulate cortex, the insula, and secondary somatosensory cortex areas, are activated, as well as centers of the limbic system. Notably, the most visible feature of cerebral activation patterns after itch-inducing stimulation is the activation of the motor areas for the scratch response [165].

For a long time, the search for the classical itch mediator substance has been going on (Table 5.4).

Another clinical condition going along with extreme itch is cutaneous amyloidosis, where deposits of amyloid and apoptotic keratinocytes are found in the papillary dermis. In the rare variant of the familiar primary localized cutaneous amyloidosis (PLCA), it was found that the OSMR gene (oncostatin-M receptor beta) may play a major role since it is involved among others in interleukin-31, possibly then acting as major itch inducer [756].

Unfortunately, itch research is far behind pain research. There are different qualities of itch. It is a well-known clinical experience regarding the morphology of skin lesions as well as the typology of scratch behavior. Using various questionnaires [159, 851], with the Brest "questionnaire" the

Table 5.4 Mediators of itch sensation ([113]; Buddenkotte and Steinhoff [897])

Histamine
Serotonin
Acetylcholine
Neuropeptides (e.g., substance P)
Cytokines
• Interleukin 2
• Interleukin 8
• Interleukin 31
Neurotrophin-4
Nerve growth factor (NGF)
Tryptase
Kallikrein, cathepsin S
Platelet-activating factor
Prostaglandins
Leukotrienes
Opioid peptides

authors found significant differences in quality of itch between atopic dermatitis, non-atopic eczema, urticaria, psoriasis, and scabies. There were also similarities that itch occurred more frequently over night time, following certain eliciting factors such as stress, dryness, and hot water. While application of cold was normally found to be beneficial in atopic dermatitis, the qualities of "stinging," "pincing," or "stabbing" were significantly more common than in the other dermatoses.

A major problem of pruritus research is its subjective character and the difficulty to be objectively measured. Usually visual-analog scales (VAS) are used; however, they do not necessarily correlate well with the clinical appearance and intensity of the skin lesions [165]. A new scale, the "5D itch scale," has been proposed, registering the five dimensions of duration, degree, direction, disability, and distribution of pruritus as a better outcome measure for clinical trials [212].

Therefore, mechanical devices have been developed to measure the scratching behavior with the so-called "itch watch" [228].

Other so-called actigraphic methods have been developed and found suitable to assess pruritus over night time [531].

The scratch response may considerably contribute to the pathophysiology of itch-induced skin damage, as has been shown by early "inhuman" studies in putting a limb into plaster or fixing a child in the bed so that it could not move [821] (see above).

In murine experiments with NC/Nga mice—atopic dermatitis induced by repeated application of house dust mite—the contribution of scratch behavior to the induced eczema was remarkable. In the light of modern findings regarding IgE autoantibodies against epidermal proteins possibly liberated from keratinocytes by the scratch trauma, these observations gain new importance [898].

There is a strong psychosomatic interaction in the itch sensation. Therefore, also psychological processes have to be considered in evaluating patients suffering from chronic pruritus. Personality factors, life events, and psychological stress may have an as important role as external stimuli. Therefore, biopsychosocial models have been proposed to better understand the vicious cycle of the itch-scratch response [821].

In a cross-sectional study investigating the impairment in quality of life, 138 patients with chronic pain were compared to 73 patients with chronic pruritus with otherwise similar demographics. The authors used the health utility score as a measure of how much lifetime a person would be willing to give from his or her life expectancy to live without the condition and found that pruritus had a substantial impact on quality of life that may be comparable to that of pain [397].

A specially developed and validated pruritus-specific quality of life instrument; the ItchyQol was developed [177].

In specially designed itch questionnaires (e.g., "Eppendorf Itch Questionnaire") these differences can be measured [159]. We even found that itch-related sensations may be better expressed in dialect than in high language [911].

With new imaging techniques like positron emission tomography (PET) or functional magnetic resonance imaging (fMRI), the activation of central nervous areas in the brain during itch can be visualized [592] (Fig. 7.10). It is interesting that besides sensory areas, which transmit the itch sensation, and the motor areas, which mediate the scratch reaction, also areas of the limbic system are activated, which points to an involvement of emotional reaction patterns.

Everybody knows that looking at an individual who scratches vehemently may also induce a scratch response in observers such that there is anecdotal evidence of a "contagious" itch. This susceptibility to visual effects seems to be increased in atopic dermatitis. In a study, healthy volunteers and eczema patients were asked to watch a 5-min movie showing individuals suffering from obvious itch and scratching. The study participants received either saline or histamine as an itch-inducing stimulus on the volar side of the forearm. Patients with atopic dermatitis scratched more frequently and reported a higher severity of itch while watching the movie compared to controls [581]. Pruritus can be so severe that inpatient therapy becomes necessary. The establishment of special "itch clinics" has been proposed [539].

The psychosomatic involvement in pruritus is immense [484]. Therefore, application of psychopharmaceuticals may be indicated in severe conditions, starting from doxepin, which also has a combined histamine H1 + H2 antagonistic effect, to tricyclic antidepressants such as mirtazapine [347].

Furthermore, there are differences between various ethnic groups in itch perception and response (see Chap. 4).

5.10 Psychological Influences in Atopic Dermatitis

Already in 1891, the French dermatologists knew about the close connection between nerves and eczema when they coined the term "neurodermite," which nowadays is used commonly in Germany (see Chapter "Terminology"). It is a well-known clinical experience that nerval or psychological factors can play a role in triggering or maintaining atopic eczema. The German term "Neurodermitis" illustrates the involvement of nerval reaction patterns in the pathophysiology of this disease. The sentence "without nerval interaction there is no eczema" contains a lot of truth [513].

I myself (JR) have fought against this term since I did not like my patients to become stigmatized as having a "neurologic" or "psychiatric" disease when they were suffering from a clear-cut skin disease [638]. However, we admit that looking at recent research in the field of psychoneuro-allergology [546, 612, 773] it is a fact that psychological influences play a role in the actual clinical course of the disease; whoever denies this will not be a good doctor for these patients. However, it is crucial not to give the patient the feeling to be "put into the psychological corner." It is annoying how often the term "psychiatric" is used to only describe psychological effects on certain diseases; it is as essential to know about the influence of a somatic disease—especially with such a tormenting itch—upon the psychological condition of the patient. We always should keep in mind that psychosomatic is not a one-way street, it always has also a somatopsychic moment in a complex interplay [139]!

Immune system and nervous system are the two systems of our organism to interact with the environment (Fig. 5.11). They cooperate in manifold ways, e.g., mast cells and nerves (Fig. 5.12). The group around J. Bienenstock has done seminal work studying this interaction and shown that there are direct contacts—almost synaptic—between nerves and mast cells or basophil leukocytes in tissue culture; furthermore, they showed that it is possible, in a Pawlowian setting, to induce anaphylactic shock in ovalbumin-sensitized rats by just applying the conditioning audiovisual stimulus (Rolling Stones music and flashlight) [73].

The analogy of nervous and immune system describes not only the high degree of specificity but also a large amount of diversity of specific reactions together with a long-lasting memory.

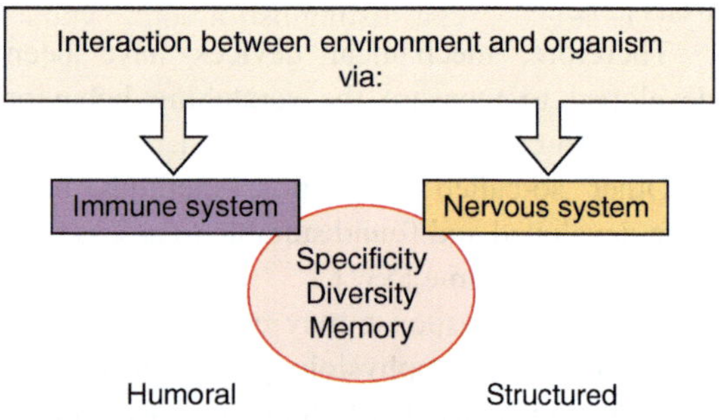

Fig. 5.11 Analogy of nervous system and immune system in the reactivity of the organism with its environment

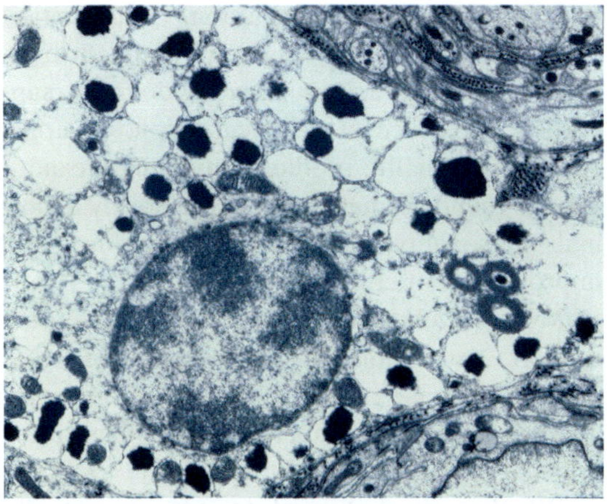

Fig. 5.12 Electromicroscopical picture of a mast cell in close contact with a sensory nerve (with friendly permission of H. Behrendt)

The difference can be seen in the nervous system as sensory, and we can feel most of its actions, and it does its function via clear cellular and tissue structures; the immune system on contrary cannot be felt when it is active; it works in the blood and in the organs with only a few specific structures (thymus, lymph nodes).

5.10.1 Psychology and Pruritus

Itch as a major symptom of atopic dermatitis actually occurs in the brain—it initiates in the skin! There is no itch under anesthesia; the new methods of imaging like, e.g., positron emission tomography (PET) or functional magnetic resonance imaging (fMRI) allow objective examination of the itch sensation in the brain; itch can be visualized [592] (Fig. 7.10).

There is a clear-cut influence of stress on symptoms of atopic dermatitis by increased expression of nerve growth factor-reactive cells in epidermis and dermis, and intensity of neuropeptide Y-positive cells as a parameter of anxiety and stress inducing pruritus [565].

5.10.2 Autonomic Nervous System Dysregulation

Due to the rapid progress in immunology, some aspects of atopy and atopic dermatitis have been forgotten which are a well-known clinical fact and had been studied in the early 50s, namely that these patients show an altered reactivity in several autonomic nervous system functions. These aspects have been studied intensively by G. W. Korting in his thesis "Endogenous Eczema" [418]. Much of this work has been forgotten.

In asthma, Szentivanyi developed the theory of beta-adrenergic blockade in the pathophysiology. In summary, atopic patients and also eczema patients exhibit weaker beta-adrenergic reactions while alpha-adrenergic and cholinergic responses seem to be increased [634, 781].

Patients with atopic dermatitis show altered responses to certain pharmacological stimuli which can be shown in vivo [912] and in vitro: These phenomena can go along with altered activity of phosphodiesterase (PDE) and alterations of the cyclic nucleotide metabolism [120, 130]. In vitro stimulation with cholinergic stimuli can enhance histamine release [635].

Altered reactivity patterns in the autonomic nervous system not only affect immune reactions but quite normal physiological phenomena such as pupillary reaction in the eye, orthostatic cardiovascular reaction (Schellong-Grote test), and sweating [912]. In a Japanese study, atopic eczema patients suffered less frequently from hypertonic blood pressure than controls (Uehara, personal communication).

In a Swedish study, heart rate variability, deep breathing, and orthostatic tests were performed in patients with severe atopic dermatitis, who showed to have an autonomic dysbalance with higher values for parasympathetic modulation than controls [79].

Elevated intracellular phosphodiesterase levels lead to the development of specific PDE inhibitors in the treatment. For a long time, theophylline was also used in eczema treatment; papaverine was used with a clear-cut activity against itch. All these agents are no longer used because of limited specificity and small therapeutic index (see Chap. 7).

The well-known white dermographism and the abnormal delayed blanch reaction to acetylcholine may also be regarded as signs of altered autonomic nervous system reactivity.

Weakened beta-adrenergic reactions can lead to an enhancement of allergic phenomena [319]. It is a well-known fact that beta blockers increase asthmatic reactions and anaphylactic reactions.

Patients with atopic dermatitis may release vasoactive mediators to minimal stimuli leading to elevated plasma histamine levels, but also to increased secretion of other mediators like leukotrienes [674]. These mediators not only have effects as pro-inflammatory agents but also act via histamine receptors on lymphocytes, especially regulatory T cells [375] in a way that increased IgE, increased mediator releasability and decreased regulatory T cell function can form a vicious cycle [636].

On the basis of this autonomic nervous system dysregulation, one may also understand some of the abovementioned psychological influences both positive and negative for the clinical course of eczema since stress or anxiety are able to release the same mediators (histamine) which also are involved in itch and inflammation [264, 276, 624].

5.10.3 The Problem of an "Atopic" Personality (or "Atopic Eczema Personality")

Many doctors—probably on the basis of some remarkable experiences with certain patients—have the prejudice of a typical "atopic eczema personality" [612, 656, 657], especially prominent also for mothers of an atopic eczema child; however, this prejudice is not really evidence-based. Each of us can tell a story about a very unpleasant meeting with a mother (or a father) of an eczema child—especially when being a teacher and member of the Green Party, she or he knows everything better than a doctor and nurse and is maximally demanding—all in all a very subjective and wrong prejudice. There is abundant literature regarding characteristic personality profiles in allergic individuals; when studied closely however it is surprising how controversial the descriptions are with attributes such as "lack of ability to surrender," "shy," "passive," "introverted" at the same time go along with "hyperactive," "need for recognition," "pedantic," "hypercorrect," and "outgoing" (quoted from [864]). Recent literature however does not support the existence of a typical atopic or atopic eczema personality profile. Longitudinal examinations found normalization of previously abnormal personality profiles going along with improvement of clinical symptoms.

More psychoanalytically oriented literature supports—sometimes in early childhood—sexual conflicts as causal for the development of allergy; they see an autoerotic component in the orgiastic scratching against itch [491].

Whether psychological factors are actually causal, i.e., relevant in the development of the disease, is still a matter of scientific debate. However, there is no doubt that psychological influences like stress or emotional excitation can trigger and exacerbate eczema flares.

Half of the patients are reporting this experience without doubts.

There are studies showing that parental partner problems may be a risk factor for the development of atopic dermatitis (see Chap. 2 "Risk Factors").

5.10.4 Parent-Child Relation ("Family Dynamics") in Atopic Eczema

Family dynamics are of special importance when dealing with children with atopic eczema. Several studies have shown that atopic dermatitis in childhood goes along with a very negative impact on family life by inducing physical and mental health problems in mothers, especially of severely affected children [344].

In psychodiagnostic tests, we investigated personality profiles of children with atopic eczema and found no statistically significant differences between children with atopic dermatitis and children with other skin diseases with regard to the parameters "neuroticism" or "extraversion" [656]. In the tests according to the Freiburg personality inventary FPI, mothers of children with atopic eczema were found to be a little "less spontaneous," "more controlled," and "less emotional" than normal. Fathers of atopic children however showed no significant differences. There was a trend of increased "irritability."

Since chronic disease and especially the itch/scratch cycle sometimes is used by the child as a "weapon" in order to get his or her will against parental education, it is of interest to study the parental educational style in this disease. Using the educational tables according to Stang, we found that, in the educational style perceived from the eyes of the children, the parameter "strictness" of the mother was stronger noted than in controls, while the educational style of the fathers was equal. Looking in detail, it was interesting that, from the eyes of the eczema children, mothers of eczema children more often would reward "adult behavior," while the parameter "affective warmth" or "shared joy" was less strongly expressed [656].

When we made the children draw the family—either as persons or as animals—eczema children in their drawings showed a less friendly atmosphere than was normally seen in control children (note: they suffered from other skin diseases leading to hospitalization!) (Fig. 5.13). Of special interest was that the body size of the

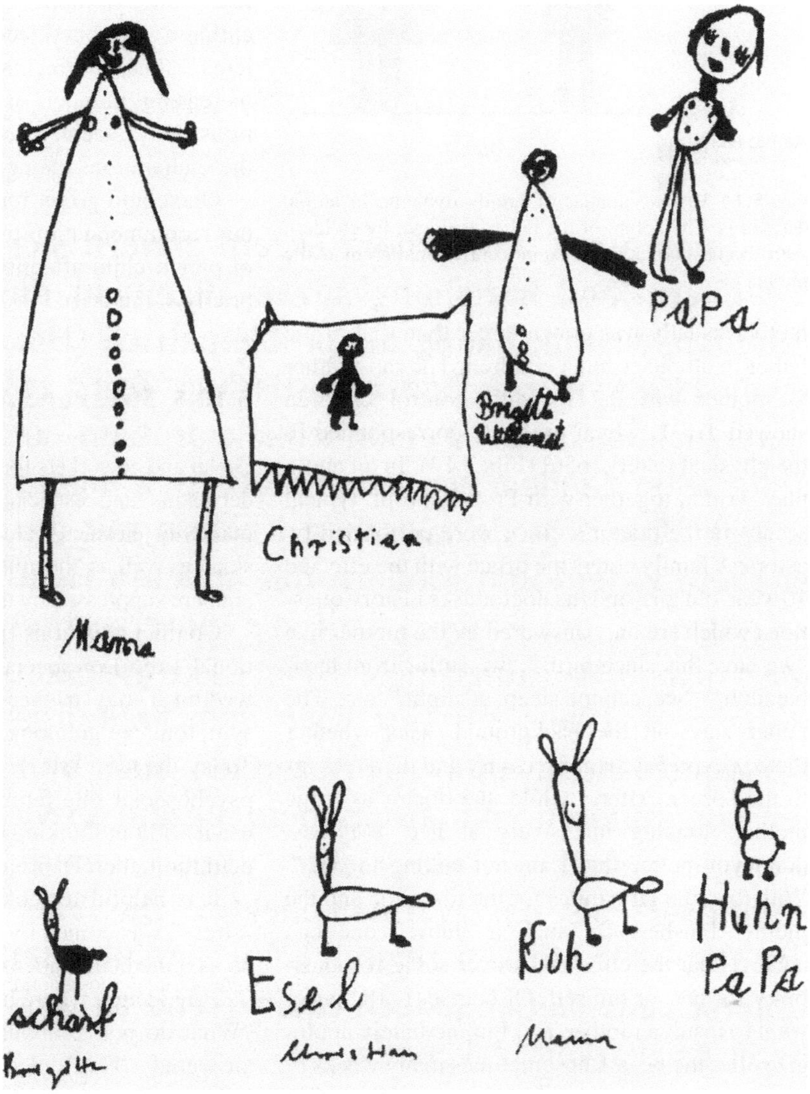

Fig. 5.13 Children's drawing of a family comprising persons and animals showing little contact [657]

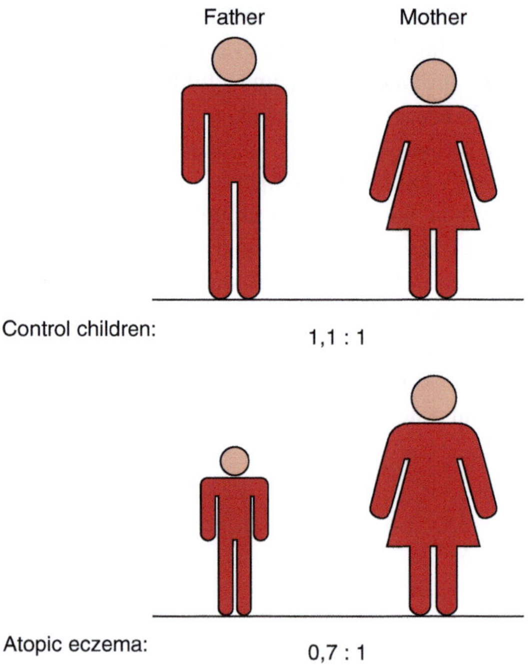

Fig. 5.14 Psychosomatics of family dynamic in atopic dermatitis. The height of the father as drawn by children with atopic dermatitis is significantly smaller than the mother's

mother usually was drawn larger than that of the father in atopic eczema children: The ratio father to mother was 0.7–1, while control children showed 1.1–1, which probably corresponded to the physical reality [656] (Fig. 5.14). In an audio play written together with Prof. Schröpl, typical scenes in the doctor's office were performed by actors: A family enters the office with the affected 10-year-old girl, and the doctor asks history questions which are only answered by the mother like "we have this since birth," "we suffer from terrible itch," "we cannot sleep at night," etc. The father stays in the background, asks whether there is extra payment necessary and then retreats to the corner. After a while, the doctor asks the mother, looking intensively at her: "Mylady, don't you notice that I am not talking to you?" With that, the girl smiles for the first time and the mother blushes. By such a "blow," one can achieve that the child takes over some responsibility for her- or himself. Of course, I (JR) never want to insult a mother, and I immediately apologize after the visit. But sometimes many weeks or months later a mother comes to me telling "this was really tough, doctor, at the first visit in your office—but you were so right, it's not my skin. I should be more relaxed!"

Table 5.5 Ways of parental affection and educational style of particular relevance in atopic dermatitis

Bad		Good	
Tenseness	No	Concern	Yes
Rigorousness	No	Consequence	Yes
Dominance	No	Strength	Yes
Overpowering	No	Motivation	Yes
Indifference	No	Relaxedness	Yes
Ambition	No	Love	Yes

In a study investigating the psychosocial adaptation in Korean schoolchildren, it was found that allergic children had more problems when they had acute symptoms of atopic dermatitis; these children exhibited more "internalizing problems," this was increasingly observed with an increasing number of IgE-mediated sensitizations. Boys seemed to be more prone to show these alterations than girls [136].

One could go on for hours with these stories; our recommendations regarding various attitudes of parent-child affection in atopic dermatitis are briefly summarized in Table 5.5.

5.10.5 Stress and Atopic Eczema

Gieler and coworkers found that patients with atopic dermatitis and especially some subgroups show markedly elevated values for "anxiety," "depression" as well as "hostility" which however, in general, are suppressed by the patients [267, 893].

Conflict situations (private problems, occupational stress) or special situations (examination, wedding) may trigger eczema flares. Itch as a symptom can go along with aggressive behavior. Today the term "stress" is used to describe these psychosocial interferences. Doctor and patients use it without thinking however when asked for a definition, there is often silence or stuttering.

It is helpful to look at the history: The term "stress" was coined by Hans Selye in 1936 when he as a medical student was asked by a professor in a big lecture where he was presenting a patient "What do notice about the patient?," and Selye answered "He looks sick," arousing general laughter in the audience. However, then Selye wanted to describe better this phenomenon so obvious as "looking sick." In trying to do this, he created a new term which meant an "unspecific response of the body to some challenge."

For many years the phenomenon was regarded to be purely biological; however, over the decades, it has also been used for psychological phenomena.

Based on various authors [207, 904], we define

> Stress as a "primary unspecific psychobiologic reaction to a threat for the individual physico-chemical or psychological well-being" (1998).

It does not make sense to talk of "stress reaction" since the reaction is already contained in the term stress. Elicitors of stress are also called stressors and can be of various origin (Table 5.6):

Regarding the timely course, one can distinguish between acute and chronic stress. Especially the latter may induce psychosomatic complaints, such as anxiety, loss of activity, impairment of self-confidence, but also vasovagal reactions and hyperventilation [682].

Stress also can alter skin barrier function. Studies have shown that the local production of corticotropin-releasing factor (CRF) may influence the integrity of stratum corneum. Stress may act via various mechanisms and induce physiologic or pathophysiologic changes which lead to symptoms in the nervous or endocrine system or in several organs (Table 5.7).

Also, modulation of the serotonergic neurotransmitter system may play a role. In patients with severe atopic dermatitis, increased expression of several serotonin receptors have been found in the epidermis [465].

Also, the expression of nerve growth factor (NGF) discovered 50 years ago has been found altered in inflammatory skin diseases, such as psoriasis, but most expressly in atopic dermatitis, where it was found to correlate with the severity of itch and objective signs of eczematous inflammation [897].

There are different methodologies to measure and quantify stress (Table 5.8).

Stress is also dependent on sociocultural aspects since many stressors come from psychosocial environment. Alexander Solschenizyn criticized the culturally accepted drive for profit of the Western world which leads to exaggerated competition, personal isolation and beyond to a

Table 5.6 Various kinds of stressors

Physical	Chemical	Biological	Psychosocial (life events)
Trauma Pain Exhaustion Heat Cold Noise	Environmental pollution	Nutrition Infection Allergy	Grief Anxiety Depression Emotional excitation

Table 5.7 Possible mechanisms of stress influence upon allergic reactions

Tissue	Cells/mediators	Clinical consequences
Nervous system	Nociceptors Neurotransmitters Autonomic impulses (weak beta-adrenergic, increased cholinergic)	Effects upon immune and inflammatory cells as well as manifestation organ
Endocrine system	Hypothalamus (CRF) Adrenal glands (catecholamines)	Hormone effects
Immune system	Th1 NK cells Th1/Th2 deviation Inflammatory cells	Immunodeficiency Susceptibility to infection IgE formation (allergy) Mediator release
End organ (airway, skin)	Mucous secretion Bronchoconstriction Vasodilatation Itch	Rhinopathy Asthma Urticaria Eczema

Table 5.8 Techniques to measure and quantify stress

Chemical	Physiological	Psychological
Determination of hormones or autacoids • Adrenaline • Noradrenaline • Metabolites • Adreno-corticotropic Hormone ACTH • Corticotropin-releasing • Factor (CRF) • Neurotrophin • Nerve growth factor NGF • Aldosterone, renin • Angiotensin • Histamine	• Pulse • Blood pressure • ECG • Muscle tension (electromyogram) • Skin temperature • Skin perfusion • Electrical resistance • EEG changes	• Cognitive activity • Affect resonance • Psychodiagnostic tests (e.g., STAI etc.)

more and more egoistic attitude with a vicious circle of stress (quoted in [904]).

Observations from Japan after the big earthquake in Kobe (Hanshin) of 1995 have shown that 38% of patients with atopic dermatitis showed marked deterioration of eczema compared to 7% in a control group without earthquake. Nine percent of the patients from the earthquake region experienced marked improvement in eczema [412].

In a multivariate regression analysis, the subjective stress was the best indicator to predict an eczema flare. Everyday stress situations can influence atopic dermatitis considerably. Many studies show that stress can trigger exacerbations of atopic eczema [393, 446].

Especially in adult atopic eczema, psychosomatic interaction and psychological problems are common. In a case-control study, affective- and stress-related behavioral and psychiatric conditions were investigated; it was found that the eczema was independently associated with several of these conditions [527].

Münzel and Schandry [527] have investigated several types of stress in patients with atopic dermatitis and healthy controls with regard to physiological effects on pulse rate, electrical skin resistance, and skin temperature. Thereby, patients with atopic eczema reacted stronger to emotional stress (when they were asked to express an opinion in front of a group) than to mental stress (counting backward).

There are several psychodiagnostic test procedures to evaluate various stress situations: There is the State-Trait Anxiety Inventory (STAI) as well as the "social readjustment rate scale." High values in these tests mean an increased risk for future disease.

When talking about psychological influence upon disease, one should never forget that the question of what is cause and what is the consequence of a disease often remains open. It is a characteristic of skin diseases that they not only represent a disturbance of the function of one organ but that they always also have a psychological component since the skin is an expression organ of the psyche and has an eminent esthetic function..

5.10.6 Hormonal Influences

It is surprising that hormonal influences upon allergy development are only little investigated. It is common knowledge that some allergic diseases like asthma or atopic dermatitis in early childhood are more frequent in boys than in girls, while in adults the female sex is much more often affected. This gives rise to the speculation that sex hormones may play a role [136].

Indeed male patients with severe atopic eczema may more frequently show signs of testosterone deficiency [849]. Substitution of testosterone in a patient with gonadal dysgenesis and concomitant severe nummular eczema led to a marked improvement of the previously therapy-resistant eczema [543].

Mast cells have shown to carry androgen receptors, and androgenic hormones may inhibit mediator release [136]. Estrogens seem to have an enhancing effect upon B cells with regard to transformation in IgE-secreting plasma cells [9].

5.10.7 Summary

Itch is the major symptom of atopic dermatitis, in some cases also pain. Due to the subjective nature of these symptoms, they are difficult to measure which makes research complicated. Several questionnaires have been developed registering not only the quantity of the itch sensation but also qualitative aspects. New imaging techniques like Positron Emission Tomography (PET) or functional magnetic resonance imaging (fMRI) allow visualization of itch phenomena in the brain. The neuroimmune axis plays an important role in the pathophysiology of this disease.

There is no doubt that patients with atopic dermatitis show altered reactivity patterns in the autonomic nervous system in the sense of a weaker beta-adrenergic and increased alpha-adrenergic and cholinergic reactivity. This not only holds true for cellular functions of lymphocytes and mast cells, but also for cardiovascular parameters.

There is no specific "atopic" or "atopic eczema" personality as is often quoted in prejudice of many doctors. However, psychological influences play a distinct role in the elicitation and maintenance of allergic and eczematous skin reactions. Stress can influence allergic reactions and lead to the triggering or worsening of atopic dermatitis. Psychological influences can also be observed within families with atopic eczema children. Family dynamics are therefore important to be studied and considered in the management, which is part of some educational programs in "eczema school."

5.11 The Heterogeneity of Atopic Dermatitis Pathogenesis with Regard to Clinical Course (Acute Versus Chronic) and Ethnicity

The clinical heterogeneity of atopic dermatitis is diverse regarding severity, location, morphology, and temporal dynamics (see chapter clinical symptomatology). Furthermore, immune-active medication such as type 2 immune-targeting biologics do not show the same degree of efficacy across the patient population, leaving a substantial number of patients that do not respond sufficiently, but in contrast also achieve a complete clearing of all symptoms in other patients (see chapter therapy). This may very likely be related to the complex pathogenesis of atopic dermatitis, in particular to distinct atopic dermatitis endotypes.

Unfortunately, the clinical heterogeneity cannot directly be linked to differences in the pathogenesis of atopic dermatitis—and, more relevant, it neither can be linked to the therapeutic response. This is why the field of objective biomarker research to answer clinically meaningful questions is among the most important and heavily studied in atopic dermatitis currently (see chapter future).

Although the overall link to clinical phenotype or therapeutic response prediction is not well established, there is progress made in biomarkers identifying the correct diagnosis or correlating with disease severity. These will be discussed in Chap. 6. Regarding biomarkers identifying different aspects of the pathogenesis of atopic dermatitis, several studies have made an attempt to correlate immune parameters, barrier function, or microbiome colonization with patient endotypes. Most of these studies however do not clearly reveal whether observed differences are secondary, e.g., related to disease severity, or in fact stable and distinct endotypes. This is the case for studies that investigated different patient clusters according to inflammatory mediators in serum or the skin as well as according to *S. aureus* density on the skin.

While acute eczematous lesions are dominated by massive infiltrate of type 2 lymphocytes and spongiosis, other immune cells enter lesional atopic dermatitis skin in the course of inflammation. In particular, type 3 immune cells secreting IL-22 lead to acanthosis (Fig. 5.15).

Historically, one of the best investigated question is whether the level of IgE might define distinct endotypes of patients with atopic dermatitis. An interesting report states in that context that there is a subgroup of patients with rapid exacerbation of atopic dermatitis after pollen exposure in an allergen provocation chamber. On the other hand, drugs targeting B cells and soluble antibod-

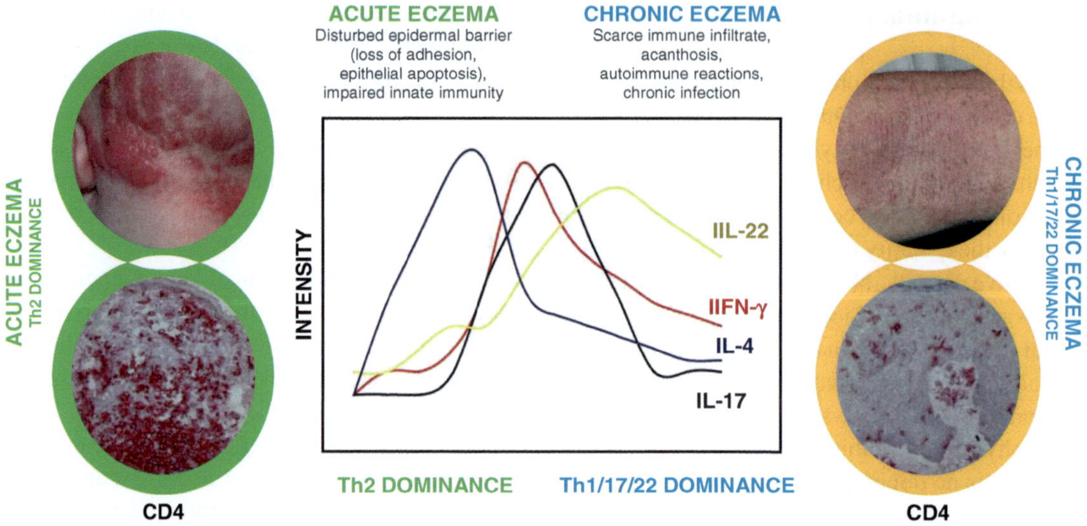

Fig. 5.15 Differences in the T cell infiltrate during the course of atopic dermatitis. Modified from

ies such as omalizumab, rituximab, or selective immune apheresis are not highly efficient when judged at the overall patient population's level (see chapter therapy). A meta-analysis of the potential of allergen-specific immunotherapy in atopic dermatitis showed that there is a slight tendency to favor immunotherapy over placebo, but no substantial clinical improvement of atopic dermatitis (see Sect. 7.7). In summary, it is still controversial whether IgE defines a clinically meaningful endotype. Potentially, more sophisticated approaches to identifying the meaningful endotype will result in a clearer picture and tailored symptomatic as well as causative therapeutic approaches.

Also, the question of whether the genetic phenotype might cause differences in the pathogenesis of atopic dermatitis has been investigated. While no qualitative differences were observed in *filaggrin* null mutation carriers, children with such a mutation showed earlier onset of the disease and higher disease severity than *filaggrin* wildtype children suffering from atopic dermatitis in a birth cohort.

Another dimension that is frequently discussed regarding differences in the pathogenesis of atopic dermatitis is ethnicity (see Chap. 2). A hallmark paper described similarities and differences between the European-Asian and the Japanese/Korean pathogenesis of atopic dermatitis, with the latter showing a mixed type 2 and type 3 (Th17) immune phenotype. As a consequence of the Th17 influx, the authors describe more frequent parakeratosis and the presence of neutrophils in lesional skin of Japanese/Korean atopic dermatitis patients. Follow-up studies suggest the Chinese atopic dermatitis population shows a similar pattern as the Japanese/Korean one. Whether the observed differences are exclusively related to ethnicity, stable, and eventually relevant when it comes to therapeutic decision-making remains unclear till present.

Finally, a population of interest regarding a potentially distinct pathogenetic mechanism are children. Here, studies suggest that while childhood atopic dermatitis shows a stably upregulated type 2 inflammation just as adult atopic dermatitis, early-onset lesions lack type 1 immune markers that might be observed in adult patients. Again, these interesting findings do not lead to translation into distinct endotypes or personalized treatment schemes. One recent report addresses the question of what the difference between self-limited atopic dermatitis of early childhood might be as compared to chronic childhood atopic dermatitis progressing toward a full phenotype in adults. Using machine-learning algorithms, prediction of the future course of the disease was possible with an accuracy of more than 80% according to the factors severity at 3 years of age, trigger factors such as stress, and levels of VEGF. Here, low levels of VEGF in infancy were associated with chronic atopic dermatitis. Whether these factors can be translated into clinical use has to be investigated in larger controlled trials.

In summary, multiple approaches to stratification of atopic dermatitis according to differences in the pathogenesis of individual patients have been and still are followed. All results confirm that type 2 immunity seems to be central, but there might be additional pathogenic events driving individual patients toward clinically meaningful outcomes such as phenotype, severity, risk of adverse events under therapy, and therapeutic response. As it has enormous consequences for the individual patient and our socioeconomic society, this field is heavily researched at the moment.

5.11.1 Summary

Atopic dermatitis is a heterogeneous disease. This holds true from a clinical perspective—primary efflorescences and distribution may vary; from a laboratory perspective, there are patients with and without elevated IgE levels; the disease varies regarding age association, associated comorbidities, and clinical course (relapsing-remitting versus continuous versus isolated flares). The clinical and molecular phenotype may also vary depending on the ethnicity, and not the last on therapeutic response. It is likely that different endotypes explain this heterogeneity however to date no clinically meaningful distinction of atopic dermatitis endotypes has been identified.

6 General Management of Patients with Atopic Eczema

Many patients with atopic dermatitis are desperate, change doctors, visit "witchcraft," and "shaman" gurus because they have heard that atopic dermatitis is incurable. Many physicians use this sentence to finally be left in peace by demanding patients or parents. Of course, they feel correct with this sentence stressing the genetic predisposition which is inborn and which cannot be altered at the moment. However, one has to clearly distinguish: The genetic disposition of atopy or atopic dermatitis cannot be changed today; however, molecular genetics may soon be valuable in predictive diagnostics.

These genetic markers however are not the disease; the disease "atopic dermatitis" can very well be treated and very often disappear over long periods or for lifetime. Therefore, we never use the term "incurable," we prefer to tell the patients that they are born with a problem and a tendency to develop hypersensitivity reactions of the skin and maybe elsewhere, but that these clinical conditions can very well be treated. We tell them that streptococcal tonsillitis cannot be called "incurable" just because there may be a relapse. Angina can very well be treated.

Based on the complex etiopathophysiological mechanisms involved it becomes clear that therapeutic management in most patients requires a complex program including aspects of diagnostics, actual treatment, and prevention.

Therapeutic procedures focus on the one hand on the acute treatment of the inflammatory skin disease, on the other hand, and at the same time, they have to include preventive aspects regarding the disturbed barrier function and individual provocation factors which can be avoided [3, 11, 96, 211, 454, 713]. The acute eczema flare can be treated very well; it is difficult to predict the intensity and frequency of new flares.

The tendency to hypersensitivity reactions of the skin requires special care and may be time-consuming.

Thus, management of atopic dermatitis is much more than writing a prescription for a tablet or an ointment. Rather it requires intense diagnostics including allergy diagnosis for individual provocation factors and needs confidential cooperation between physician and patient so that behavioral changes can be induced. The motivation of the patient or the parents to take responsibility for the disease has to be slowly developed (patient "empowerment") and often needs special educational programs. These aspects will be covered in Chap. 8 (Eczema School). We like to call the whole bunch of procedures to be done in order to improve the clinical condition "patient management" [650]. These procedures comprise much more than diagnostics and treatment and comprise recommendations regarding clothing, nutrition, style of living, leisure activities and occupational counseling, etc.

The general management of this disease contains also aspects of diagnosis, especially allergy diagnosis in order to detect individual trigger factors which then can be avoided. For this several diagnostic procedures are used.

K. Eyerich, J. Ring, *Atopic Dermatitis - Eczema*, https://doi.org/10.1007/978-3-031-12499-0_6

6.1 Diagnostic Procedures

There are few diseases where diagnostics and therapy are so closely connected as in allergy and especially atopic dermatitis.

This chapter does not deal with the actual diagnosis "atopic dermatitis" and considerations for differential diagnosis, but it reflects the ongoing diagnostic procedures necessary in the individual patient after the diagnosis "atopic dermatitis" has been made. Like in all other allergic diseases, the procedure can be classified into four steps [161, 338] which are connected to each other [644] (Fig. 6.1):

- History.
- Skin test procedures.
- In vitro allergy diagnosis.
- Provocation tests.

At the moment there is no standard routine procedure for provocation testing with aeroallergens in atopic eczema such as an exposure in a standardized chamber (pollen chamber) with varying concentrations of aeroallergens. Thus, provocation tests at the moment are restricted to food and food additives (see below).

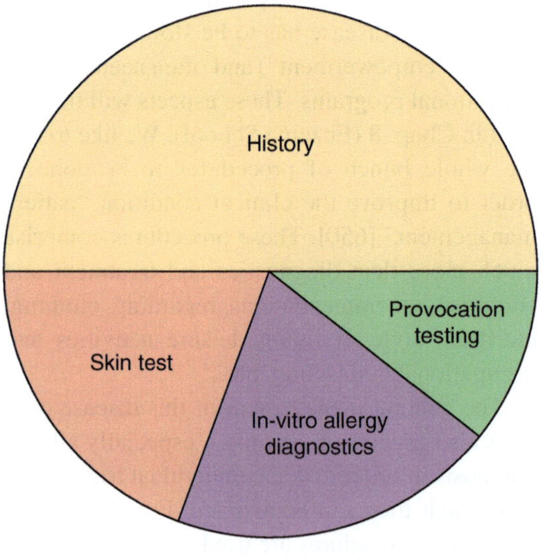

Fig. 6.1 The four major columns of allergy diagnostics

6.1.1 History

A very careful history not only considers the clinical course of the disease but also includes questions regarding the symptoms, the onset, the duration, the timely course, the circumstances with regard to possible triggering factors like seasonal, local, occupational conditions. Activities in holidays or leisure, application of drugs, hormonal situation, stress, all have to be included in a careful history in atopic dermatitis [104] (Table 6.1).

Table 6.1 Contents of a good history in atopic dermatitis

Symptoms
• Onset (first onset, acute disease)
• Duration
• Timely course (circadian, around the year, seasonal)
• Intensity (severity)
• Frequency
• Response to therapy
• Exacerbation by therapy
• Hospitalization
Concomitant diseases
• Personal history (atopy)
• Family history (atopy)
• Other diseases (gastroesophageal reflux, skin or airway diseases)
Eliciting factors and environmental aspects
• Season
• Local environment (indoor, outdoor)
• Occupation
• Holiday
• Hobby
• Drugs
• Foods
• Exercise
• Stress, emotional excitement
• Common cold (viral infection)
• UV light
• Hormonal situation (menstruation, pregnancy)
Lifestyle
• Living, apartment
• Animal contact (also passive)
• Tobacco smoke (active, passive)
• House dust mite, molds
• Chemicals
• Plants
• Cosmetics
• Snarling, breathing through the mouth

6.1.2 Skin Test Procedures

Among various skin test procedures, primarily those which are done percutaneously (scratch test, skin prick test) as well as patch test procedures are discussed.

6.1.2.1 Skin Prick and Intradermal Test

The most commonly used skin test is the skin prick test where a drop of an allergen extract is applied to the skin and pricked with a special lancet, preferably without bleeding. After 15 min it is read. Positive prick test reactions are typical for atopic diseases, occasionally they are exclusively used for the diagnosis of atopy. It is estimated that 90% of atopics show positive skin prick test reactions against common aero- or food allergens (especially cat, house dust mite, and grass pollen) [693]. In the intradermal test, which is nowadays not so common, 0.02–0.05 ml of an allergen dilution is injected strictly intradermally, using a small needle. Intradermal tests are necessary when prick tests remain negative in spite of a suggestive history.

The interpretation of the test results has to be done with regard to possible clinical relevance from detailed history or provocation test (see below).

6.1.2.2 Atopy Patch Test (ATP)

Positive skin prick tests or specific IgE antibodies against aeroallergens or foods almost routinely can be found in atopic dermatitis. The relevance of these sensitizations was controversial for decades. In the philosophy of this disease in the last 100 years, the estimation of allergy playing a role went up and down like modes of fashion. Decades where merely the dry skin or the psychological influence was in the focus alternated with phases where the role of allergy was put forward strongly. Mainly due to lack of methods this uncertainty continued. It is a clear clinical experience that many patients develop flares after contact with animal dander or in dusty environments while they experience improvement in allergen-free rooms or under high-altitude conditions [84].

At the end of the 70s of the twentieth century, several working groups wanted to develop a test procedure as a correlate for these clinical observations, since the skin prick test alone was not suitable. It correlated much better with the allergic airway reactions of hay fever or asthma than with the atopic dermatitis symptoms.

We first tried the intradermal test with a late reading (6–10 h) and believed to find a correlate in the so-called late-phase reaction (LPR) similar to severe cases of bronchial asthma [192]. This late cutaneous reaction (LCR) was regarded as a model of atopic eczema; however, the absence of epidermal involvement, which is so characteristic of the eczematous inflammation, was an argument against (see Chap. 1).

Therefore, we and other groups tried to induce eczema by epicutaneous application of aeroallergens; we used intradermal and prick test extracts and remained unsuccessful for many years. Others tried to come to positive test reactions by manipulation of the test areas through tape stripping or preceding irritation by scratching. The breakthrough was done by the group of Thomas Platts-Mills [512] who were able to induce eczematous skin reactions after application of house dust mite extract on rather large skin areas. Therefore, in the future, we used larger Finn chambers than normally used for the classical patch test in contact allergy and were equally successful in the procedure which we called "atopy patch test" (APT) [166, 167, 390].

In the 90s, we standardized the APT with regard to methodology, skin test site, influence of medication, etc., extracts used, especially also considering the vehicles [158, 162, 166]. Today we can say that the atopy patch test represents a standard procedure in allergy diagnostics for patients with atopic dermatitis (Fig. 6.2). Contrary to our theoretical considerations, where we thought that a hydrophilic emulsion would be better for the application of protein allergens, petrolatum proved to be the most reliable means as vehicle also for the atopy patch test (Fig. 6.2a) [166].

Differences in Classical Patch Test

Apart from the methodology (use of larger diameter Finn chambers), there are differences between the atopy patch test and the classical patch test in

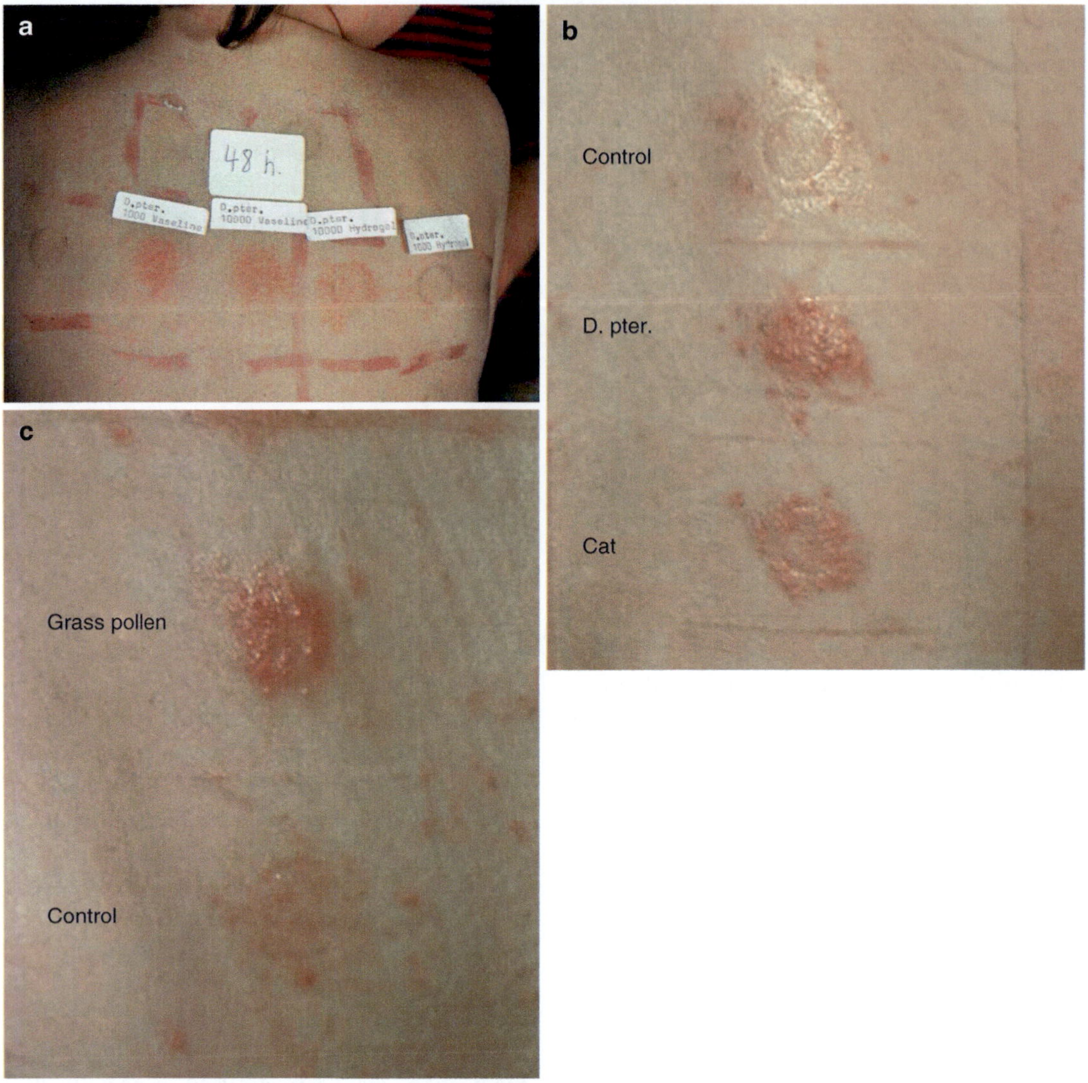

Fig. 6.2 Positive atopy patch test after 48 h. (**a**) Comparison of petrolatum and hydrogel as vehicle. (**b**) Allergen 200 IR/G (Index of Reactivity) in petrolatum. (**c**) Grass pollen and petrolatum control

contact allergy also in the reading of the test results. In the atopy patch test, the substances used are protein allergens, while in the contact allergy patch test small chemicals (haptens) are used. Furthermore, there are differences in morphology, dermatohistology, and time course. The classical patch test shows a typical crescendo pattern with a maximum of the reaction after 72 h, in atopy patch test often a maximum is already reached after 48 h (Table 6.2). The reproducibility of the atopy patch test is very good with 80–90%. In histopathology, an early influx of eosinophils and eosinophil products can be seen in the atopy patch test more commonly than in contact allergy. Clinically, often follicular patterns are observed, real vesicular or bullous reactions are extremely rare. The European Task Force on Atopic Dermatitis ETFAD has come up with a special reading guide for APT reactions [158, 169].

Unfortunately, test reagents are in many countries not routinely available; they have to be self-made by best using lyophilized allergens in petrolatum to be mixed by an experienced pharmacist [166].

Table 6.2 Difference between classical patch test in contact allergy and atopy patch test

Criteria	Patch test contact allergy	Atopy patch test
Nature of allergens	Low molecular chemicals	Proteins
Kinetic of the reaction	Maximum after 72 h (crescendo)	Often after 24 h
Morphology	Papulovesicular with spreading	Often follicular, rarely vesiculous
Dermatohistology	CD4 lymphocytes, Th1	CD4, Th2 Eosinophils
Indication	Allergic contact dermatitis	Atopic dermatitis

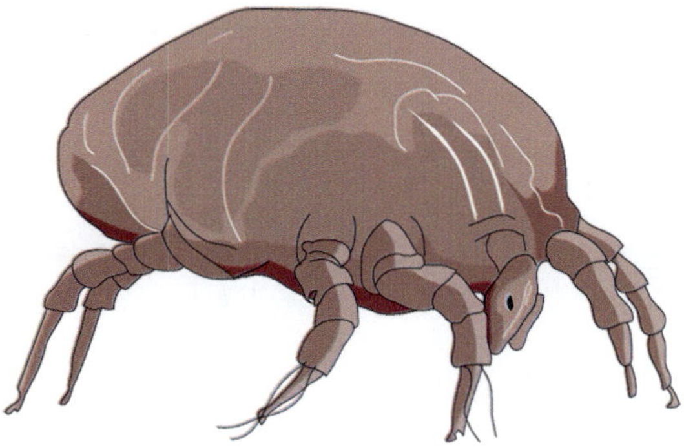

Fig. 6.3 The most common allergen positive in atopy patch is house dust mite Dermatophagoides pteronyssinus

Pathophysiologically, the atopy patch test represents an artificially induced atopic inflammation after penetration of high-molecular-weight allergens into the epidermis. These are recognized and taken up by dendritic cells (see Chap. 5). IgE, as well as IgE-binding receptors, have been recognized on the surface of epidermal dendritic cells partly in colocalization with house dust mite allergen [479, 788]. From atopy patch test biopsies, specific T cell clones could be isolated which characteristically show a Th2 cytokine pattern. At a later point of time—after 48 h or in more chronic lesions—also in atopic inflammation Th1 patterns become visible [111, 414, 619, 873].

In a common study of the European Task Force on Atopic Dermatitis ETFAD, the atopy patch test was further standardized. Petrolatum was chosen as vehicle, the protein allergens from lyophilized extracts, together with minimal concentrations of an emulsifying agent, cetylpyridinium chloride, were mixed with petrolatum. In large Finn chambers (1 cm in diameter) they are applied to uninvolved and unaltered skin, preferably on the back. For the most common aeroallergens in central Europe, eliciting allergen doses between 5000 and 7000 protein nitrogen units (PNU) were used.

The most common positive APT reactions were found with aeroallergens like house dust mite [176, 275] (Fig.6.3), but also cat epithelium and pollen allergens are often positive [160]. The APT is dose-dependent and especially positive in patients where the eczematous skin lesions occur

Table 6.3 Sensitivity and specificity of various test procedures in patients with atopic dermatitis using clear-cut personal history as the gold standard [168]

Test	Sensitivity (in %)	Specificity (in %)
Grass pollen ($n = 79$)		
Skin prick test	100	33
Specific IgE	92	33
Atopy patch test	75	84
European Multicenter Study ($n = 314$)		
Skin prick test	68–80	50–71
Specific IgE	72–84	2–69
Atopy patch test	15–45	64–91
German Multicenter Study ($n = 253$)		
Skin prick test	69–81	44–53
Specific IgE	65–94	42–64
Atopy patch test	42–56	69–92

in air-exposed areas, e.g., face, hands, or forearms. In a comparison of various test procedures, the clear-cut history in disease exacerbation after allergen contact was taken as the gold standard; the following sensitivities and specificities could be calculated (Table 6.3). In 75% of patients who had an exacerbation during the last preceding pollen season, atopy patch test against grass pollen was positive compared to only 16% in eczema patients without seasonal exacerbation.

Compared to skin prick test and in vitro specific IgE, APT showed a lower sensitivity (75%) compared to almost 100% for the skin prick test, which is natural when we regard the atopy definition (see Chap. 1). However, the specificity was

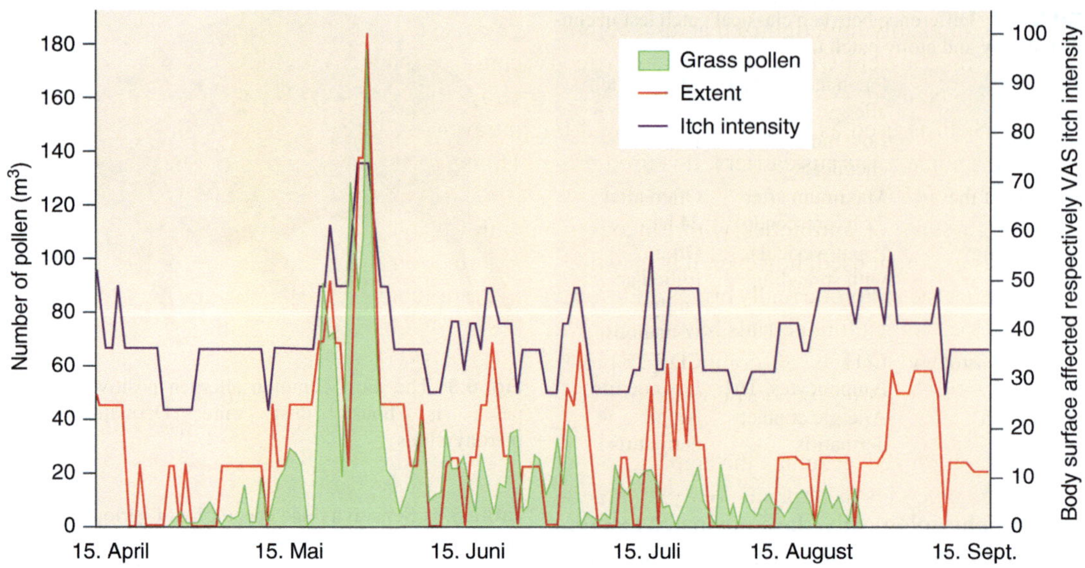

Fig. 6.4 Relevance of pollen exposure for exacerbation of atopic dermatitis in children (MIRIAM panel study [429])

much higher (80–90%) for the atopy patch test compared to 40–60% for skin prick test or specific IgE. It is possible, using the APT, to evaluate the relevance of an IgE-mediated sensitization for the actual eczematous skin changes and not for general allergy (see Fig. 6.4).

Considerations regarding the concordance of the various test results are of special interest. There are patients with negative prick test and without specific IgE and positive atopy patch test [391]. In 53 of 314 patients (14%), at least one allergen was positive in APT without corresponding sensitization in skin prick test or in vitro IgE (Table 6.3). This is interesting with regard to the question regarding intrinsic versus extrinsic atopic eczema (see Chap. 1). According to our understanding, positive atopy patch test reactions should be regarded as a sign of extrinsic atopic dermatitis, even if skin prick test and IgE are negative. Possibly the IgE reaction takes place without the involvement of mast cells or circulating IgE antibodies but with the involvement of IgE on the surface of dendritic cells [63].

The atopy patch test meanwhile has become a routine diagnostic procedure starting with a merely scientific instrument. We only recommend house dust mite avoidance with corresponding living and bedroom changes when the atopy patch test is positive.

Problem Food Allergens

The use of the atopy patch test with food allergens remains difficult [857]. While some years ago there was the big hope that, by using APT, one could replace time-consuming provocation tests in eczema [547, 807], the nature and quality of food allergen extracts seems to be problematic. Direct application of native wheat flour, e.g., may be irritative. Atopy patch test with food is still a matter of scientific studies. However, in our and others' experience, (Taieb et al., personal communication), there are clear-cut positive APT reactions with foods, especially in children who are negative in skin prick test and in vitro specific IgE and where this reaction is of clinical relevance (Table 6.4).

6.1.2.3 Classic Patch Test for Contact Allergy

While some years ago allergic contact dermatitis was not regarded to be a problem in atopic eczema or was expected to occur much less frequently, newer studies have shown that contact allergy also represents a problem in atopic dermatitis. One study showed that in 6% of over 600 patch-tested children with atopic dermatitis, positive epicutaneous tests were found especially for topical preparations, such as emollients and anti-

Table 6.4 Positive atopy patch test in patients with negative prick test and negative RAST (43 out of 314 patients)

N	Allergens
31	Dermatophagoides pteronyssinus
7	Cat epithelium
8	Grass pollen
16	Birch pollen
11	Hen's egg
16	Celery
18	Wheat flour

septics, particularly in children with severe atopic eczema [480].

Many studies have shown that allergic contact dermatitis can occur in patients with atopic dermatitis, especially in chronic hand dermatitis [461, 675, 714] (see Chap. 4). There are numerous studies showing that patients with atopic eczema also suffer from contact allergy. In our own study, we found 41% [214] positive patch test reactions in atopic eczema patients. This also holds true for children who have been rarely tested epicutaneously so far. Also chronic foot eczema can be due to contact allergy against shoe materials.

Testing of Corticosteroids

It is recommended to test patients with atopic dermatitis also with classical patch tests in order to rule out contact allergies. Special consideration should be given to the testing of topicals used, especially corticosteroid topicals which in chronic eczema can also act as contact allergens. This is often not easy to diagnose, since the pharmacologic effect of anti-inflammatory cortisone acts against the inflammation, while at the same time the steroid molecule as contact allergen maintains the inflammation. Therefore, in therapy-resistant eczema, the testing of topical corticosteroids is recommended also in children [480, 675, 777].

6.1.3 In Vitro Allergy Diagnostics

In vitro allergy diagnosis plays an important role in the management, especially in cases of severe atopic eczema with generalized skin lesions or under systemic medications, when skin tests are not possible.

6.1.3.1 Specific IgE Antibodies

The determination of specific IgE antibodies in serum is the focus and represents the major progress in allergy diagnostics in the last 50 years. Since the introduction of radioallergosorbent test (RAST), a variety of procedures has been developed to measure circulating specific IgE antibodies in the serum in a quantitative or semiquantitative way (RAST or Immunocap classes or units kU/L).

Total serum IgE also should be determined; however, it is of less relevance. In extremely high serum IgE levels (above 1000 kU/L)—as can be found in severe cases of atopic eczema—the interpretation of specific IgE has to be modified because of the high background noise. Probably the ratio-specific IgE to total IgE may have a better diagnostic relevance with regard to the specific sensitization [348]. Total IgE elevations can be regarded as general marker of the atopic diathesis. Atopic eczema is one of those diseases with the highest serum IgE levels measured, higher than in respiratory atopy [658].

6.1.3.2 Cellular In Vitro Allergy Testing

In rare cases, when no specific IgE is detectable in serum, the determination of basophil activation after allergen stimulation can be helpful, either as activation of basophil leukocytes by expression of CD63 (Basotest) or CD203 (flow CAST) [681]. Also, the measurement of histamine or sulfidoleukotriene secretion from basophil leukocytes after allergen stimulation can give information (CAST-ELISA). With regard to delayed reactions of eczema exacerbation, also lymphocyte transformation tests have been used. The group around Thomas Werfel found food-dependent allergen-specific T cell clones [616, 856, 861]. All these methods are scientific in nature and have not found entrance into daily clinical use.

6.1.4 Oral Provocation Test in Food Allergy

Many patients with atopic eczema suffer from food hypersensitivity with variable manifestation, either as urticaria, angioedema, anaphylaxis

[640, 651] or as exacerbation of an existing atopic dermatitis. The frequency of food allergy in atopic eczema is estimated around 20–30% in childhood and considerably lower among adults [691]. The most frequent food allergens in childhood atopic eczema are ovalbumin, cow's milk, soy, wheat, as well as also peanut, and tree nuts.

In diagnostics of food allergy, the real art is—as general in allergy diagnosis—to evaluate the relevance of sensitization for the clinical disease. Many children have positive skin prick tests to various foods without ever noticing any deterioration of the symptoms after intake. Therefore, especially in this area, dietary recommendations should be very well considered [403]. We recommend the avoidance of a food only when the relevance of a sensitization for atopic eczema or for another allergic disease is certain.

6.1.4.1 Double-Blind Provocation Test

The determination of relevance can be done by clear-cut history (rather rare) or by oral provocation test best performed in double-blind procedure. The groups around Werfel and Niggemann found, in studies with double-blind, placebo-controlled oral provocation test, clear-cut positive reactions in over 50% of the children [100, 548], similar to the results of Sampson 2001 and 2003 [679].

The timely appearance of skin lesions occurred in a majority of cases relatively rapidly (30 min to 2 h). Ca. 15% react only after 12–48 h, which sometimes is difficult to recognize under daily life conditions. A rather large number of patients also experience immediate-type reactions together with delayed-type reactions to foods.

6.1.4.2 Practical Performance

The performance of a placebo-controlled oral provocation test needs good blinding of foods which mostly are applied in porridge form [67]. The selection of the vehicle has to be done on the basis of previous allergy tests (skin prick test, RAST) since occasionally there are also allergies against unsuspicious foods like St. John's bread. The foods to be tested are mixed with the placebo ground substance together with unsuspicious colorings and flavors (e.g., black currant juice) for blinding.

In the oral provocation test, food additives should not be forgotten since they also can trigger exacerbations in atopic eczema, especially in adults [817, 826]. According to the schedule of the oral provocation test for idiosyncrasy (OPTI), as it is performed in chronic urticaria [644] also in patients with atopic dermatitis, the detection of a pseudo-allergic hypersensitivity against food additives can be achieved [889], especially against sulfites.

With a history of severe anaphylaxis and positive skin prick test or RAST results, one can refrain from oral provocation.

In order to estimate the relevance of sensitization for atopic dermatitis however provocation is often mandatory. The double-blind, placebo-controlled oral provocation test until now remains the gold standard and is usually done in specialized centers. It can be further improved by the measurement of mediators in plasma during the provocation procedures [566]. For daily practice, a nutrition diary is recommended where the patient or the parents record the symptoms, together with the food intake.

6.1.4.3 Skin Test Versus Specific IgE Testing

Unfortunately, the predictive value of skin prick test and specific IgE quantification with regard to food allergy in atopic eczema is limited. The positive predictive value (PPV) of food allergen-specific IgE is only around 30% for eczematous skin reactions, while it is 60% for clear-cut immediate-type reactions [841]. Also the nature of the eliciting food allergen plays a role: The relevance of sensitization against hen's egg or peanut is much higher than that of positive test against cow's milk or cereals.

The role of atopy patch test in the diagnostic procedure for food allergy is controversial (see atopy patch test).

6.1.5 Microbiological Diagnostics

Based on the considerations regarding pathophysiology (see Chap. 5 "Microbial Factors"), microbial factors with colonization or infection of the skin surface should also be considered in the diagnostic procedure.

Microbiological examination makes sense and should cover the following aspects:

- Bacteriological swabs of lesional and uninvolved skin as well as nasal mucosa (especially S. aureus).
- Mycological examination of squamous material especially in the head/neck region (Malassezia furfur).
- Virus detection of HSV when eczema herpeticum is suspected.

In infants and small children and oozing skin lesions, superinfection is common not only by staphylococci but also by streptococci (impetiginized eczema). These considerations will also find entrance into the therapy (see Chap. 6 "Antimicrobial Therapy").

6.1.6 Psychological Diagnostics

The obvious influence of psychological factors upon the clinical course of atopic dermatitis should be considered also in the diagnostic steps and, if there is an indication, psychosomatic counseling together with the use of validated questionnaires is recommended [767].

In particular, the following instruments have proven helpful:

- Marburg Skin Questionnaire (Marburger Hautfragebogen MHF).
- Cognitive itch questionnaire (Juckreiz-Kognitions-Fragebogen JKF).
- Dermatology Quality of Life Index DQLI [234].
- Deutsches Instrument zur Erfassung der Lebensqualität bei Hautkrankheiten DIELH [695] (German Instrument for Quality of Life in Skin Diseases).
- Eppendorf Itch Questionnaire [165].

In addition, there are specific questionnaires for children [615], as well as the AESEC (atopic eczema severity and emotional consequences) [660].

Often the motivation to write a diary for self-observation is very helpful for the patient in order to recognize the influence of psychological factors.

The most common psychological provocation factors comprise stress of any kind, both mental, but also emotional in nature [660]. Furthermore, memories of significant life events which have not adequately been coped with, also too intensive concern with regard to the own skin disease, may have an enhancing or prolonging character. The naive and well-meant question: "How feels your skin?" can occasionally trigger an intense itch crisis. Parents and relatives should know about this!

6.1.7 Summary

There are only a few diseases where diagnostics and therapy are so closely connected as in allergy and eczema. Careful allergy diagnostics is standard in the management of atopic dermatitis and comprises the four steps from history, skin test, to in vitro allergy diagnostics and provocation testing. The atopy patch test (APT) deserves special consideration; with this procedure, it is possible to evaluate the relevance of an IgE-mediated sensitization for patients with atopic dermatitis for the actual skin disease. The most common positive atopy patch test reactions are found against house dust mite, animal epithelia, and pollen. Also classic contact-allergic patch test reactions should not be overlooked; contact allergy patch testing belongs to the standard diagnostic repertoire also in atopic dermatitis, also in childhood. Food allergy can often only be evaluated by placebo-controlled oral provocation tests. This also holds true for food additives which equally can elicit exacerbations of atopic dermatitis. We do not recommend an allergen avoidance diet unless the relevance of this food for triggering an exacerbation of the disease has been clearly established.

6.2 Use of Biomarkers in Diagnostics of Atopic Dermatitis: New Aspects

6.2.1 New Aspects in the Diagnosis of Atopic Dermatitis

All abovementioned criteria are sufficient for the expert dermatologist or allergist to make the diagnosis of atopic dermatitis and the trigger factors in the majority of cases. However, these criteria are largely subjective in nature, and every single criterium only gives a hint to the diagnosis atopic dermatitis. Thus, it is only logical that there are substantial diagnostic gaps in our current workflow. These gaps relate to the diagnosis itself (e.g., differentiation from atopic dermatitis and psoriasis at special locations such as the palms, differential diagnosis atopic dermatitis versus early mycosis fungoides) as well as to prediction of clinically relevant outcomes, e.g., the natural clinical course of atopic dermatitis, development of comorbidities such as rhinoconjunctivitis or allergic asthma (allergic march, Chap. 1), or prediction of response to a given therapy.

The answer to these gaps might lie in two novel diagnostic developments, namely artificial intelligence-guided imaging analysis as well as molecular diagnostics. The following paragraph on novel diagnostic tools is modified from (Fig. 6.5).

As for the first, immediate advantages are that imaging methods are minimally or noninvasive and can be performed repetitively. There are several examples of imaging techniques used to improve diagnostics of atopic dermatitis. In a small cohort of 21 patients, it was shown that dermoscopy can be helpful in distinguishing eczema and psoriasis. Namely, in psoriasis there were more orange-brownish dots, while eczema serum crusts were frequently detected. However, dermoscopy requires a lot of experience and the criteria mentioned were only approximations and could not be applied prospectively to individual patients. Other imaging techniques may play a role in the future; for example, opto-acustics, a combination of laser and ultrasound, was shown to be useful to discriminate psoriasis from eczema. However, this technology is just at the beginning. Confocal microscopy has already been used to detect correlates of the inflammatory reaction after patch testing of allergens. It is still unclear however to what extent confocal microscopy could be useful to aid the diagnostics of atopic dermatitis. Taken together, imaging techniques are very promising for the diagnostics of atopic dermatitis, but currently easy-to-adapt tools are missing. This represents a barrier to implementing such strategies in the daily clinical routine. In the near future, though, machine learning algorithms might be used to design software tools that can overcome these problems. This is already a reality in the field of melanoma, where dermoscopy analysis by using AI software is equal to or better than expert dermatologists.

Besides imaging-based analysis, molecular diagnostics has made great advances in the field of atopic dermatitis diagnostics. Molecular diagnostics is basically any detection of a specific molecule that correlates with the diagnosis of a certain disease—or the risk of developing certain comorbidity or the individual therapeutic response (see below). Serum, skin swabs, tape strips/squamae, or lesional skin can be used as test material.

There are several proposed biomarkers that may help to diagnose atopic dermatitis in a reliable and objective way. Italian colleagues propose IL-36a as a possible biomarker for (hand) eczema in the differential diagnosis of psoriasis. On the basis of 30 patients with suspected hand eczema, they first showed the diagnostic gap in the standard procedures described above. Out of 30 patients, only eight could be clearly diagnosed based on anamnesis, patch tests, and clinical examination; on the other hand, according to histology and clinical features, psoriasis was suspected in 9 patients; In 13 patients however the

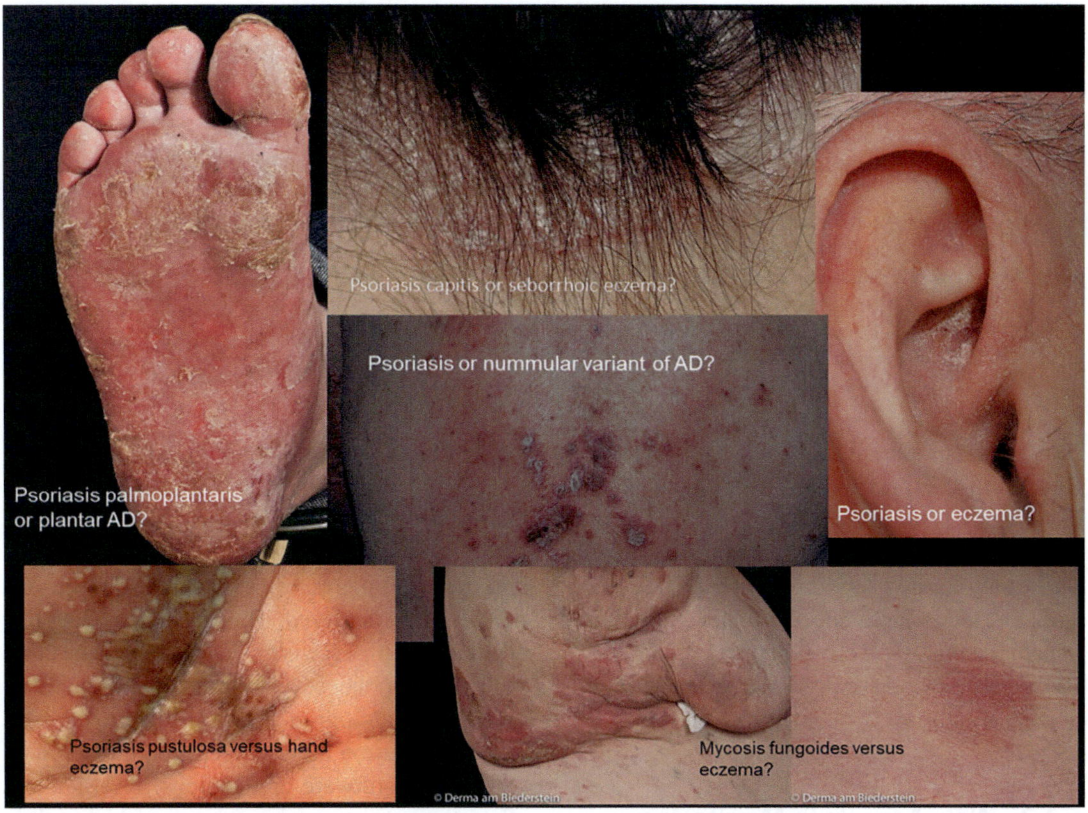

Fig. 6.5 New aspects in the diagnosis of atopic dermatitis

suspicion of idiopathic hand eczema was more likely to be expressed. The group then examined a number of markers from the IL-1 cytokine family; of these, only IL-36a was able to distinguish psoriasis from hand eczema. This small study has not yet been validated.

Another member of the IL-1 family, namely IL-36 g, has been suggested by other groups as a possible biomarker for differentiating between psoriasis and eczema. Early studies have shown that IL-36 g is particularly elevated in psoriasis lesions and psoriasis can possibly be differentiated from other inflammatory skin diseases by immunohistochemistry. This might even be possible from skin tape strip analysis. However, in the study, only 15 biopsies out of 21 could be correctly assigned here and this method has not yet been prospectively validated.

This lack of prospective validation is also relevant for other proposed markers (Table 6.5). In a small collective of Han Chinese, CCL26 was identified as a marker for differentiating between psoriasis and eczema one of the first studies in the field of molecular diagnostics suggested CXCL9 as a biomarker for lichen planus against psoriasis and eczema.

One problem of all these studies is that they investigate only one individual biomarker: since the method of determining biomarkers is not standardized, the probability is very high that no uniform upper or lower limit values can be established—depending on the reagents and machines used the absolute values fluctuate substantially, which can lead to contradicting results in different laboratories.

In order to circumvent this problem and at the same time avoid high costs and effort, we have developed a classifier in our working group that reliably differentiates psoriasis from eczema based on the ratio of two biomarkers, namely NOS2 and CCL27. These genes were identified in a special collection of patients who suffer from

Table 6.5 Diagnostic molecular biomarkers of atopic dermatitis. Modified from Garzorz-Stark N et al. Molecular diagnostics of hand eczema. Hautarzt. 2019; 70:760–765. https://doi.org/10.1007/s00105-019-4466-9. PMID: 31468073

Marker	Indication	Performance	Reproduced?	Reference
NOS2/ CCL27	Discriminates atopic dermatitis and subtypes from psoriasis and subtypes	Sensitivity and specificity >97%	Yes	
IL-36a	Discriminates atopic dermatitis from psoriasis	Correlation coefficient: 0.6	No	
IL-36 g	Discriminates psoriasis from atopic dermatitis and other inflammatory skin diseases	n = 15 patients	No	
CCL26	Discriminates atopic dermatitis from psoriasis in Han Chinese patients	n = 33 patients	No	
CXCL9	Distinguishes lichen planus from atopic dermatitis and psoriasis	19/20 Lichen patients correct	No	

both psoriasis and eczema at the same time. Based on the expression of NOS2 and CCL27, a molecular test was then developed which proved to be superior to the methods currently available. This test was also verified for clinical subtypes of atopic eczema, including hand eczema or nummular eczema as well as guttate psoriasis or erythroderma and showed consistently highly reliable results.

6.2.2 New Aspects in Monitoring Severity of Atopic Dermatitis

Just as the diagnostic workflow, our current assessment of the severity of atopic dermatitis is objective. It is usually performed by a combination of composite severity scores such as the SCORAD or the EASI (Chap. 4) as well as by interviewing the patient about his or her quality of life and symptoms of atopic dermatitis, ideally through validated patient-related outcome measurements (Chap. 4). In parallel to the development of novel tools to diagnose atopic dermatitis, both image analysis tools and molecular diagnostics are currently investigated for their potential to improve the severity monitoring of atopic dermatitis.

Imaging analysis basically means training a computer to assess disease severity in a so-called machine learning approach. This has been done, for example, by a Korean group that fed a computer with 8000 clinical images of atopic dermatitis together with the severity information as assessed by EASI score given by three dermatologists for each of these images. This resulted in the accuracy of the calculated severity items by the algorithm of 92–99%, respectively. It is the nature of machine learning that these algorithms will become better over time, with more and more images analyzed. Thus, we can expect that artificial intelligence is or will quite soon be competitive with the severity assessment done by expert dermatologists. The translation of these algorithms into a daily clinical routine could be realized by software applications or APP's that allow the patient to take pictures of him or herself. Some of these APP's already exist and even allow to integrate daily assessment of PRO's and a symptom's diary the patient can fill out. For assessment of the total body severity, standardized camera systems are already available. However, they are quite costly at the moment and require GDPR-conform storage of large data amounts. Furthermore, for special locations, such as area of hair, it will take much longer to get meaningful algorithms. But overall we can expect that image-based objective severity monitoring will become a part of our diagnostic workflow of atopic dermatitis in the near future.

In parallel to this development, molecular biomarkers have been suggested to correlate with eczema severity. The majority of studies have been performed on serum of atopic dermatitis patients as it is easily accessible. Early studies suggested a moderate correlation of TARC (CCL17), a chemokine involved in the recruitment of type 2 immune cells to the skin, with atopic dermatitis severity. This was confirmed in several independent studies, together with the observation that IL-22 in the serum correlates modestly with disease severity. To improve correlations, combinations of distinct serum proteins were investigated. In fact, these combinations markedly improved the correlation to atopic dermatitis severity. One of these marker combinations is TARC, IL-22, and soluble IL-2 receptor. This combination has been shown to correlate with therapeutic response to cyclosporine or dupilumab also. However, none of these tools but one have been prospectively validated in independent cohorts without changing the formula, and this one validation resulted in a standard error of the algorithm of 8 points on the SCORAD scale. Of note, this is the same standard error that occurs if many expert dermatologists assess patients with the SCORAD. Thus, biomarkers from the serum do not represent an improvement in objectivity as compared to standard clinical assessment at the moment. It can be expected however that also these algorithms will improve. Furthermore, minimally invasive molecular diagnostics can also be done from lesional skin, e.g., by investigating inflammatory or barrier parameters using the tape strip method. Here, sticky tapes are repetitively pressed and detouched from lesional skin, and the adherent material is subsequently analyzed by PCR methods or protein measurement. It has been shown that biomarkers reflecting both barrier abnormalities and inflammation can be measured from tape strip material, and that these correlate with improvement of the clinical severity to therapeutic interventions such as topical therapy.

Taken together, molecular diagnostics has the potential to improve the severity assessment of atopic dermatitis by introducing a reliable and objective measurement tool with minimally invasive techniques. To implement molecular diagnostics in dermatology, several barriers need to be overcome, namely reimbursement and feasibility to include assessments in the clinical routine. Companies such as Dermagnostix or Biocartis develop point-of-care devices that could overcome these barriers, so we can expect that in addition to image-based algorithms we might have easy-to-access and economic test devices in our diagnostic workflow in the near future.

6.2.2.1 New Aspects in the Prediction of Clinically Relevant Outcomes of Atopic Dermatitis

Our current understanding of atopic dermatitis finishes with the question of the individual development of atopic dermatitis over time—we can not predict with any current tools which patients will have a rather benign course of their disease as opposed to a severe life-long phenotype, potentially with development of further comorbidities. Thus, for these relevant questions, novel diagnostic tools are desperately needed.

The first question of clinical relevance is in which patients atopic dermatitis might be self-limited, where it might be self-limited but come back at higher age, and where it might have a constant and severe phenotype (see Chap. 4). In a study investigating around 300 children with atopic dermatitis, persistence could be predicted with a sensitivity and specificity of more than 80% by a combination of skin severity at 3 years of age, certain trigger factors such as stress and low VEGF serum levels. Another study identified positive family history, high socioeconomic status, female sex, asthma, and a positive skin prick test as predictors of persistent atopic dermatitis Thus, a combination of clinical phenotyping and novel diagnostic tools might help to answer the question of the natural clinical course of atopic dermatitis in early childhood.

Regarding the development of comorbidities, novel insights into the trajectories of atopic dermatitis patients on epidemiological level as well as insight into the pathogenesis justify optimism. In a large epidemiological trial investigating children with atopic dermatitis, development of atopic comorbidities was associated with race and more specifically genotype. While the majority of patients of Afro-American origin developed allergic asthma (61%), development of rhinoconjunctivitis was associated with the European-Asian race (33%), and IgE-mediated food allergy to the Asian population (6%). Specific SNP's were identified for each of these groups. At the same time, we understand that the development of comorbidities might be associated to an altered immune reaction to allergens if they encounter the body via the skin as compared to mucosal membranes. While cutaneous sensitization seems to result in a preferential type 2 immune induction, mucosal membranes are rather prone type 1 and type 4 immune responses. While this is not relevant in clinical practice today, the hope is that a combination of precise genotyping together with immune-related biomarkers might identify patients at risk to develop atopic and further comorbidities in the future.

The third relevant question is a prediction of the therapeutic response at an individual patient´s level. This is the holy grail in translational research in atopic dermatitis today. Numerous large consortia work on this question as it has an enormous socioeconomic impact. However, overall no reliable biomarkers have been identified as of now. Early suggestions such as level of LDH in the serum that might correlate to dupilumab response, IL-22 baseline levels that might correlate with response to the IL-22 antibody fezakinumab, or CD23 levels on B lymphocyte populations that allow early prediction of an immune response to immune-apheresis all need to be validated in the future. However, with more sophisticated techniques, larger registries and better clinical phenotyping paralleled by coordinated research initiatives we can expect that valid biomarkers will be identified that truly change the clinical decision-making of when and which therapy to what patient in atopic dermatitis.

6.3 Avoidance of Individual Provocation Factors

Often patients complain that there would be no "causal" therapy for this disease. However, in the individual case one has to think about "cause" and "trigger factor" in daily life. The latter can very well be diagnosed and often be avoided in the sense of a causal therapy. This procedure, often called allergen avoidance, relies upon the results of careful allergy diagnostics (see Sect. 4.1). The recommendations regarding avoidance of individual provocation factors comprise much more; unspecific and specific stimuli often go together in the maintenance of severe eczema (Fig. 6.6).

6.3.1 Avoidance of Unspecific Irritants

Various influences and noxious substances from the environment are able to irritate the sensitive skin of patients with atopic dermatitis compared to healthy persons and trigger eczema flares (Table 6.6).

There are leaflets explaining these phenomena which should be given to the patients although this information is often regarded as trivial (Table 6.7). Very often we see that especially in this so simple field of avoidance of irritants heavy mistakes are made. People very early choose strong and possibly risky drugs before they even tried to start with simple avoidance of irritants and skincare. In our leaflet for patients, we try to explain the importance of many so-called trivial things. A leaflet never replaces the dialogue which is very time-consuming and practically not achievable in the average office time of a practicing physician.

Therefore, this is a domain of eczema school and educational programs (see Chap. 6 "Prevention").

Apart from adequate skincare using basic therapy of disturbed skin barrier function, the consideration of certain principles regarding hygiene and clothing plays an important role.

The so-called wool hypersensitivity of many patients is rarely based on a true allergy against sheep wool, but rather a typical marker of patients with atopic diseases showing the increased sensitivity of the skin to the mechanical stimulus of the small fibers.

Negative influences of environmental pollutants are also to be considered, like environmental tobacco smoke (also passive) as well as traffic exhaust. Also chemicals in indoor air, like volatile organic compounds or formaldehyde, can lead to deterioration of eczema [199, 349].

Mechanic traumatization or exsiccation as well as contact to solvents are risky for atopic individuals. This also has a component with regard to occupational counseling and early diagnosis of occupational disease (see Chap. 8 "Prevention").

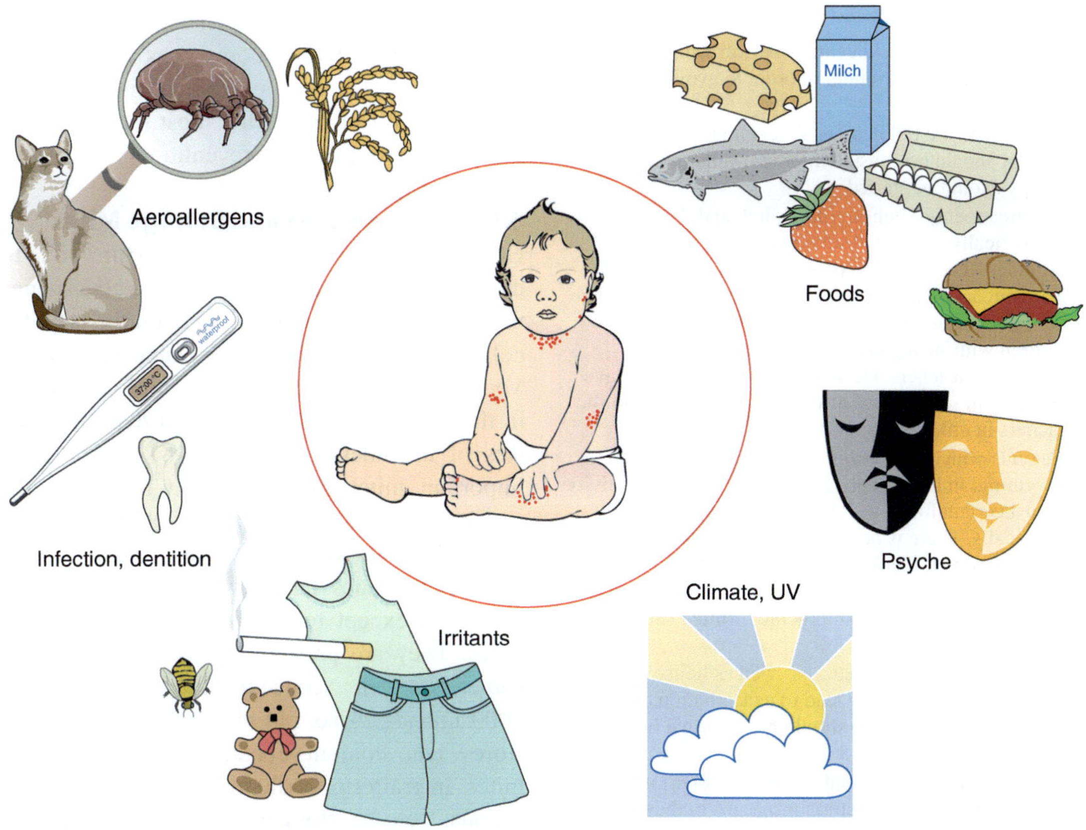

Fig. 6.6 Individual trigger factors for flares of atopic eczema

Table 6.6 Atopic dermatitis: nonspecific irritants

Physical	E.g., mechanical, exsiccation, UV light, temperature
Chemical	Detergents, solvents, acids, alkali
Pharmacologic	Vasoactive substances (alcohol, nicotine, amines)
Immunologic	Allergens, superantigens
Psychologic	Stress, emotional conflicts

Vasoactive substances (e.g., alcohol) can trigger itch crises and thus contribute to eczema deterioration. In this context also psychological stress can be an unspecific irritant (see Chap. 5).

A special method for treatment of atopic dermatitis which considers both unspecific and specific stimuli is climate therapy which can be performed at sea level (e.g., North Sea) or at high altitude (above 1500 m, e.g., Davos, Switzerland) [84, 198, 217, 232].

Table 6.7 Information leaflet for patients with atopic dermatitis

The disease is based on a genetic predisposition which can become manifest either as eczema, bronchial asthma or allergic rhinoconjunctivitis, e.g., hay fever.
The skin of patients with atopic dermatitis is dry, the hair relatively brittle.
There is an increased tendency to develop eczema, that is, red, squamous, itchy, sometimes oozing skin changes (the latter predominantly occur on the elbows, knee joints, hands, neck, and face).
The skin of children or adults with atopic dermatitis needs continuous care. The following aspects have to be considered:
Use mild detergents or soaps or syndets for cleaning
Avoid too often or too hot showering, no foam bath
Before showering or bathing, an emollient additive (bath oil) should be given
After bathing or showering, the skin has to be creamed with emollients (lotion cream) prior to using the towel which should only be used as a mild touch, not as an intense rubbing!
Wool or irritant textiles never should get in direct contact with the skin (preferably use cotton or silk)

(continued)

Table 6.7 (continued)

It is important that skin care is performed in the morning and in the evening in order to avoid itchy eczematous reactions
When there are red itchy or eczematous skin reactions, a doctor should be consulted, or anti-inflammatory therapy should be started
The treatment of itch is crucial. Itch and the automatically connected scratch reaction cannot be forbidden! The side effects of an anti-inflammatory treatment are definitely less damaging than the damage through injuring the skin by scratching. Especially children with strong itch should find sympathetic parents and teachers. Occasionally children who have problems in school need a special colloquium with the teachers in order to get the necessary understanding
Patients with atopic eczema principally can eat everything. In individual cases, there is hypersensitivity against certain foods which have to be tested specifically. There is no general anti-eczema or anti-allergy diet. Obesity should be avoided. Newborns at risk should be breastfed if possible over 4 months. If this is not possible, hypoallergenic formula should be given
Pets (cats, dogs, birds, etc.), as well as house dust (old carpets, skirts, etc.), may lead to exacerbation of the disease. The living room should have normal humidity (less than 55%)
Sea or high altitude climate (above 1500 m) is well tolerated. Some rehabilitation programs in these climate zones can be helpful

6.3.2 Aeroallergens

The role of aeroallergens in eliciting eczema flares in atopic dermatitis has been covered in the Chapter Atopy Patch Test. Thus, it makes sense that avoidance of these allergens should be recommended. The most common airborne allergens leading to eczema exacerbation derive from house dust mites of the species Dermatophagoides pteronyssinus and Dermatophagoides farinae [806].

When talking about indoor air improvement, many measures are discussed leading to a decrease in allergen concentration in living rooms. Many of these procedures are scientifically not well investigated although they are based on rational considerations [181].

Thus, the avoidance of molds with its growth and spore formation belongs to general prevention measures not only for atopics. From epidemiological studies, it is known that dampness and mold growth in living rooms goes along with a higher prevalence of atopic dermatitis, which has also been considered in the most recent recommendations for primary prevention.

6.3.2.1 House Dust and Storage Mites

House dust is a poorly defined mixture of sedimenting particles from the air whose consistency varies considerably depending upon the way it is collected. Only in 1964 the Dutch researchers Voorhorst and coworkers discovered small mites in the house dust and recognized them as elicitors of the allergic reactions [832]. The most important mites in this context belong to the family of the Pyroglyphidae, like Dermatophagoides pteronyssinus and Dermtophagoides farinae which occur all over the world except for the arctic and alpine altitudes. They are present in bed and upholstery, sometimes in concentrations of up to 4000 mites/g. Also, old textiles, furs, and grain stores can contain considerable numbers of mites. In grain stores (flour, grains from different cereals, etc.), storage mites are common (Lepidoglyphus destructor, Acarus siro, etc.). The living conditions of house dust mites depend upon a complex ecosystem with factors like air humidity, concomitant mold growth, temperature, presence of human dander or organic fibers, etc. [181]. These mites are companions of humans and live from human dander.

In order to get rid of house dust mites, acaricides (benzyl benzoate, tannic acid, or hyperosmolar saline) are used, but these are of limited efficacy. The ecosystem has to be changed, e.g., by washable (60 °C) encasings of mattresses [787]. Bedding and linen should be washed once a week at temperatures around 60 °C.

Stuffed animals, teddy bears, or textile toys can be kept for several hours in a deep freeze. Not only mattresses and beddings should be miteproof, but there are also miteproof pyjamas ("eczema overalls") which can be used over night in severe atopic dermatitis [629]. Also, adequate basic therapy with emollients under closed conditions (wet wraps) and tube bandages have proven valuable.

The normal living room cleaning with vacuum cleaning or moist procedures (wiping) usually only minimally reduces the mite concentrations. While carpets were not recommended some years ago, today, with the development of new materials and adequate care, carpet floors are no longer definitely forbidden. However, there is a consensus that the bedroom floors which can be moistly cleaned are preferable when there are atopic diseases in the family.

There are several methods to detect house dust mite concentration or house dust mite allergen in a quantitative way which help in avoidance procedures (guanine coloring test "Acarex" or ELISA for house dust mite allergens [445].

Possibly other allergens are of relevance also for atopic dermatitis compared to airway atopy like allergens der p 2 and der f 2 [444, 549, 805].

6.3.2.2 Animal Epithelia

Many patients know from their own experience that contact with pets leads to an exacerbation of their skin symptoms. However, many patients do not know how to suppress this. When giving avoidance recommendations with regard to pets, it has to be distinguished strictly between primary prevention in order to avoid sensitization and development of atopic disease in risk families or individual prevention in an already sensitized or affected individuals (for primary prevention see Sect. 6.1). It is of interest that pets of allergic individuals may be allergic themselves [688]. Affected individuals with animal dander allergy usually avoid animal contact; however, eczema does not improve after removal of the pet (e.g., cat). This may be due to the fact that cat allergen is kept over long periods in the indoor air since it is not connected to large particles which sediment faster, like house dust mite allergen. Therefore, it is typical that cat-allergic individuals realize the presence of a cat in the indoor air much faster than other persons.

Allergies against dog seem to play a less important role, especially with regard to primary prevention. On the other hand, there are dog-allergic individuals with atopic dermatitis where eczema exacerbates immediately after dog contact. These persons have to avoid dogs. By disciplined educational programs which are possible in dogs (control by education) it is often possible to reserve certain areas of a house to humans and keep them "dog-free." These strategies however need discipline from humans and animals.

Principally allergies can occur against all animals; however. With variable frequency. Bird or amphibia in terraria are less often allergy inducers than furry pets. Fish in aquaria may be kept; however, there is an allergy against fish food like red larvae of the species Chironomus [43]. Rodents (like mice, rats, or hamsters) which are increasingly common in Western households (in Germany probably already in one million households) seem to be especially sensitizing. Against these animals, allergic reactions develop rapidly and abrase not only the skin, but also airways, and induce severe asthma attacks.

6.3.2.3 Pollen

It has been shown that pollen can trigger atopic eczema [859], as is reported by many patients during summer months, and has been shown in a nested case-control epidemiological trial [429]. It can be shown in a positive atopy patch test. Therefore, it makes sense to avoid pollen in patients with atopic dermatitis and grass pollen sensitization (Table 6.8) [141]. It is important to know that closing the window does not guarantee absence of pollen in the indoor air; to achieve this, air conditioning with adequate filters is mandatory.

6.3.2.4 Foods

There is no general anti-allergic diet which could be recommended in atopic dermatitis [171, 573, 605]. Since the early experiments by Prausnitz and Küstner, it is known that food allergens can be absorbed after oral intake and elicit systemic reactions, e.g., flare-up at test sites [600]. Specific avoidance measures in the sense of a true allergy diet are recommended when they are specific and relevant. Temporarily general elimination diets can be recommended for diagnostic procedures [32, 327]. However, they also go along with some risk [173, 661] when persons avoiding cow's milk inadvertently were exposed to cow's milk and developed anaphylactic shock.

Table 6.8 Recommendations to reduce aerogen pollen exposure in patients with atopic dermatitis

Avoid staying in outdoor air at high pollen counts (see pollen information service broadcasting, newspaper, internet)
In cool weather or long-lasting rain, pollen counts are markedly lower
Daily exposure maxima (in rural environment) are early morning and evening. During this time, windows should be closed. The optimum time for ventilation of rooms is 0.00 h–4.00 h at night
With the use of pollen-protective foils, windows can be opened
On days with longer exposure to open air, persons should shower before going to bed (inclusively washing of hair). Then consequent skin care
Clothing should not be kept in the bedroom since by this many pollen will come into the room
Utmost care should be given to keep the bedroom cool and with a low amount of dust
Regular vacuum cleaning with a vacuum cleaner with a fine particle filter and wet wiping and cleaning of surfaces in the living room during the pollen season is important; this work should not be done by the affected individual himself or herself
The use of skin care preparations prior to exposure in the open air on air-exposed skin areas makes sense
Textiles should not be dried in the open air
Pets can carry considerable amounts of pollen into the living rooms
Use of cars: When cars are parked outside or under trees, there may be a massive aggregation of pollen in the car ventilation which is then released when the motor is started. Pollen filters in cars are available and recommended
If possible, affected individuals should consider the pollen season when they make plans for vacation. Intelligent choice of time and location of holiday makes a partial or complete avoidance of allergen contact possible

Another situation is given in prevention: Breastfeeding and hypoallergenic formula are indicated [220, 226, 302, 315]. Normal nutrition avoiding vitamin or element deficiencies is crucial [179, 430, 697].

Knowledge about the content of foods has been improved by better declaration rules which are very helpful for affected patients [827].

6.3.3 Summary

The avoidance of individual provocation factors is central in the management of patients with atopic dermatitis. Apart from nonspecific irritants, which have to be avoided generally like irritating textiles (wool), mechanical trauma or pollutants, allergen-specific avoidance measures have been helpful in house dust mite, but also in pollen allergy. Detailed counseling is mandatory and represents part of educational programs. In mite-free high-altitude climate, many patients experience improvement.

6.4 Basic Therapy of Disturbed Skin Barrier Function

All procedures to restore the disturbed skin barrier function which can be clinically regarded as "dry," "rough," or "sensitive" are often called "skincare," which has the consequence that they are not reimbursed by many insurances in many countries. Therefore, semantically it is better to talk about "basic therapy of disturbed skin barrier function" to help in understanding the basic defect. Unfortunately, for this type of treatment often the term "use of 'drug-free' vehicles" has become widely used in order to distinguish this type of treatment from specifically efficient pharmaceuticals like glucocorticosteroids or immunosuppressives. However, there is no doubt that these vehicle substances also have distinct effects on the organ skin.

The major principle of this basic emollient therapy is the application of lipids in order to restore the skin barrier. The composition of these lipids is crucial for the effect.

6.4.1 General Considerations for Topical Dermatotherapy

6.4.1.1 How to Select Galenics

Galenics is the art to bring effective substances together with the desired vehicles into the correct mixture so that they reach the respective tissue. It is the most important aspect of topical dermatotherapy. It is the art of the experienced dermatologist, allergist, or pediatrician together with the pharmacist [855, 874].

In principle, there are different physicochemical characteristics of topical preparations which can be classified according to their nature with the so-called phase triangle according to Polano (Fig. 6.7) as

- Solid phase (e.g., powder),
- Lipid phase (lipids of various origin) or.
- Fluid phase (e.g., aqueous or alcoholic solutions).

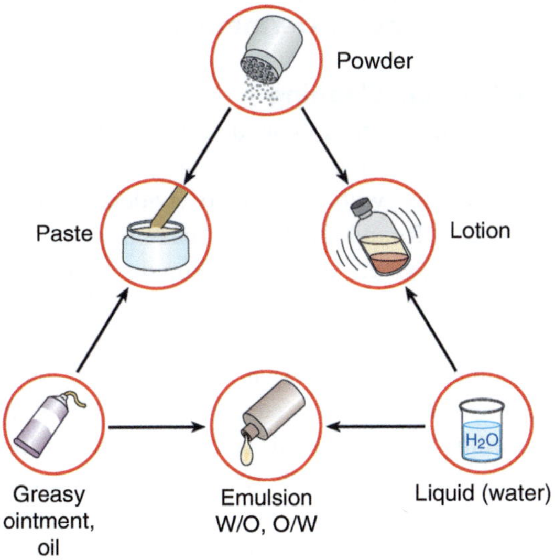

Fig. 6.7 Triangle of phases—Liquid, solid, lipid—according to Polano for selection of vehicles in topical dermatotherapy

By the mixture of these three different basic conditions, a variety of preparations with very different characteristics with regard to efficacy and acceptability can be derived [260].

Unfortunately, the common language does not patent exact scientific terms. The term "ointment" is used for any substance which can be spread on the skin. In dermatological use, ointment describes a more greasy preparation while cream has more hydrophilic constituents and lotion is even more aqueous in nature. Therefore, many preparations are advertised under dermatologically incorrect names.

The term "lotio" means a suspension of a solid, e.g., zinc oxide or titanium dioxide in a solution like water or alcohol, and lotio alba aquosa is an excellent topical preparation in acute skin inflammation or itchy conditions.

The contents of topical therapeutics can be of animal, plant, or mineral origin (Table 6.9), and show their effect already in the upper layers of the epidermis. It has to be considered that fatty materials form an occlusive film over the skin surface which prevents the loss of humidity, but also the exchange of substances occurring normally through the skin barrier. This can be a dis-

Table 6.9 Vehicles for topical dermatotherapy

Fluid phase	Solid phase	Fatty phase/lipid phase
Water (aqua), Alcohol, Ethanol, Isopropanol Ether Acetone	Mineral Zinc oxide, Titanium dioxide Talcum Plant Starch (amylum), Wheat starch (Amylum Tritici), corn starch (Amylum maysi)	Mineral Paraffin, petrolatum (petrolatum album/flavum) Synthetic lipids Polyethylene glycol Propylene glycol Plant Olive oil (oleum olivarum) Peanut oil (oleum arachidis) Animal Adeps suillus Beeswax (cera alba) Cod liver oil (oleum iecoris) Wool wax (adeps lane)

advantage in very acute inflammatory conditions so that too greasy ointments should not be given in acute stages. The dermatological paradox describes that the opposite of "dry" is not "moist," but "fat"; a very moist preparation like an aqueous solution will—by increasing evaporation—lead to further dryness of the skin, while the application of a greasy ointment will contain humidity and moisture in the upper skin layers.

In this, the probably most famous physician in world history, Claudius Galenus (second century AD), who impressed medicine over a time of thousand years, is still considered modern today. In our more and more rapid and accelerating world, this art may be lost; however, it allows, with simple means and limited side effects and low costs, to achieve long-lasting improvement and avoidance of risky pharmaceutics. All you need is some patience and experience. We tell our patients: "The skin is not an organ which can be cured at the flick of a switch or at the push of a button."

The secret of every topical preparation is how to bring water and fat together to form a suitable emulsion. This amphiphilic system can be regarded on a spectrum between pure fatty constituents like petrolatum or paraffin and pure liquid solutions like water or alcohol and are characterized according to their nature constituent as either water-in-oil (W/O) or oil-in-water (O/W) emulsion. Creams are oil-in-water emulsions, while ointments in the dermatological terminology are water-in-oil emulsions. The larger the aqueous part of an emulsion, the more emulsifiers have to be used, which means that these are rather complex systems containing more substances than a rather fatty ointment with only petrolatum. Today patients seem to prefer more hydrophilic preparations. When I compare old prescriptions of the ancestors in dermatology, we wonder how patients were able to tolerate these!

The best protection of the skin can be achieved by water-in-oil emulsions which form a fatty film on the skin surface and provide protection also in occupational context (itchy hand dermatitis). Maybe also the general shortage of time plays a role since creams or lotions can be applied faster than greasy ointments. We recommend our patients to take the time, every morning after the cleaning procedures (bathing or showering with adequate showering oils), for 5 min skincare in the bathroom, let the ointments go in after application; one can read a newspaper during this time where the fatty fingerprints do not disturb. This finally saves a lot of costs, time, and adverse reactions and is a good prevention in atopic dermatitis.

In the selection of the right galenics, several aspects have to be considered, namely

- The tissue inflammation which tells you how deep the effective substance should penetrate,
- The type of inflammation, whether infectious or non-contagious,
- The duration, i.e., chronicity,
- The individual skin type (dry skin, sebostasis, or greasy skin),
- The localization (extensor sides versus flexures or intertriginous areas).

The intertriginous areas where skin touches skin, like in the anogenital area or the axilla, are not a good place for too fatty topicals. Here powders or pastes should be preferred (Fig. 6.8).

6.4.2 Basic Skin Barrier Therapy in Atopic Dermatitis

6.4.2.1 Skin Cleaning

Skin hygiene measures are discussed with respect to prevention. However, there are limited scientific studies with regard to evidence. In a European Round Table on "best practice for infant cleansing," an expert group discussed and reviewed the literature with regard to bathing and cleansing of newborns in the first year of life. Alkaline soaps have been found to have some disadvantages compared to liquid cleansers regarding skin surface pH and lipid content. Mild liquid cleaners for newborns should be used, and preferably those which also contain some emollient. Bathing was regarded to be generally superior to washing also with regard to some emotional and psychological interactions between infants and parents [74].

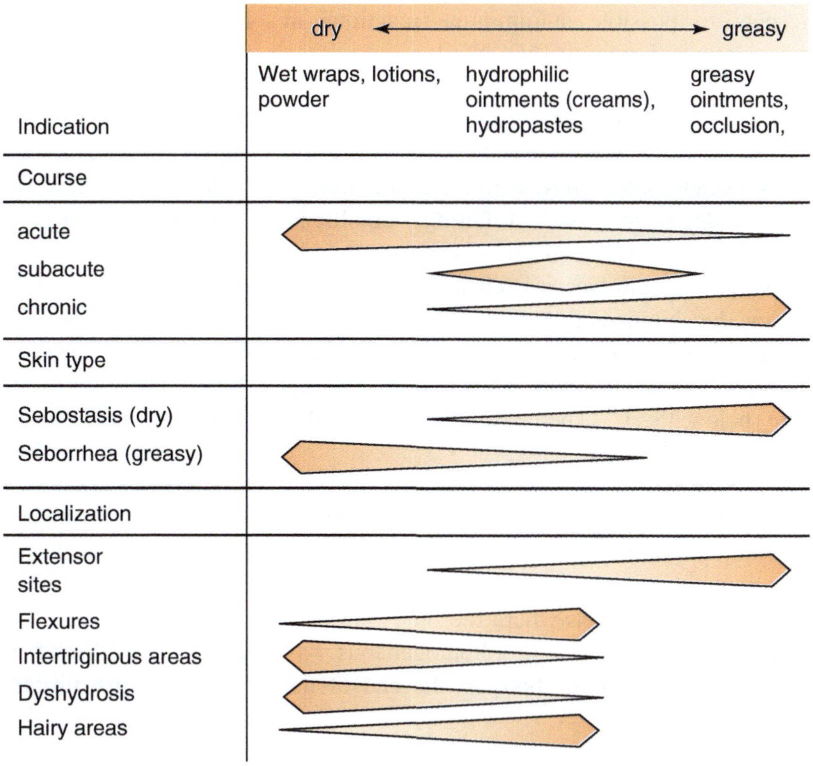

Fig. 6.8 Optimal selection of vehicle according to duration of disease, localization of skin lesions, and individual skin type [652]

Hardness of Water

For skin cleaning procedures, the degree of hardness of water is of relevance. A study from the UK showed a significant dependance of atopic dermatitis prevalence and the degree of water hardness [500]. With very hard water, decalcifying procedures are recommended [793].

Soaps and Detergents

Gentle cleansing procedures are essential, especially when the skin is inflamed [420]. One problem is the selection of adequate soaps and detergents. For a long time, alkali soaps were not recommended or forbidden because of the irritative effect due to the alkalic nature of their constituents on the acid mantle of the skin surface [487, 813].

However, in recent decades new detergents have been developed, better termed surfactants, which keep the acid pH and are also usable in hard water and available as liquid soaps. Chemically one can distinguish among syndets between anionic, non-ionic, and amphoteric substances:

- Anionic surfactants contain sulfates or sulfonates (sulfosuccinate) or carboxylate (sarcosinate) or alkyl phosphate.
- Nonionic surfactants consist of polyglycol ethers or esters and fatty acid alkanolamides. Amphoteric syndets contain alkylbetaine among others [95].

The debate about the advantages and disadvantages of syndets versus soaps has been less intense over the last few years. There is consensus that skin cleansing is an essential part of topical therapeutic management in skin diseases, also in atopic dermatitis. We are no longer "hydrophobic" in treating our patients! [74, 262]. The removal of superficial microbial flora or epidermal proteins like crusts or dandruff represents a major factor in preventing further stimulation of immune reactions in the epidermis, also with respect to possible autoimmune reactions in severe atopic dermatitis [664, 816].

6.4.2.2 Oil Bath or Showering Oils

While many dermatologists forbade showering some decades ago, today, with the production of better detergents and refatting emollient-containing showering oils, there is no contraindication [342]. However, it is clear that showering makes the skin drier than an oil bath. Therefore, in acute conditions or in very dry skin, we still recommend oil baths with not too high temperature (below 35 ° C). There are different oil baths, namely

- Emulsion oil baths where the lipid part is emulated in the form of small droplets in the aqueous face and.
- Spreading oil baths where the lipids are contained on the surface in a homogeneous way and spread over the body at the end of the bath.

It is important that, after the bath or shower, patients do not rub themselves totally dry, but rather just take away the outer moisture of the moist skin and apply the necessary emollients, creams, or ointments on the humid skin [477].

NaCl

Some authors recommend sodium chloride as an additive to baths together with oil for the keratolytic and skin-softening effect. Salt concentrations up to 5% are recommended. Sodium chloride bath oils in higher concentrations, sometimes also with the addition of magnesium, should increase the effect of balneotherapy mimicking the Dead Sea situation, also together with UV treatment [190] (see also Chap. 7 “Phototherapy”).

6.4.3 Emollients Used for Basic Dermatotherapy

Basic dermatotherapy is the essence of every treatment of atopic dermatitis and should be performed over a long time [463, 915]. In the acute flare however anti-inflammatory substances are needed, mostly glucocorticosteroids which then can be slowly reduced in the sense of a “tandem” therapy or interval therapy.

Most producers of corticosteroid-containing topicals also offer the corresponding “basic therapeutics” with the same vehicles, but without the specific drug.

The mixture of several substances in basic therapeutics is not a trivial matter, not everything can be mixed with everything. Pharmaceutical expertise is necessary since several mixtures can “break” and no longer be stable and homogeneous for the skin [272, 717]. The use of emollients is generally safe, except for the occasional occurrence of contact allergy [188, 243].

6.4.3.1 Emollients with Specific Ingredients

Emollients containing vehicle substances alone have to be distinguished from emollients containing additional possibly helpful substances, they are called “emollients plus” [876, 877]. Such substances may be urea, flavonoids, saponins, out of plantlets, or microbiota like Aquaphilus dolomiae [288, 506]. Dry skin is a cardinal symptom of atopic dermatitis; therefore, adequate moisturizing of the upper layers of the epidermis is an absolute requirement. Under natural conditions, the skin itself produces so-called natural moisturizing factors (NMF) consisting of low-molecular-weight substances like amino acids as degradation products of proteins. Low-molecular-weight compounds such as urea or glycerol may be added to emollients.

Urea is used in various conditions of dry skin or exaggerated keratinization as keratolytic [874] in concentrations up to 20% and higher. In atopic dermatitis, usually 5% urea is enough and better tolerated. Especially small children do not like urea because of a mild burning sensation. Glycerol and urea are used in creams and improve the hydration of stratum corneum considerably thus adding to a protective effect. Care should be given when there is damaged skin because of burning sensation [464].

By using emollients with urea, the consumption of anti-inflammatory substances, especially topical glucocorticosteroids, can be reduced significantly [14].

A variety of other ingredients are used not only for galenic reasons but also because of specific effects such as antipruritic effects (see Chap. 7 "Antipruritics"). A new topical emollient containing a unique lamellar matrix including palmitoyl ethanolamide—a cannabinoid agonist—was studied in a multinational multicenter prospective cohort study in over 2000 patients. There was a substantial relief of objective and subjective symptoms of atopic eczema after regular use of the cream [763, 766, 901].

A well-accepted ointment for atopic dermatitis skincare is the so-called atopy ointment ("Atopikersalbe") (Table 6.10). If it is found too greasy, we use the well-known unguentum emulsificans aquosum (aqueous hydrophilic ointment of general prescription formulas of the German or European Pharmacopoeia) or a lipophilic cream according to Gehring [260].

Table 6.10 Selection of self-prepared emollients for basic skin care in atopic dermatitis

"Atopy ointment"	
Solutio acidi citrici 0.5%	30.0
Glycerini	15.0
Unguentum Cordes	ad 100
"Basic skin care cream" of the German Pharmacopoeia	
Glycerol monostearate	4.0
Cetyl alcohol	6.0
Medium-chain triglycerides	7.5
Petrolatum album	25.5
Macrogol (100 glycerol monostearate)	7.5
Propylene glycol	10.0
Aqua purificata	ad 100.0
Lipophilic cream (according to Gehring)	
Triglycerol diisostearate	3.0
Isopropyl palmitate	2.4
Hydrophobic basic	24.6
Potassium sorbate	0.15
Acidum citricum	0.1
Magnesium sulfate heptahydrate	0.5
Glycerol 85%	5.0
Aqua purificata ad 100.0	ad 100.0

Unfortunately, not everywhere in the world these emollients are accessible because of rather high price [331]. The use of pure oils (olive, sunflower) is not recommended, since afterward the skin will dry out.

6.4.4 Summary

Under the name "basic therapy," all procedures are comprised which are used to repair the disturbed skin barrier function. This also includes adequate skin cleaning measures as well as the application of emollients to restore lipids in the skin, be they used as shower oils or oil baths. One has to keep in mind that patients with atopic dermatitis are very individualistic also with regard to the selection of their skincare products. What is good for one patient may not be liked by the next one. Therefore, it is recommended to test skincare products possibly at different body sites prior to prescribing larger volumes. Certain ingredients with effects of natural moisturizing factors have proven helpful in adults, such as urea and glycerol.

6.5 Practical Tips in the Treatment of Atopic Eczema in the Acute Flare

6.5.1 Practical Management of an Acute Eczema Flare

In the management of atopic dermatitis, a stepwise procedure has proven practical (Fig. 6.9) which includes the acute treatment, the basic dermatotherapy of the disturbed skin barrier, and the special treatment of chronic, lichenified, lesions. These steps can be used in an overlap and in parallel. As soon as there is improvement of the acute skin lesions, detection of individual provocation factors by using allergy diagnostics should be done [169, 855].

The acute treatment procedures comprise a stepwise approach (Fig. 6.9)

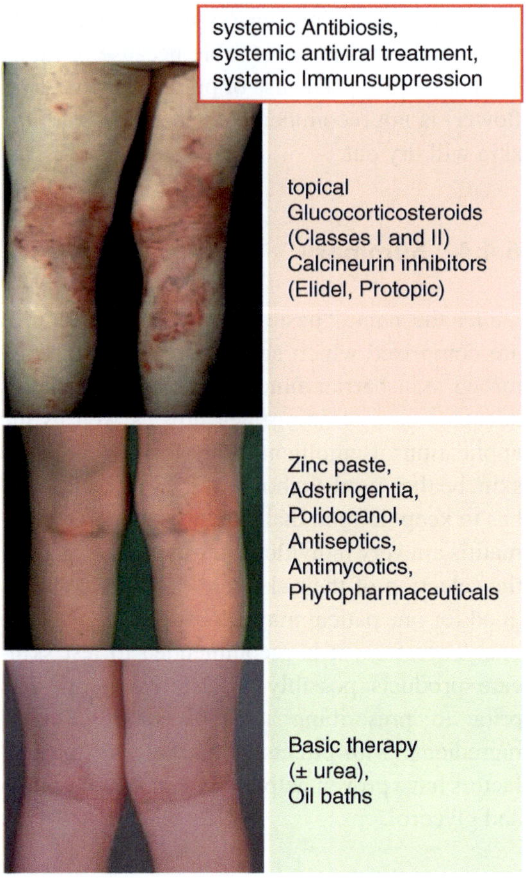

Fig. 6.9 Stepwise approach for different stages of therapy of atopic dermatitis

- Anti-inflammatory treatment.
- Antipruritic treatment.
- Prevention of further skin damage.

6.5.2 Anti-inflammatory Treatment

In the focus of anti-inflammatory treatment of acute eczema flares are topical glucocorticosteroids (TCS) (see Sect. 7.1 "Glucocorticosteroids") and topical calcineurin inhibitors (TCI). Rarely, systemic application of glucocorticosteroids (very short time!) is required [321]. The correct choice of vehicle in the sense of adequate galenics is crucial (see above).

6.5.3 Antipruritic Treatment

In order to fight the itch, moist preparations should be used which however may at the same time lead to further drying of the skin. Therefore, they should be combined with occlusion, i.e., as wet wraps (fat-moist in combination).

With this procedure, first an ointment-covered textile is applied which then is covered with a moist layer in an occlusive bandage (tube bandage; this has the additional advantage to prevent direct scratching). If the whole body is affected, one can use the same principle with the so-called wet pyjama or ointment cloth (Salbentuch). Lukewarm baths with the use of bath oils can support the acute anti-inflammatory and antipruritic effects. Even lotio alba can be used with an antipruritic effect. The most effective antipruritic treatment however is the application of topical glucocorticosteroids. Also, TCI has a direct antipruritic effect.

Often also systemic antihistamines are used, mostly those with sedating side effects, sometimes as intravenous infusion (see Chap. 7).

This acute treatment with medium-strong glucocorticosteroid topicals usually brings rapid improvement of skin lesions.

6.5.4 Inpatient Treatment

In the acute flare, patients can benefit greatly from a short inpatient therapy, since not only the adequate treatment procedures can be better performed, but also the change of environment including psychosocial factors often brings improvement (e.g., aeroallergens like house dust mites).

It is important that this phase of acute treatment is followed by consequent further treatment according to the stepwise management.

6.5.5 Amount of Topicals

One of the most common mistakes made by patients or inexperienced doctors is to prescribe and apply not enough emollients and specific topicals. Therefore, we usually ask the patients to bring back the empty tubes for the next visit, so we can immediately see how much has been really used.

A simple guide is the so-called fingertip rule: The amount of ointment on a fingertip of an adult corresponds to approx. 0.5 g ointment (tube opening 5 mm). This amount is good for an area of two adult palms (1% of body surface).

This makes clear how much ointment has to be used with regard to body surface involved at different ages, namely 250 g/week for a 12-year-old child.

With the use of specific anti-inflammatory substances, one has to consider that penetration of substances differs greatly between various body areas (Table 6.11).

Although it is actually simple, it is the topical dermatotherapy where most mistakes are made which explains very often the "unresponsiveness to treatment" in many patients. Therefore, educational programs also cover this aspect; special courses for dermatology or pediatric dermatology nurses, which then teach parents to correctly apply topical dermatotherapy, are offered in some countries.

Also, the application of wet wraps has to be trained [366, 713].

Table 6.11 Absorption of topically applied drugs is different, depending on body sites

Body region	(related to volar fore-arm)
Volar forearm	1
Head	5
Face	13
Abdomen	2.5
Back	2.5
Legs	0.5
Genital area	40

6.5.6 Summary

In the acute eczema flare, general management with using topical dermatotherapy (e.g., wet wraps) with the correct choice of the galenics is crucial. Topical glucocorticosteroids (mild to medium) are the strongest antipruritic agents, followed by topical calcineurin inhibitors. Most mistakes are made in topical dermatotherapy with regard to the way and the amount of ointment applied. The fingertip rule can help in practice to learn how much ointment is needed for which size of body surface involved.

7 Special Therapeutic Options and Substances in the Treatment of Atopic Eczema

7.1 Glucocorticosteroids

The introduction of topical glucocorticosteroids into dermatology may be regarded as the greatest progress in the treatment of numerous skin diseases in the second half of the twentieth century [776].

Only rarely systemic glucocorticosteroids are necessary in atopic dermatitis (see Sect. 7.8). It is almost always possible to treat an acute flare (see above) with topical treatment, maybe supported by intravenous antihistamines.

Still today—in spite of increasing skeptical and critical attitude of many patients—topical glucocorticosteroids are in the focus of treatment of atopic dermatitis [11, 333, 855, 880]. In the physician's desk reference of Germany ("Rote Liste"), there are over 100 preparations under the heading "Dermatica/Corticosteroids" in various applications forms, among them ca. 50 combination preparations with various galenic characteristics (systemic corticosteroids are not enlisted here).

7.1.1 Effects

The pharmacological effect of glucocorticosteroids is bound to specific molecular structures (Fig. 7.1). By the introduction of halogen atoms (e.g., fluor or chlorine) in position 9 alpha, the biological activity is considerably increased, similarly in position 6 alpha. Furthermore, esters or acetonides lead to a stronger efficacy of topical glucocorticosteroids.

Glucocorticosteroids have numerous effects on the skin (Fig. 7.2). The steroid molecule after absorption is bound to a cytoplasmic receptor in the keratinocyte which then is included in the nucleus where it influences the transcription of messenger RNA. Steroids have both stimulating and inhibiting effects. The name derives from the best-known effect, namely the mobilization of muscle glycogen and enhancement of neoglucogenesis from amino acids. In fatty tissue, glucocorticosteroids induce lipolysis, in various tissues they induce an involution in the direction of atrophy, especially in lymphatic cells, bone and skin. These effects are mainly due to an inhibition of DNA synthesis [316].

Via a gestagen-like effect, similar to progesterone, they also can induce sometimes serious

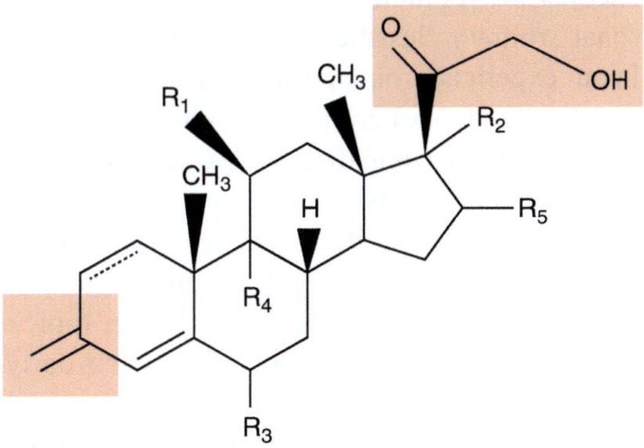

Fig. 7.1 Chemical structure of glucocorticosteroids

K. Eyerich, J. Ring, *Atopic Dermatitis - Eczema*, https://doi.org/10.1007/978-3-031-12499-0_7

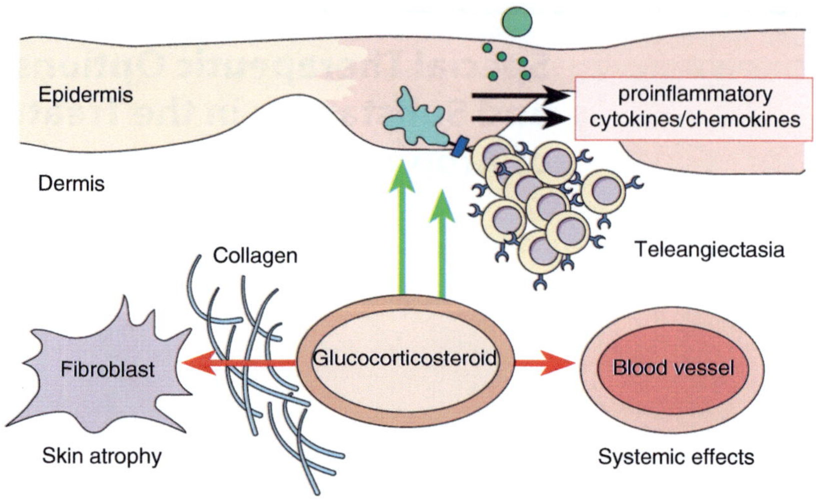

Fig. 7.2 Effects of glucocorticosteroids in the skin with intrinsically connected undesired side effects

psychologic alterations such as sleep loss, depression, euphoria, or nervosity.

Among the many variants of glucocorticosteroids, several substances have been developed with the aim to improve absorption efficacy while, on the other hand, minimizing side effects. Modifications include hydroxylation, or adding further carbon side chains, or adding halogenides. Methylprednisolone aceponate with double esterification increases the lipophilicity and thus the penetration into the epidermis. In several preclinical and clinical studies, this substance has shown to have a good efficacy and safety profile [471].

These differences in strength of efficacy have to be considered in practical use [474]. Most commonly used is the classification acc to Niedner [474] (Table 7.1). Table 7.2 shows a personal arbitrary classification for daily use [644]. In our experience, only products from class 1 or 2 (mild to moderate) are necessary for atopic dermatitis; for other skin diseases we very well need stronger preparations!

More important than the selection of the substance is the choice of adequate galenics (see above Chap. 6). In the acute phase, topical glucocorticosteroids can be used twice daily, later on, the application once daily is enough [844]. In the acute phase, the application of wet wrap has proven helpful [178, 329, 366].

Table 7.1 Classification of corticosteroids

Class I (mild)
• Dexamethasone (0.02–0.05%)
• Hydrocortisone (0.25–1.0%)
• Hydrocortisone acetate (0.25–1.0%)
• Prednisolone (0.4–0.5%)
Class II (moderately strong)
• Alclometasone dipropionate (0.05%)
• Betamethasone valerate (0.05%)
• Desoximetasone (0.25%)
• Flumethasone (0.02%)
• Flumetasone pivalate (0.02%)
• Fluocortolone (0.25%)
• Flupredniden-21-acetate (0.1–2.5%)
• Hydrocortisone-17-butyrate (0.1%)
• Hydrocortisone acetate (0.1%)
• Hydrocortisone buteprate (0.1%)
• Methylprednisolone aceponate (0.1%)
• Prednicarbate (0.25%)
• Triamcinolone acetonide (0.05–0.1%)
• Dexamethasone (0.1%)
Class III (strong)
• Amcinonide (0.1%)
• Betamethasone-17,21-dipropionate (0.05%)
• Betamethasone-17-valerate (0.1%)
• Desoximetasone (0.05%)
• Diflorasone-diacetate (0.01%)
• Diflucortolone-21-pentanoate (0.1%)
• Fluocinolone acetonide (0.025–0.1%)
• Fluticasone propionate (0.025–0.1%)
• Mometasone furoate (0.1%)
Class IV (very strong)
• Clobetasol propionate (0.05%)
• Diflucortolone valerate (0.3%)

Table 7.2 Classification of topical glucocorticosteroids according to their strength and side effects [644]

Class	Substance
I (not halogenated)	Hydrocortisone, hydrocortisone butyrate, hydrocortisone acetate, desonide, methyl prednisolone aceponate, prednisolone, prednicarbate
II (weakly fluorinated)	Fluorcortinbutyl ester, clobetasone butyrate, fluticasone propionate, mometasone furoate
III (medium strength)	Betametasone valerate, triamcinolone acetonide, flumethasone pivalate, fluocortolone dexamethasone
IV (strong)	Betametasone propionate, fluocinolone acetonide, diflucortolone valerate
V (very strong)	Fluocinonide, halcinonide, clobetasol propionate

In therapy-resistant chronified lichenified lesions, occlusive treatment can be necessary. One should be careful with the application of glucocorticosteroids in intertriginous areas (axilla, anogenital area) because side effects will appear faster (e.g., striae distensae) [249].

7.1.2 Side Effects

7.1.2.1 Skin Atrophy

Systemic side effects of topical glucocorticosteroids are extremely rare in the treatment of atopic dermatitis (Table 7.3) [76]. Very little—if at all—absorption has been observed. However, patients continuously are confused by these phenomena through wrong information by newspapers and other patients. There seems to be sometimes a real "corticophobia" which takes away a lot of time in the daily physician/patient interaction [170, 194, 235, 520, 524, 835].

More important are side effects of topical glucocorticosteroids on the skin (Table 7.4). Besides very rare cases of cortisone allergy, all these side effects more or less are directly connected to the pharmacological effect of the substance. The disturbance of the osteofollicular keratinization leads to the formation of comedones and steroid acne. The inhibition of proliferation and regeneration of epidermis induces atrophy, the degeneration of collagen and elastic tissue induces senile elastosis as well as the formation of teleangiectasia, purpura, and ecchymosis as well as striae distensae (stripes of pregnancy). Many patients are afraid of cortisone side effects [448, 525] (Figs. 7.3 and 7.4).

Table 7.3 Side effects of systemic glucocorticosteroids

Endocrinologic	Diabetes mellitus Catabolic metabolism Osteoporosis Disturbance of liquid metabolism Electrolyte disturbance Hypophyseal suppression (Cushing) Hypertonia
Gastrointestinal	Gastritis, ulcus ventriculi
Immunosuppression	Weakened defense against infections
Neurologic	Myopathy (muscle weakness) Neuropathy Psychic alterations (behavioral change, sleep loss, nervosity, "withdrawal symptoms")
Ophthalmologic	Cataract Glaucoma
Hematologic	Thromboembolic complications

Table 7.4 Side effects of topical glucocorticosteroids

Striae distensae
Atrophy (all skin layers) ("pseudo-cicatrices stellaires")
Embolia cutis (after intramuscular injection)
Increased light sensitivity
Cutis punctata linearis colli
Teleangiectasia, rubeosis steroidica
Pigmentation alteration
Hypertrichosis
Purpura and ecchymoses
Acne
Hair loss
Disturbance of wound healing
Perioral rosacea-like dermatitis
Granuloma gluteale infantum (Fig. 5.4)
Contact allergy

7.1.2.2 Perioral Rosacea-like Dermatitis

A special side effect of topical glucocorticoids is the so-called perioral or periorbital rosacea-like dermatitis (perioral dermatitis) which occurs after application of mostly halogenated glucocorticosteroids and—mostly in atopics—

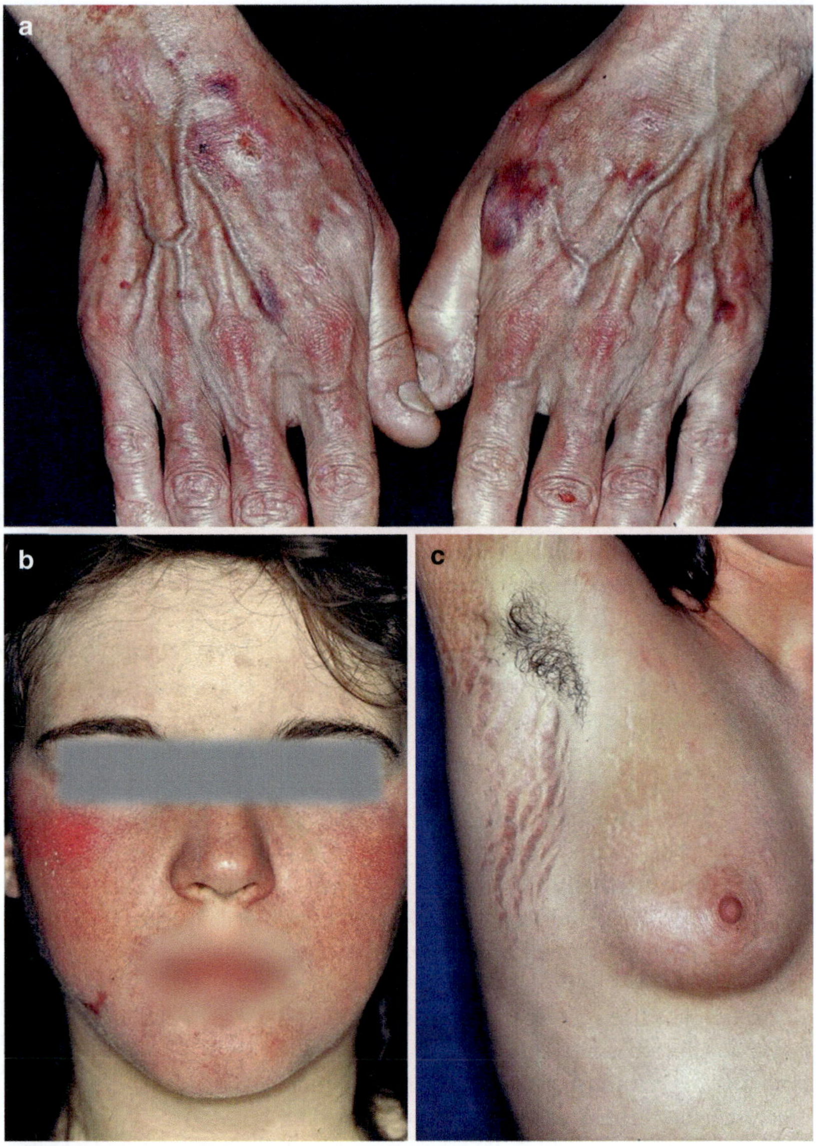

Fig. 7.3 Common side effects of topical corticosteroids in the skin. (**a**) Atrophy of the skin in atopic dermatitis. (**b**) Corticoderm after topidal corticosteroids in atopic dermatitis. (**c**) Striae distensae after short-time application of topical corticosteroid

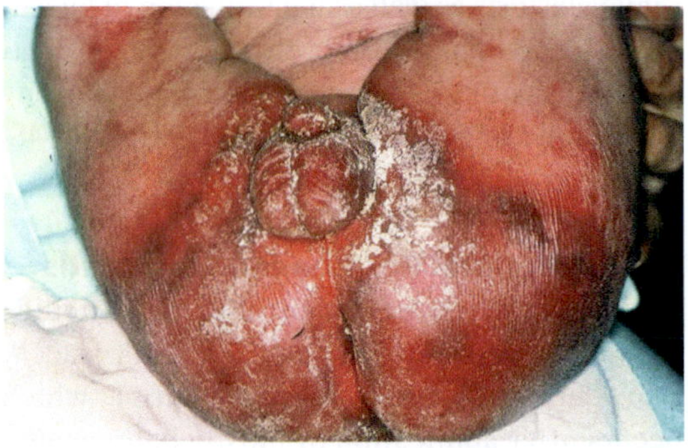

Fig. 7.4 Granuloma gluteale infantum in atopic dermatitis

becomes manifest in the face as fine acute pointed papules and redness with burning sensation (little itch) (Fig.7.5). In infants this can be seen in the diaper area as granuloma gluteale infantum (Fig. 7.4). Often the initial indication for the steroid treatment is no longer known, and the patients believe that the steroid is the only cure. Indeed, whenever the steroid is withdrawn, there is a rapid exacerbation which disappears immediately when the steroid is applied again. We explain our patients—not quite scientifically—this phenomenon "your skin is

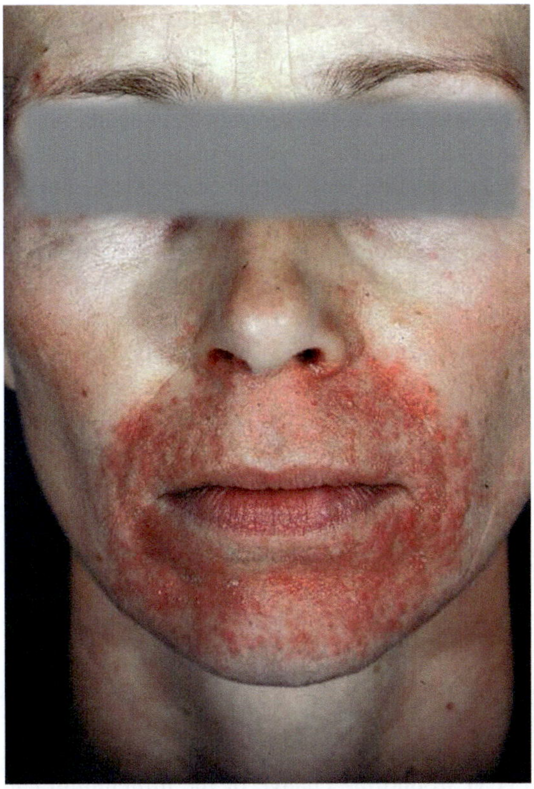

Fig. 7.5 Perioral rosacea-like dermatitis in atopic dermatitis

addicted to cortisone, we have to make a withdrawal procedure." The condition is also known as "red-face syndrome" or "cortisone addiction" [299].

7.1.2.3 Ocular Complications

Glaucoma and cataract development has to be named first as possible ocular complications [180, 298, 677]. This risk with topical glucocortical steroids was studied in 88 patients with facial and eyelid involvement. There was one patient with transient ocular hypertension and one patient with optic disc cupping as well as seven patients with the diagnosis of cataract, two corticosteroid-induced and four age-related ones, and one in relation to atopic dermatitis itself. These patients also had used systemic corticosteroids. The authors concluded that topical application of topical glucocorticosteroids per se is not related neither to the development of glaucoma nor of cataract; however, systemic glucocorticosteroids may lead to these complications [298]. These conditions should not be mixed with conjunctival reactions after some biologics, e.g., dupilumab (see below).

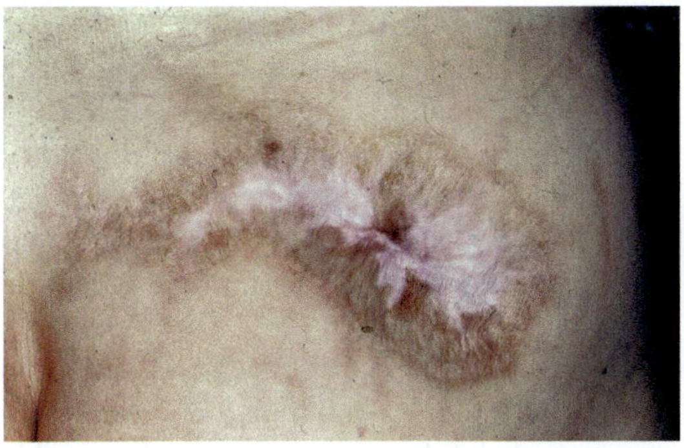

Fig. 7.6 Lipoatrophy after intramuscular cortisone injection

7.1.2.4 Lipodystrophy

Furthermore, the rare, but very unpleasant lipodystrophy after intramuscular injections of glucocorticosteroid crystal suspensions which can also lead to muscular atrophy has to be mentioned (Fig. 7.6).

7.1.2.5 Diminishing the Dose (Tapering)

Corticosteroid therapy never should be stopped abruptly since this might lead to a rebound of the skin disease. A slow dose reduction until the final stop is indicated. Either the efficacy strength of the steroid can be lowered by choosing different classes of substances or the frequency of application can be lowered (tandem therapy). This can be done by alternating the steroid application with basic emollients in increasingly rarer steroid applications (4 days steroid, 3 days basic emollient until 2 days steroid, 5 days emollient or steroids only once a week). This regimen can be prolonged over longer time periods in order to prevent new exacerbations [58, 303, 589]. Similar principles have also been described for topical calcineurin inhibitors (see Sect. 5.2) and have been called "proactive therapy" [879]. For this regimen it is helpful that many steroid producers also offer steroid-free skincare basic emollients with the same ingredients.

7.1.2.6 Combination Therapy

The use of combined glucocorticosteroids with antibiotics or antimycotics is seen critically; however, sometimes such a combination can be useful. What should be avoided is the uncritical "triple therapy" (corticosteroid, antibiotic plus antimycotic) instead of performing adequate diagnosis!

Specific prescriptions (magistral prescriptions) with individual mixtures of certain substances are helpful, especially also with regard to the individual estimation by the patient. However, a good pharmacist has to guarantee the galenic compatibility of the final emulsion; not everything can be mixed with everything.

There were no major serious adverse events in the study group. Furthermore, there was no influence of topical pimecrolimus on the development of normal immune responses after standard vaccination programs; thus, no clinically relevant systemic immunosuppressive effect was noted [473].

It makes no sense to combine TCS with TCI when treating the same body areas; however, it is not uncommon to use TCI in the face or other sensitive areas and TCS on the rest of the body [885].

7.1.3 Summary

The introduction of glucocorticosteroids in dermatology was the greatest progress for eczema patients in the second half of the twentieth century (Fig. 7.1). Systemic glucocorticosteroids only rarely have to be given in atopic dermatitis. The selection of the substances depends on the strength of efficacy, but more upon the galenic characteristics. For atopic dermatitis, mostly mild to moderate strength steroids are adequate. The application of topical glucocorticosteroids in the correct vehicle should be timely limited and ended via a "tandem therapy." Proactive strategies with once or twice weekly applications of the effective substance have proven helpful. The most important side effects of topical glucocorticosteroids comprise several steps of skin atrophy as well as the common manifestation of perioral rosacea-like dermatitis which occurs especially in young women after topical corticosteroids.

7.2 Topical Calcineurin Inhibitors

The introduction of topical calcineurin inhibitors (TCI) around the change of the millennium can be regarded as major progress in the treatment of atopic dermatitis. At the moment, two topical TCI are available, the substance tacrolimus from the mushroom Streptomyces tsukubaensis (brand name Protopic) and the semisynthetic ascomycin derivative pimecrolimus (brand name Elidel). Those substances also are sometimes called macrolactams because of their similarity in structure with macrolide antibiotics (Fig. 7.7).

Fig. 7.7 Chemical structure of tacrolimus and pimecrolimus

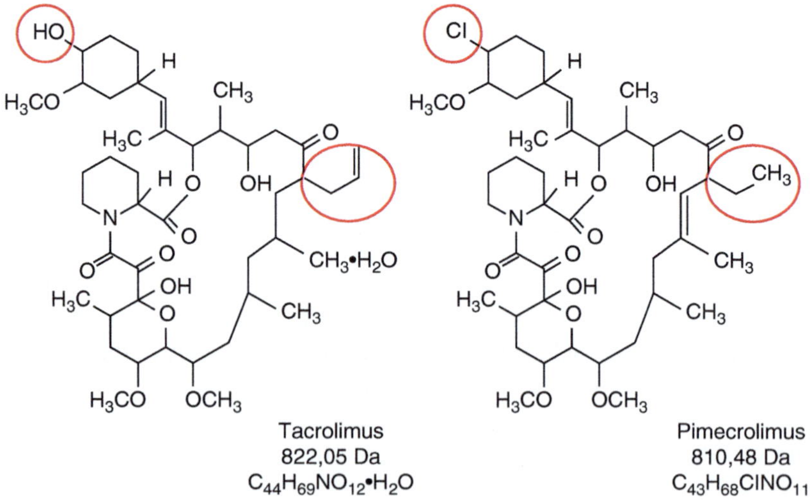

7.2.1 Pharmacologic Effects

TCI have similar effects as Cyclosporin A (see Sect. 7.8) with inhibition of T cells by binding to the cytosolic immunophilin (FK506 binding protein) and inhibiting calcineurin phosphatase (Fig. 7.8). Thereby, signal transduction and transcription of several proinflammatory cytokines in lymphocytes is inhibited [87, 878]; furthermore other inflammatory cells, like mast cells or basophil leukocytes, are inhibited. Contrary to glucocorticosteroids, TCI do neither inhibit the proliferation of keratinocytes nor fibroblasts, i.e., they have no atrophy-inducing side effects [622].

In addition to the anti-inflammatory effects, TCI seem to have a direct effect on skin nerves, and becomes manifest in a strong antipruritic activity independent of the anti-inflammatory effect [504, 771].

Tacrolimus is also in systemic use for organ transplantation. Newer developments include rapamycin (Sirolimus) as well as everolimus. Different from TCI, they act via a cytosolic protein mTOR (molecular target of rapamycin) and induce immunosuppressive effects in the nucleus (Fig. 7.8).

Numerous studies have shown the efficacy of tacrolimus and pimecrolimus in atopic dermatitis [578, 579, 620, 621, 672]. They are significantly effective compared to basic therapy, tacrolimus seems to be stronger than pimecrolimus [579]. Overall, the efficacy is comparable to mild topical glucocorticosteroids of class I and II. Tacrolimus is available in two concentrations (0.01% and 0.03%) and in a relatively greasy ointment (Protopic). Pimecrolimus is available as 1% cream and is well accepted by the patients. For practical application of TCI, a similar procedure as used with glucocorticosteroids is helpful. One should not stop abruptly. From twice daily application, one goes down to once daily and finally in a way of interval therapy to twice or once weekly, which can be performed over longer time periods and has been called "proactive therapy"; for this procedure, tacrolimus has a special registration in Europe [884].

Unfortunately, both preparations are only registered for children over 2 years, although according to the opinion of many experts they are extremely helpful in infants, especially with facial involvement, because of their safety profile [206, 469].

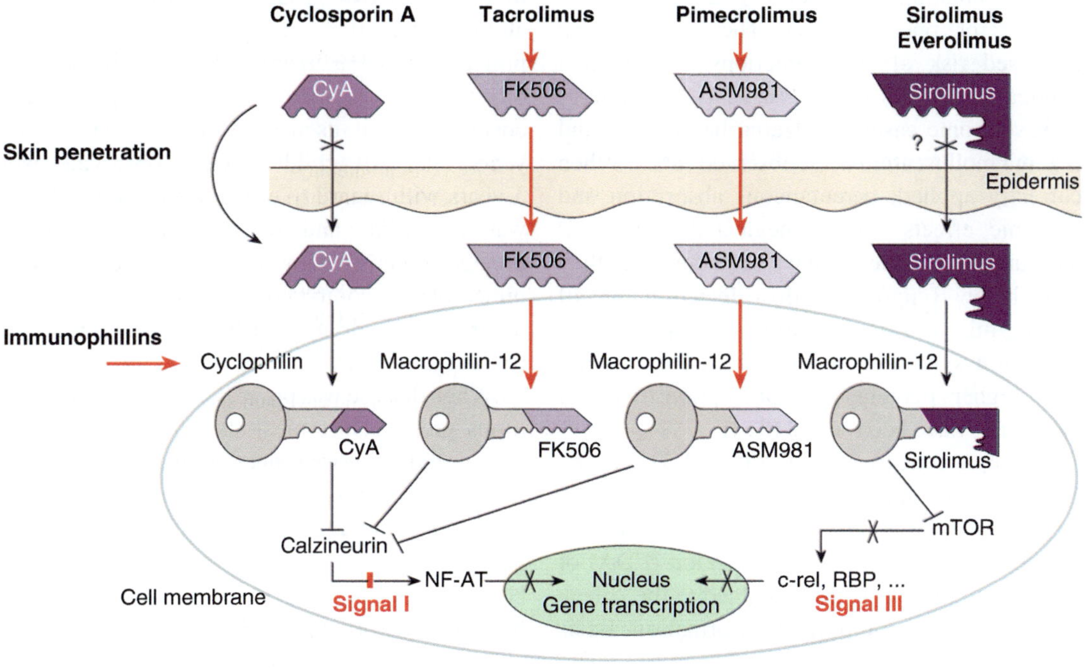

Fig. 7.8 Mechanism of action of calcineurin inhibitors and mTOR antagonists [87]

TCI can also be used in the treatment of side effects of topical steroids, such as perioral dermatitis [727].

7.2.2 Side Effects

TCI have advantages compared to glucocorticosteroids since they do not show the well-known side effects of topical glucocorticoids. They even can be used in perioral rosacea-like dermatitis or pityriasis alba [633].

Acute side effects consist of burning sensations after the first application (more common with tacrolimus), which mostly subsides during prolonged treatment. Occasionally patients observe severe burning dysesthesia when they drink alcohol; the mechanism of this reaction is not clearly established [510].

The transient warmth and tingling disappears usually after some days [508]. Contrary to topical glucocorticosteroids, pimecrolimus does not deplete Langerhans cells in the epidermis and thus seem not to influence the local immune response. Therapy with TCI in children did not show inhibitory effects on antibody responses after vaccination (diphtheria, tetanus, measles, rubeola, or pneumococci). There is also no increased risk of skin infections after topical application of TCI [382, 740, 834]. There have however some cases of eczema herpeticum and eczema molluscatum been observed [862]. When correctly applied, percutaneous absorption and systemic effects can be neglected. Whenever measurable blood levels have been detected, they were below 1 μg/mL, with a detection rate of 0.5 μg/mL. However, patients with the rare Netherton syndrome seem to be an exception; here higher percutaneous absorption rates of tacrolimus have been found [814].

A major concern with the use of TCI is the risk of cancer induction, which on the basis of theoretical considerations has been mentioned by the Food and Drug Administration (FDA) of the USA in the spring 2005 and led to the "black box warning" in the product information. Basis of this decision was an animal experimental study in hairless mice with well-known increased susceptibility to UV light effects and possible photocarcinogenicity, which was found for a higher (never commercially used) tacrolimus concentration in the sense of a shortened time until the appearance of undefined "skin tumors" [646].

This model has been very controversially discussed; the study has not been reproduced by other groups. Therefore, most expert committees or societies have recommended avoiding exaggerated sun exposure during treatment with topical TCI (but also glucocorticosteroids).

In large and long-term observation and clinical studies of patients treated with TCI, no increased incidences of malignant tumors have been observed, neither lymphoma nor melanoma or non-melanoma skin cancer [25]. In some studies, there were decreased prevalences of skin cancer in patients under TCI treatment [29, 125], maybe due to better sun protection in this patient group [472].

In a prospective randomized open trial in over 2000 infants the efficacy and safety of pimecrolimus was investigated. Infants were attributed randomly to two groups at first appearance of atopic dermatitis: one group was treated with pimecrolimus 1% cream as first-line therapy, the other group was treated with topical glucocorticosteroids as it used to be the standard some years ago. All children were observed over 5 years with regard to efficacy and safety. There was a similar and fast response to topical pimecrolimus therapy in infants treated with pimecrolimus compared to steroids. A rather high number of children never had to use topical steroids at all [740].

When disease was progressing, in the pimecrolimus group also topical steroids were used, in the steroid group stronger preparations or systemic treatment was applied.

TCI are not registered for use during pregnancy or lactation; however, they may probably be used off-label, so far no teratogenic effects have been reported [152, 824].

7.2.3 Summary

The introduction of specific anti-inflammatory treatments like topical calcineurin inhibitors tacrolimus and pimecrolimus was major progress since they do not exert atrophy-inducing side effects like topical glucocorticosteroids. In addition, they have a specific antipruriginous effect. TCI are especially valuable in eczema treatment in problem areas like the face or the anogenital area. They seem to be weaker in efficacy than topical glucocorticosteroids. TCI can also be used in a proactive regimen over long time periods in order to prevent exacerbations.

7.3 Antimicrobial Therapy

One of the pathophysiological characteristics of atopic eczema with definite practical clinical relevance is the high density of bacterial or otherwise microbial colonization of the skin surface, even in clinically uninvolved skin (see Chap. 5 "Role of Infection and Microbial Factors"). Apart from acute superinfections (e.g., impetiginized eczema, eczema herpeticum which can be difficult to treat [18], the mere colonization of the skin surface with pathogenic germs may contribute via various mechanisms to maintenance of inflammatory skin reactions. Scratching favors Staphylococcus aureus binding to the skin and contributes to the diéstruction of the skin barrier [18].

In the treatment, one has to distinguish between general antiseptic therapy and specific antimicrobial treatment by antibiotics, antimycotics, or virostatics.

7.3.1 Antiseptics

Antiseptics are substances which kill microbes of any kind or inactivate them; chemically, they belong to quite different structural classes.

Chlorhexidine is a cationic bis-biguanide with a relatively low potential risk of allergic sensitization which shows good effects in a 1% solution as chlorhexidine digluconate. It is useful for application in intertriginous areas and skin folds [761].

Povidone iodine can be used on large surfaces of infected or burnt skin; for eczema, it plays a minor role; however, it is used in small areas when they are eroded and superinfected.

Triclosane is effective in vitro against S. aureus, Klebsiella, and Proteus species and also has antimycotic activity. It exerts mild antibiotic effects which may give rise to the development of resistance. Triclosan can be mixed well in a water-in-oil emulsion and has anti-inflammatory effects. It can be used for a long-term treatment combined with adequate basic therapy (see Sect. 4.3 "Basic Therapy of Disturbed Skin Barrier Function").

Polyhexanide is a polymerized form of chlorhexidine which originally was used as surface disinfectant in the food industry. Its antimicrobial effect is due to disturbance of membranes and denaturation of microbial proteins. It is used for antisepsis in wound treatment; rare cases of allergies have been reported. It is also effective against methicillin-resistant Staphylococcus aureus (MRSA) .

Octenidine is used for disinfection in surgery and as an antiseptic cleansing agent for oral hygiene with good compatibility. It is hard to dissolve in a cream however there are some formulations with or without steroid (hydrophilic prednicarbat cream, NRF11.144/11.145 of the German National pharmaceutical formulation catalog).

Colorings have been used in topical antimicrobial therapy for decades; most of them are triphenylmethane dyes with broad antimicrobial activity [105]. Due to difficulties to produce large amounts in adequate purity and decreasing commercial interest, colorings often are no longer offered by the producers. The most commonly used colorings are Gentian violet (Crystal violet, pyoctanin) which is used in intertriginous areas in low concentrations (0.1–0.5%). The red substance Eosin can be used as 1% solution in oozing eczema lesions. The disadvantage is the intense staining potential on skin and textiles, which has to be discussed with the patient before treatment.

Clioquinol is effective in combination with topical glucocorticosteroids, especially in combination with color therapy in nummular variants of eczema.

Essential oils have a high representence and popularity in the lay press. As a matter of fact, they contain natural antimicrobial substances with also anti-inflammatory properties. However, some of them have a rather high potential for allergenicity, especially tea tree oil (Melaleuca alternifolia).

Silver nitrate (AgNO3) has been used for decades in wound treatment and in high dilution as an antiseptic.

Sodium hypochlorite is used in the USA as so-called bleach bath and it is popular for skin cleaning; small amounts of sodium hypochlorite are added to the tap water in the bathtub and induce an antimicrobial effect [343].

7.3.2 Antimicrobial Textiles (Functional Textiles)

New development can be seen in silver-coated textiles where the fiber—e.g., cotton—is coated with antiseptic substances, e.g., silver. Silver textiles have been used in atopic eczema and were able to significantly reduce colonization of skin with S. aureus, leading to a marked improvement of eczematous skin lesions as measured in the SCORAD without additional therapy [257] in a placebo-controlled trial.

Silver ions have a broad spectrum of antiseptic properties and do not induce the development of resistance. Allergies against silver are almost unknown. One problem that has not quite been finally solved yet is the eventual absorption of silver ions in inflamed skin. The acceptance of silver textiles from the side of the patients is very good [256] (Fig. 7.9).

Apart from silver ions, also other antiseptic substances or detergents have been bound to textile fibers in order to produce antimicrobial textiles like, e.g., benzalkonium chloride [363].

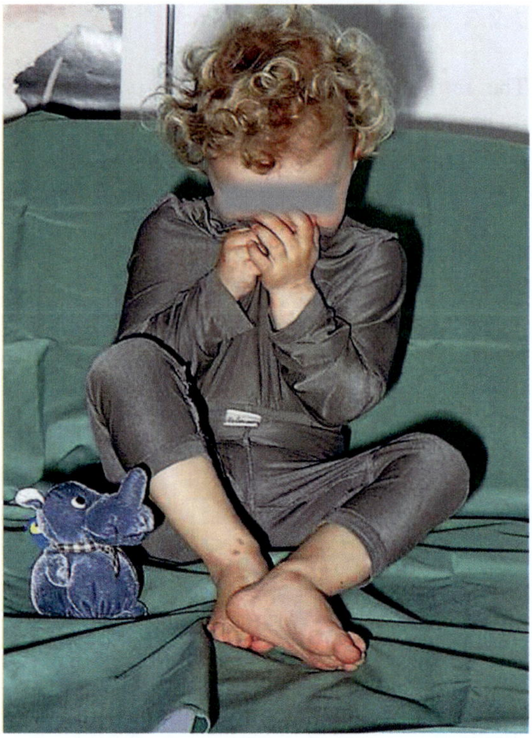

Fig. 7.9 Child with silver-coated textile

7.3.3 Antibiotic Therapy

7.3.3.1 Systemic Antibiotic Therapy

As long as there is only colonization of the skin surface without clinical signs of an infection, there is no indication for systemic antibiotic therapy in eczema [855]. In impetiginized eczema, especially with large surfaces involved, a short-time systemic antibiosis has proven helpful, especially with cephalosporins of newer generations (cefuroxime, cefadroxil, cefotiam) or penicillinase-resistant penicillins (oxacillin, flucloxacillin, dicloxacillin) [81, 219, 876, 877]. The use of systemic antibiotics have been studied in a recent systematic review [263]. In cases of penicillin allergy, macrolide substances or clindamycin can be used.

7.3.3.2 Topical Antibiotics

A topical antibiotic therapy is always connected with the possible risk of development of resistance and therefore has to be particularly indicated. First antiseptic measures should be used. There is also the risk of a contact sensitization especially for neomycin, tetracycline, or polymyxin [865].

Fusidic acid is the substance of first choice when topical antibiosis is required; it inhibits staphylococci in low concentrations and is also active against MRSA. Unfortunately, there is an increasing resistance against fusidic acid to be observed. In visibly impetiginized areas a combination of fusidic acid with topical glucocorticosteroids can be used.

Mupirocin is used as a nasal ointment and is effective against S. aureus carriers. It is used prophylactically [457].

Combinations of antibiotics with glucocorticosteroids are often used; however, it is questionable whether the antibiotic really brings additional effects. Most of the clinical trials have not shown a significant advantage of combined topicals compared to the pure glucocorticosteroids [263, 453].

In impetiginized eczema, the application of topical therapeutics is crucial. We recommend the procedure of "wet wraps" (see Chap. 6). An antiseptic substance like polyhexanide 0.2% or chlorhexidine 0.5% is applied in a wet wrap. This, together with a wet wrap of basic treatment or steroid is placed on top and fixed by a commercially available tube bandage. Over this, a second dry tube bandage is fixed. The substances should remain for several hours, and the wet wraps should be continually moisturized [2].

7.3.4 Antimycotic Therapy

In seborrheic skin areas, sometimes patients have a predilection for eczema together with the growth of the opportunistic yeast Malassezia furfur (head and neck dermatitis). Here a therapy with antibiotics, e.g., ketoconazole or itraconazole, but also ciclopirox olamine is effective and leads to improvement of eczematous skin lesions [103, 497, 699, 757]. Systemic antimycotic therapy is rarely indicated. Some authors recommend combined antimycotic and antibacterial therapy in all forms of severe atopic dermatitis. It is natural that superinfection with Candida albicans, especially in intertriginous areas, or dermatophytes (Trichophyton) should be treated with antimycotics.

7.3.5 Antiviral Therapy

Herpes simplex infection in atopic eczema can give rise to the serious disease of eczema herpeticum (see Chap. 4). In these cases, systemic antiviral therapy, best with three times daily intravenous infusions of acyclovir 5 mg/m^2 or 15 mg/kg body weight, is the method of choice [887]. In cases of relapses, long-term prophylaxis with valacyclovir is recommended [733].

Infections with molluscum contagiosum are not rare in atopic dermatitis and may give rise to the involvement of large skin surfaces and special localizations (genital area), which makes treatment difficult. Careful removal or cryotherapy is the most commonly used treatment options.

Also, exacerbation of eczematous skin lesions has been observed with Coxsackie virus infections "Eczema coxsackium" [476, 542] and is treated symptomatically.

Also, varizella-zoster virus infection can be a complication of eczema [712]; vaccination in early childhood but also in the elderly is recommended [431].

7.3.6 Vaccination and Atopic Dermatitis

It is one of the most commonly asked questions whether patients with atopic dermatitis should be vaccinated like normal children. While this was a debate some decades ago, this question can now be answered clearly with "Yes." There is not only no increased risk but it is recommended to perform vaccination programs especially carefully in patients with atopic dermatitis since they are more at risk than other persons [365]. The only caution which has to be observed is the time point of vaccination: One should not immunize during an acute eczema flare.

This also holds true for the new opportunities of vaccination against human papillomavirus (HPV); there have been single reports of exacerbation of eczema after vaccination with Gardasil or Cervarix, which however were spontaneously resolving.

Patients with atopic dermatitis have an increased risk after smallpox vaccination with scarification to develop eczema vaccinatum. That is why this classic vaccination against Variola Vera with scarification was contraindicated in atopic eczema (see Chap. 4). With a newly developed vaccine using the modified virus Ankara (MVA) injected subcutaneously, it is possible to achieve immunogenicity with good compatibility also in patients with atopic eczema [163]. Should a catastrophe occur by bioterroristic attacks effective vaccination strategies would be possible for doctors and nurses working in intensive care units.

7.3.7 COVID-19 Infection and Vaccination

At the moment there is little evidence that SARS-CoV-2 infection increases the risk for eczema development or exacerbations—although this would not be too surprising. Other inflammatory diseases have shown exacerbations after COVID-19 [555] (see also Chap. 4).

The situation regarding COVID-19 vaccination is a matter of discussion in lay people. However, several societies have given clear recommendations and position statements on the risk of anaphylaxis or severe allergic reactions in patients with atopic eczema or other allergic diseases [405, 555]. The message is that people with AE can well be vaccinated. Contraindications may be seen in patients with prior history of anaphylaxis to ingredients of the vaccine to be applied.

7.3.8 Summary

Antimicrobial strategies are not only important in the treatment of acute infections, but also generally in the prophylaxis with regard to the high density of colonization of the skin surface with pathogenic germs in these patients. Generally, antiseptics are used like triclosan, in the acute treatment also colorings or clioquinol. Functional textiles coated with silver or other antiseptics represent an elegant method without using systemic or topical drugs ("textiles as drugs"). In severe cases, systemic antibiosis or antimycotic treatment in head and neck dermatitis can be used. The commonly discussed question of whether patients with atopic dermatitis can be vaccinated like normals can be answered with a clear "yes." There are only considerations with regard to the time point. One should not vaccinate during an acute eczema flare. Patients with anaphylaxis to ovalbumin should be tested with the vaccine before treatment.

Atopic eczema is not a contraindication for COVID-19 vaccination [659].

7.4 Antihistamines

Histamine is the best-known mediator substance of IgE-mediated allergic reactions [156, 746]. After its release from activated mast cells or basophil leukocytes, it exerts the well-known proinflammatory effects rapidly on vessels, superficial skin nerves, and smooth muscles. When injected into the skin, the classic Lewis trias can be observed:

- Increase in capillary permeability of endothelial cells (plasma exsudation, wheal formation).
- Increase of perfusion by vasodilatation (erythema).
- Axon reflex via superficial nerves (flare).

Together with these objectively visible effects goes the elicitation of the subjective symptom "itch." Therefore, it was natural to use antihistamines for the treatment of itch.

Histamine Receptors

Histamine exerts its effects via four different specific receptors; the H1 and the H2 receptor are also expressed in the skin, while H3 receptors are located in the central nervous system and H4 receptors on various leukocytes [292, 293, 746].

For most allergic symptoms, H1 effects are important, H2 receptors play a role in the effect on the gastric mucosa (acid secretion) as well as on the heart. There are also H2 receptors in the skin, facilitating flush reactions.

H3 receptors in the central nervous system allow an autocrine inhibition of histaminergic neurons, leading to increased vigilance.

Bovet and Staub introduced antihistamines into the therapy of allergic diseases in 1937 [90]. In the following, under the term antihistamines, we mainly address H1 antagonists.

Newly described Histamine H4 receptor antagonists may act against itch [528, 860]. However, clinical trials in atopic dermatitis failed to prove efficacy in improvement of cutaneous inflammation.

Generations of Antihistamines

In practice one often reads about various "generations" of antihistamines (Table 7.5); classic antihistamines with the well-known sedating side effects are the first generation. They also exert anticholinergic and antiserotoninergic effects. On the other hand, also some tricyclic antidepressants have antihistamine effects. There is a certain overlap that can be used in strongly pruritic conditions [247, 529].

As second generation, the so-called nonsedating antihistamines came into use 25 years ago [65]; they do not cross the blood/brain barrier and thus have no sedating effects in the central nervous system, at least in normal doses. Some of these substances also have other anti-allergic effects by acting on inflammatory cells such as eosinophil migration (cetirizine) or mast cell activation (loratadine), or superoxide formation of leukocytes (loratadine and azelastine) [609, 747].

Under the term "third generation," substances are comprised which are metabolites of well-known H1 antagonists which are no longer further metabolized in the liver or in the kidney such as levocetirizine, desloratadine, or fexofenadine.

7.4.1 Effects of H1 Antagonists

Antihistamines are used all over the world as standard treatment in the therapy of acute flares of atopic eczema; however, there is only limited evidence and only few well-controlled studies [492]. This holds true, especially for the older classical antihistamines with sedating properties like dimetindene, clemastine or doxylamine, or diphenhydramine. Maybe this can be explained by the fact that these substances have been introduced already 50 or 60 years ago, so before the era of randomized prospective controlled trials.

For the newer nonsedating antihistamines, there is a variety of studies which show positive effects against itch also in atopic eczema [306, 387] as well as a high number of uncontrolled pilot studies [402, 442, 529]. However, effects at skin lesions are limited or absent [880].

Table 7.5 Generations of antihistamines (H1 antagonists)

Classic sedating antihistamines	Newer, less sedating antihistamines	Metabolites of non-sedating antihistamines
Dimetindene	Terfenadine	Fexofenadine
Clemastine	Cetirizine	Levocetirizine
Diphenhydramine	Loratadine	Desloratadine
Alimemazine	Ebastine	
Bamipine	Mizolastine	
Cyproheptadine	Rupatadine	
Dexchlorpheniramine	Azelastine	
Hydroxyzine	Levocabastine	
Doxylamine	Bilaxtene	

7.4.1.1 Modes of Application

Usually antihistamines are applied systemically, most of them orally. There are only two preparations, namely dimetindene and clemastine, which are available for intravenous injection. Apart from the topical application of medium-strength glucocorticosteroids in the correct galenics, the intravenous infusion of H1 antagonists is standard therapy in treating pruritus and acute eczema flares in our department.

The sedating side effects can be neglected in the acute treatment of severe eczema flares in hospitalized patients, or when applied in the evening.

Topical use of antihistamines as cream or gels for treating pruritus after insect stings is often advertised, but probably only effective due to the cooling gel consistency of the vehicle. Due to these exsiccating properties of topical antihistamine preparations, they are not recommended in the treatment of atopic dermatitis.

7.4.2 Side Effects of Antihistamines

7.4.2.1 Classical H1 Antagonists

Here the sedating effects of classic H1 antagonists have to be mentioned first which also increase side effects of other centrally active drugs or alcohol. Patients have to be informed about these side effects which become manifest in deterioration of vigilance in traffic, but also in occupational life when difficult machines have to be operated. I recall reports about severe traffic accidents by patients who continued a therapy with strongly sedating antihistamines (e.g., cyproheptadine, hydroxyzine) without or against medical advice. When an antihistamine therapy has to be continued over longer periods in everyday life, it is absolutely required to take a nonsedating antihistamine (fexofenadine) in the morning and sedating antihistamines (dimetindene) only in the evening.

In small children, paradoxical reactions can occur if the sedating antihistamines stimulate an arousal reaction.

Due to the concomitant anticholinergic, antimuscarinergic, or antiserotoninergic effects, other side effects like difficulties in urination, attack of glaucoma, dry mouth, and others have to be considered, especially when other similarly acting drugs are given.

7.4.2.2 Second and Third Generation

The substances of the second or third generation are commonly called "nonsedating." There are marked individual differences which are at the moment not totally explained by pharmacology, but also are not due to a simple placebo or nocebo effect.

Some companies circumvent the problem of sedation in some countries by the simple recommendation to take tablets in the evening after dinner. According to my opinion, the least sedating H1 antagonists are terfenadine [65] and its metabolite fexofenadine as well as desloratadine, which are also registered in the USA and permitted for pilots of aeroplanes since they do not interfere with vigilance.

7.4.2.3 Cardiac Arrythmia

Some antihistamines of the second generation (astemizole and terfenadine) were associated with severe cardiac arrhythmias, especially prolongation of the QT time; this was due to increased levels of the substance with concomitant application of other drugs metabolized via cytochrome P450 enzymes (e.g., azole antimycotics, macrolide antibiotics), but also naturally occurring substances in grapefruit juice. These effects are no longer observed with the metabolite fexofenadine. Astemizole has been withdrawn from the market in many countries.

Several authors recommend increasing the dose of antihistamines when the effect is not sufficient up to a fourfold dose in diseases such as urticarial [494]. However, there may also be increased side effects and in atopic dermatitis, this may only be useful in a few cases given the limited efficacy.

7.4.2.4 Pregnancy

A special problem is the treatment of pregnant women. There are few convincing studies giving clear-cut evidence. For safety reasons, most companies write on their informations to avoid intake during pregnancy. We often advise patients then to take the antiemetics used for a decade with antihistaminergic effects such as dimenhydrinate which have proven safe for millions of pregnant women.

Also, preparations of the first generation which are registered for infants, like doxylamine, dimetindene, or clemastine can be used. Also, no negative reports are published regarding loratadine and cetirizine.

7.4.3 Other Anti-Allergic Substances

Other antihistamines, i.e., antagonists of H2, H3, or H4 receptors, do not play a role in the treatment of atopic dermatitis at the moment. Drugs from the group of psychopharmaceuticals with simultaneous antihistaminergic properties can be helpful in some patients with severe atopic eczema in long-term treatment like opipramol or doxepin.

Also, the mast cell blocker ketotifen with antihistamine properties can be used; its effect usually takes some weeks [225, 351]. Also topically applicable derivatives of cromoglycates which have proven to be active in respiratory allergy can be used as mast cells stabilizers after oral application in patients with atopic eczema and concomitant food allergy or mastocytosis. The oral application of cromoglycate as a capsule or powder four times a day before the meals may be beneficial in eczema patients with food allergy.

The leukotriene antagonist montelukast is known for asthma therapy and has shown beneficial effects in pilot studies in atopic eczema [899].

7.4.4 Opioid Receptor Antagonists

Since the perception of itch occurs in the brain by activation of a variety of areas in the central nervous system (Fig. 7.10), also centrally acting strategies have been tried. Opioid receptor antagonists have been tried as antipruritics, e.g., nalmefene [519] and Naltrexone [481] however they did not make it into routine use.

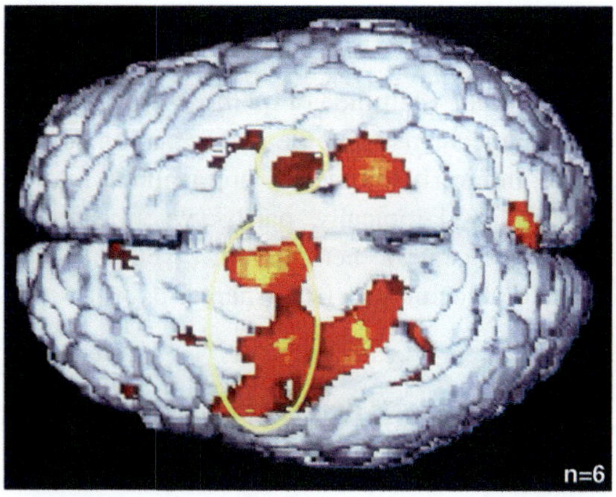

Fig. 7.10 Visualization of itch sensation in the brain in positron emission tomography (PET). Activation of motoric areas in histamine-induced itch: Gyrus precentralis and supplementary motor area

7.4.5 Summary

Antihistamines are standard therapy in the treatment of itch all over the world; however, there are few controlled studies in atopic dermatitis. Topical antihistamines can be neglected in atopic eczema. The sedating side effects of classic antihistamines may be beneficial in the acute treatment of severe flares in hospitalized patients or when given in the evening. Although increased plasma histamine levels have been found in atopic eczema, histamine does not seem to be the critical mediator of the atopic itch sensation.

7.5 Other Antipruritic and Anti-Inflammatory Substances

Itch is the central symptom of atopic dermatitis and represents a major problem for most patients and their families, impairing or destroying the quality of life. We all know the poster which went around the world with the introduction of pimecrolimus (Elidel), showing an infant with a T-shirt with the inscription: "If I don't sleep, nobody sleeps!" (Roger Allen, Nottingham) as well as the pictures of bloody linen due to nightly scratch attacks.

Due to the multitude of qualities and elicitors, but also mechanisms of the itch sensation, a variety of antipruritic strategies are available, partly to be applied topically, partly systemically, or reflecting central nervous involvement with behavioral techniques (see Chapter psyche).

7.5.1 Topical Antipruriginous Agents

In the acute itch condition, physical means are helpful in applying cool stimuli (wet wraps or lotio alba) or even punctual hyperthermia, e.g., in insect bites ("bite-away" pen). Glucocorticosteroids are the most potent antipruriginous pharmacotherapeutic topical agents (see Sect. 7.1) as well as topical calcineurin inhibitors (TCI) (see Sect. 7.2). Besides, a variety of other substances is used therapeutically in order to diminish or treat itch sensation.

7.5.2 Local Anesthetics

Since itch sensation is mediated via excitation of sensory nerve fibers in the skin, local anesthetics naturally have an effect especially after intradermal or subcutaneous injection. This is no acceptable method for larger skin areas. Yet, in treating very circumscribed, chronic lichenified, or pruriginous skin lesions, the intradermal injection of local anesthetics can be helpful.

The topical application of local anesthetics as a lotion, cream, or ointment (e.g., Emla) is of little use in treating eczema, except for small circumscribed areas which can occur in the condition of notalgia paraesthetica. The topical application of local anesthetics is connected with a rather high risk of sensitization and development of contact allergy.

7.5.3 Polidocanol

Polidocanol is a polymerized local anesthetic from dodecyl alcohol and ethylene dioxide. This substance with a molecular weight of 600 D can penetrate especially into inflamed skin and reaches sensory nerves, and thus exerts an antipruriginous effect [246].

Polidocanol is used either as lotion (5%), suspension, or cream. In very dry skin, it can be combined with 3–5% urea [915]. This treatment can be self-applied by the patients as often as they wish. Thus, one can spare topical glucocorticosteroid use.

7.5.4 Cannabinoid Agonists

Endogenous cannabinoids play a role in epidermal differentiation; receptors can be found on keratinocytes, sensory nerve fibers, and inflammatory cells. With cannabinoid agonists, antipruriginous effects can be observed. In a larger study, by the addition of the cannabinoid agonist *N*-palmitoyl ethanolamine in a differentiated basic therapeutic vehicle (Physiogel AI), a good effect in atopic dermatitis has been observed [383, 763].

7.5.5 Capsaicin

The vanilloid alkaloid capsaicin binds to the receptor TRPV1 on sensory nerve fibers and keratinocytes and leads to an inactivation of sensory nerve fibers. Acutely after application, there is a burning painful sensation [626, 853, 906]. Capsaicin, the effective substance in tabasco sauce, is better used in strongly itching circumscribed chronic lesions or in pruritus on non-altered skin than in atopic dermatitis. When used, one should carefully watch the doses and start with lower concentrations from 0.025% over 0.05% to 0.1%. Capsaicin should not be used in intertriginous areas, in the face or on mucous surfaces.

7.5.6 Tar Preparations

Coal tar is one of the oldest treatments going back into the history of dermatology. It is a not very well-defined mixture of more than 1000 substances, among them also high concentrations of polycyclic aromatic hydrocarbons (PAHs).

Crude coal tar is produced when coal is heated without oxygen. Liquor carbonis detergens is made by extracting pix lithanthracis 1:5 with alcohol.

In earlier times, tar treatment with wood, slate, or coal tar was standard, especially the coal tar extract (liquor carbonis detergens) or pure coal tar (pix lithanthracis). These preparations have an anti-inflammatory and antipruriginous effect without the mechanisms being known.

Tar is a mixture of many, partly still unknown substances which originate in the process of distillation. Tar products have antiproliferative, anti-inflammatory, and antimicrobial activities. Especially phenolic components seem to have antipruritic effects [526]. The use of tar preparations is controversial in many countries due to the carcinogenicity observed in animal experiments [594].

While there is animal data on carcinogenicity of coal tar, there is still a controversy with regard to the safety of its use in humans. Therefore, a large historical cohort study was performed studying the late effects of coal tar treatment in eczema and psoriasis, the Radboud study (LATER study) in 14,009 patients suffering mostly from psoriasis or eczema. The study covered observation periods between 13 and 43 years after treatment and found no increased values neither for skin cancer nor non-skin malignancies [663]. This supports earlier studies from Hannuksela-Svahn et al. [307], Larko, [443]. The authors concluded that coal tar can be maintained as a safe treatment in dermatological practice. We use pix lithanthracis rarely and only in hospital settings and prefer liquor carbonis detergens which can be mixed with emollients to produce acceptable preparations for the patients.

There may be a revival for tar products since it counteracts Th2/Th22 reaction via the aryl hydrocarbon (AH) receptor and STAT6 dephosphorylation and upregulates Filaggrin expression [80]. The development of substances directly inhibiting the AHR such as Tapinarof may also be interpreted as "smart tar" and seems promising as new topical treatment formulations in clinical trials [326, 587].

7.5.6.1 Sulfonates

Sulfonates differ from tar since they are neither phototoxic, mutagenic, teratogenic nor cancerogenic [187, 838]. They are produced from slant oil and represent ammonium bituminosulfonates. Effective substances have a thiophene ring structure. Sulfonates are used also in folliculitis or furuncles to attract neutrophil leukocytes.

In atopic eczema, lotions or pastes can be used which have beneficial effects in chronic lichenified skin areas.

7.5.7 Adstringentia

By alteration of superficial proteins in the epidermis, adstringentia of natural or synthetic origin can have beneficial effects, going along with exsiccation and anti-inflammatory effects. Most commonly used are preparations from oak bark or synthetic tannins on the basis of gallic acid (Tannolact, Tannosynt). Lukewarm hand baths together with tannic acid have shown to be beneficial in dyshidrotic hand dermatitis, as well as seat baths in perianal or perigenital eczema.

7.5.8 Etheric Oils and Others

Among etheric oils, especially menthol is the best-known antipruriginous agent; its effect is mediated via direct action on the cold receptor fibers thus overlaying the itch sensation. However, menthol is only available in solution, mostly alcoholic, and thereby has a very strong exsiccative effect. It is mostly used in acute conditions such as after insect bites where there is a very localized application area.

A variety of other substances is used topically against itch or against eczema. The nonsteroidal anti-inflammatory drug bufexamac was promoted for some years to be as active as corticoids. However, due to the rather strong sensitizing properties, it is no longer in wide use [140] and has been withdrawn in most countries.

Topical antihistamines which are used as gels for insect stings are not recommended for treatment of atopic eczema. This also holds true for topical preparations of doxepin or acetylsalicylic acid.

7.5.9 Summary

Itch is the most important symptom of atopic eczema and is at the center of successful therapy. The order to children "stop scratching" does not make sense since itch is defined as the unpleasant sensation eliciting the urge to scratch. The most important antipruriginous strategy is topical anti-inflammatory treatment with glucocorticosteroids or calcineurin inhibitors. Besides, polidocanol in good galenic mixtures can have an antipruritic effect, equally cannabinoid agonist, tar, and sulfonate preparations as well as tannic acid which have been used in the long-term treatment of lichenified areas and have been shown to spare topical corticosteroids. Numerous novel topical substances aiming at changing the cutaneous microbiome are currently in early clinical trials. It is too early to make a general statement whether this interesting approach is promising or not.

7.6 UV Therapy

Phototherapy is a standard procedure in the treatment of many inflammatory skin diseases [335]. There are various modalities using different spectra of UV irradiation [434, 628]:

- Heliotherapy (this is the exposure to natural sunlight).
- Broadband UVB (280–320 nm).
- Narrowband UVB (311–313 nm).
- UVA (320–400 nm).
- UVA1 (340–400 nm).
- Photochemotherapy using a combination of UV with photosensitizers, e.g., psoralens (PUVA).
- Radiation with visible light or blue light.

7.6.1 Heliotherapy

Heliotherapy uses the exposure to natural sunlight under controlled conditions. It is crucial to test the patient's photosensitivity (establishing the minimal erythema dose or checking Fitzpatrick's light sensitivity skin types) [582].

Heliotherapy is especially performed using climate conditions such as different altitudes, either very low beyond sea level as on the Dead Sea in Israel or at high altitude like in Davos, Switzerland (1560 m) [217, 310].

The patient is told to precisely watch the time of sun exposure, starting with very short periods of 2–3 min and slowly increasing the time.

7.6.2 UVB Radiation

UVB radiation is the standard treatment of psoriasis and many inflammatory skin diseases; it has also a special effect on pruritus, also on pruritus without skin alteration.

Studying the individual wavelength within the UV spectrum, it has been found that 311 nm seems to be the most effective, which is called narrowband UV radiation [285]. It has been shown that phototherapy with UVB is able to stimulate the production of antimicrobial peptides in the epidermis [271].

7.6.3 UVA Radiation

Through development of special lamps, the application of longwave UV spectrum was possible, especially through the development of infrared filters which lower the typical heat induction.

The mechanisms of UV radiation-induced immunosuppression are complex, some of them obviously occurring as a result of the repair processes induced by damage to epidermal structures, especially DNA, but also changes in membrane phospholipids and trans-urocanic acid and tryptophan [265]. Since the group of Margaret Kripke has shown that UV radiation can suppress delayed-type immunity against transplanted tumors in mice [236], photoimmunology has developed as an exciting branch of research [336]. In the epidermis, Langerhans cells (CD1d) and langerin-positive CD103 negative dendritic cells migrate to the draining lymph node and stimulate the production of regulatory T cells [728]. In experimental studies, it has been found that there are obviously two peaks within the electromagnetic spectrum which show especially marked effects with regard to immunosuppression, namely in the UVB range around 310 and in the UVA range around 370 nm [265].

Especially within the longwave spectrum of UVA, the UVA1 part (340–400 nm) has been first studied by Krutmann et al. [434]. Different doses of UVA are used [576]. Krutmann in his first studies used the high dose of 130 J/cm^2; we prefer a medium dose (50–60 J/cm^2) which is more efficacious than the low dose (10–20 J/cm^2) and is tolerated well [421].

Apart from atopic eczema, UVA1 is also used in localized scleroderma and granuloma anulare [666]. UVA1 has shown an inhibitory effect on mediator-secreting cells such as histamine from basophils or mast cells [432, 433].

In an own study on 230 patients treated with low-dose, medium-dose, and high-dose UVA1 over 6 years, we could prove the good therapeutic effects in atopic eczema, scleroderma, lichen sclerosus et atrophicus, prurigo nodularis, and cutaneous T cell lymphoma [666]. Eighty four percent of 86 patients with atopic eczema showed moderate to marked improvement after 3 weeks of UVA1 radiation while low-dose was considerably weaker [421].

UVA1, besides anti-inflammatory effects, also seems to have specific antipruritic efficacy which is well accepted by the patients. We perform UVA1 treatment in a total of 15 sessions over 3 weeks with a slow increase of dose. UVA1 has its place in acute flares of eczema and is tolerated well [411].

In actual guidelines both narrowband UVB and medium dose UVA-1 are recommended [885].

7.6.4 Photochemotherapy

There is no doubt that the most effective type of UV therapy is, together with the use of photosensitizing substances, photochemotherapy, e.g., psoralens (with UVA, PUVA). However, this also is the treatment with most side effects; it should be preserved for severe cases and can be compared to systemic immunosuppression [50].

Systemic application of psoralens is nowadays used only rarely. The topical application in a bath (balneophotochemotherapy) or in a cream (cream PUVA) is preferrable [283, 284, 336].

Psoralen is used in a concentration between 0.1 and 0.5 mg/l (methoxypsoralen 8-MOP) or 0.3% meladinine in a lukewarm bath (32–35 °C over 20 min). Alternatively, psoralen can be incorporated in a cream (0.001%) which is allowed to penetrate the skin over 30 min prior to UVA radiation. This method is preferably used in localized areas such as hand or foot eczema or nummular variants.

7.6.5 Visible Light

New developments comprise the application of visible light, especially the spectrum of the blue light, sometimes also called "light vaccine" which has been studied in pilot studies [44].

Often UV therapy is combined with the use of salt baths (photosole therapy), trying to imitate the effects of climate therapy at the Dead Sea or at other seasides.

7.6.6 Extracorporal Photophoresis

The method of extracorporal photophoresis was introduced in the 80s. Leukocytes are removed from the peripheral blood by cell apheresis and irradiated outside of the body with UV and 8-MOP [407]. This method represents a real immunosuppression and is preferably used in the treatment of cutaneous T cell lymphomas; however, also in very severe cases of atopic eczema [408, 409, 562].

7.6.7 Summary

Despite the growing options we have regarding systemic treatments, UV radiation retains its place as a standard regimen in the therapy of atopic eczema. Most commonly narrowband UVB (311 nm) or UVA1 wavelengths are used. When localized skin areas like palms or soles are severely affected, also balneo or cream phototherapy (PUVA) can be helpful.

Apart from local reactions like erythema, burning or triggering an eczema flare, there are no serious long-term risks with regard to skin cancer or Phototherapy [822], except for systemic PUVA treatment with a certain risk potential [460]. Due to the unknown risk of long-term side effects in childhood, this treatment should be reserved for very severely affected children upon special indication. In very severe cases of atopic eczema, extracorporal photopheresis can be helpful.

7.7 Allergen-Specific Immunotherapy

While allergen-specific immunotherapy (ASIT), also called hyposensitization, has a standard place in the treatment of IgE-mediated allergies of airways and insect venom anaphylaxis [644], it is surprising how relatively little we know about the effect of this causal treatment in atopic eczema. This is even more surprising when considering the clear-cut relevance of IgE-mediated sensitizations in many patients (see Chap. 5), as has been shown by the atopy patch test.

In certain recommendations for immunotherapy, atopic eczema even may be regarded as a contraindication for such a treatment; there is anecdotal evidence of acute flares of eczema after an immunotherapy injection when ASIT is performed against hay fever.

In animal experiments, it has been shown that it is possible to induce tolerance in a model of murine atopic dermatitis, either occurring spontaneously or after epicutaneous sensitization with ovalbumin. Tolerogenic dendritic cells were shown to successfully inhibit atopic dermatitis-like skin lesions induced by repeated epicutaneous exposure to antigen [385].

7.7.1 Results of Clinical Trials

Reviews of the literature on ASIT in atopic dermatitis comprise open, but also randomized and placebo-controlled studies [119, 157]. Most of the studies showed a clear-cut effect of ASIT on the eczematous skin disease.

One author (JR) performed a very simple placebo-controlled prospective trial in a pair of monozygous twins severely affected with eczema, but also suffering from hay fever, after obtaining informed consent from the parents and the two girls. One was treated with grass pollen extract, the other one with saline placebo. After the first pollen season, one of the girls was significantly better than the other one (Fig. 7.11). So we decided to break the code and found out that the girl who had improved had been treated with the verum. Then also the sister was treated with true ASIT and she also improved in the following year [639].

One of the most convincing studies has been performed by Werfel et al. on 89 patients where he could show a dose-dependent effect of subcutaneous ASIT with house dust mite allergen, regarding improvement of atopic eczema as measured in SCORAD [858]. A variety of other studies have shown similar results [153, 301, 741].

Also, sublingual application of allergen-specific immunotherapy (SLIT) can be effective [577].

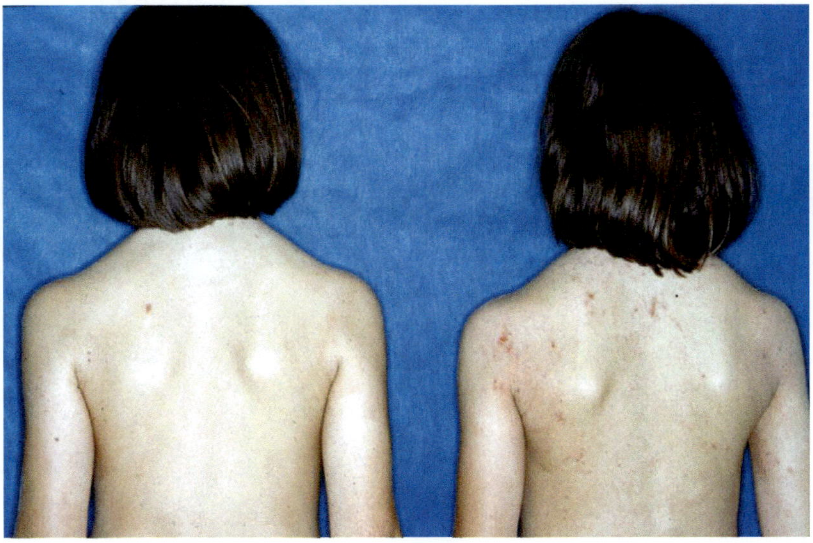

Fig. 7.11 Double-blind study with subcutaneous allergen-specific immunotherapy (ASIT) with grass pollen extract in homozygous twins with atopic dermatitis (left verum, right placebo) [638]

In pilot studies with house dust mite, also remarkable improvements in atopic eczema were seen [119].

In a recent study by Novak et al., there was no overall difference in a group of 168 eczema patients. However, there was an interesting significant improvement in a subgroup analysis of patients with very severe atopic dermatitis, namely a SCORAD over 15 [554]. Also, rush protocols (3-day dose increase) and ultrarash (build-up in 1 day) have been shown to be effective in reducing eczema symptoms [354].

The major mechanism through which allergen-specific immunotherapy works is the induction of peripheral tolerance via T-regulatory cells (Treg) which supply the balance between Th1 and Th2 immune response reactivity patterns [13].

From a time of 50 years ago, the idea came that a complex of histamine and gamma globulin might affect plasma histamine levels in a beneficial way [261]. In an animal experimental study, it was shown that this complex was able to regulate the Th1-Th2 balance in favor of Th1 cytokines [536].

In a recent pilot study, a combined treatment of allergen-specific immunotherapy with house dust mites together with the application of the histamine–immunoglobulin complex led to significant clinical improvement of eczematous skin lesions [536].

Systematic reviews have shown mixed results [36, 631].

7.7.2 Summary

Since it was shown that IgE-mediated sensitizations play a role in many patients in the elicitation and maintenance of eczematous skin lesions and several studies investigating the effects of allergen-specific immunotherapy (ASIT) have shown improvement, it would theoretically make sense to try this treatment in selected patients. However, until now, there is no recommendation in evidence-based guidelines. Contrary to earlier guidelines however atopic dermatitis is no longer regarded to be a contraindication for allergen-specific immunotherapy for other allergic diseases.

7.8 Systemic Immunomodulatory Therapy

The majority of patients with atopic dermatitis respond well to the above-mentioned treatment strategies combining avoidance of trigger factors, emollients and mostly topical application of anti-inflammatory substances, eventually together with antimicrobial ther-

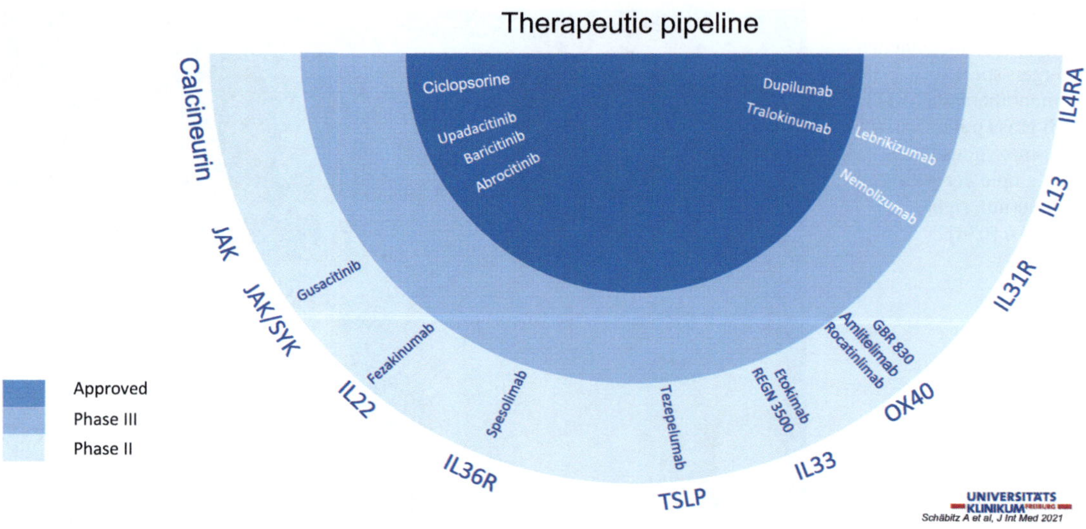

Fig. 7.12 The therapeutic landscape of atopic dermatitis. Small molecules (left side) or biologics approved (inner dark blue circle) or in late-stage clinical trials (outer rings)

apy. However, there are severe cases that do not respond and need systemic immune-modulation.

The therapeutic landscape of systemic therapies in atopic dermatitis is split into two worlds: while there are numerous conventional immune-modulating drugs historically given to patients with atopic dermatitis, the level of evidence regarding efficacy and development of side effects is poor [15]. Almost no randomized clinical trials have been performed, and the only conventional systemic drug that is approved for the treatment of atopic dermatitis is cyclosporine.

In contrast, a substantial number of smart conventional drugs, so-called small molecules, as well as biological agents became either approved since 2017 or are currently in clinical development (Fig. 7.12) [686].

7.8.1 Conventional Systemic Immune-modulators

7.8.1.1 Glucocorticosteroids

Glucocorticosteroids are mainly used as topical preparations (see Sect. 7.1); however, in rare cases, they are also given systemically. It may be surprising that in large reviews on treatment habits among general practitioners, the systemic use of glucocorticosteroids is not so rare [703]. However, there is almost no controlled study with regard to the effect of systemic glucocorticosteroids. Recently, a study has been published as investigator-initiated double-blind randomized multicenter trial in adult patients with severe eczema (SCORAD over 40 and Dermatology Life Quality Index over 10); systemic prednisolone (0.5–0.8 mg/kg) was compared to cyclosporin (2.4–4.0 mg/kg). There were an unexpectedly high number of withdrawals in this severely affected group so that finally only 38 patients were randomized and went into the study. Only in 1 out of 21 patients under prednisolone, compared to 6 out of 17 under cyclosporin, was stable remission achieved ($p < 0.03$). The authors concluded that cyclosporin is significantly more effective than prednisolone in treating severe adult eczema [708]. We personally use systemic steroids for atopic eczema very rarely and only in special cases with acute dramatic flares for some days.

Systemic steroids may be given to pregnant women with severe eczema in order to avoid other immunosuppressives with their contraindications.

7.8.1.2 Cyclosporin A

Cyclosporin A was discovered in transplantation medicine, where it is meanwhile the classic immunosuppressive to prevent rejection after organ transplantation. It exerts its effects via binding to a cytosolic immunophilin similar to calcineurin inhibitors (see Sect. 5.2) but acts only systemically. In dermatology, cyclosporin A is used in various inflammatory diseases [710, 914].

Dosage

Cyclosporin A is one of the most effective substances and is given at a dose of 2.5 mg/kg, slowly to be increased to 5 mg/kg body weight. One also can try a body weight-independent dosage of 150–300 mg/day. After marked improvement or stable remission, the dose is slowly reduced (0.5 mg/kg in 2- to 4-week intervals). Cyclosporin treatment has to be performed over longer time periods since, after withdrawal, severe "rebound" reactions can occur. Due to its side effects (see below), a maximal treatment duration of 2 years is recommended [169, 647, 648].

Cyclosporin is also effective in children and adolescents [115, 312, 313]; however, the indication has to be put very strictly, and it should be reserved for severe cases.

Side Effects

Cyclosporin A has a small therapeutic index; the side effects include frequent gastrointestinal symptoms, headache, and especially disturbance of the renal function with resulting hypertension [877]. Therefore, patients have to be checked intensively with regard to renal disease but also neoplasia, immunodeficiency, or hypertension prior to cyclosporin therapy. Under therapy, laboratory parameters regarding urea and creatinine, as well as electrolytes and differential blood counts, have to be controlled.

Rare side effects include paresthesias, hypertrichosis lanuginosa, and hyperplasia of the gingiva.

Due to possible photocarcinogenicity or due to the actual immunosuppression, patients under cyclosporin A therapy should use sun protection.

Incompatibilities with other drugs such as antibiotics and antimycotics which are metabolized via cytochrome P450 have to be considered. Cyclosporin A acts by blocking T cell activation and preventing the secretion of a variety of cytokines such as interleukin-2. Furthermore, cyclosporin A has an effect upon keratinocytes in preventing apoptosis and has a direct antipruritic effect by acting on mast cells. Possibly the place for cyclosporin is in the short-term treatment of very severe eczema patients with IgE-mediated autoreactivity (see Sect. 3.3).

7.8.1.3 Azathioprine

Azathioprine is a purine analog with a general effect on lymphocytes. It is usually used in order to spare steroids; however, it has a slow onset of action. It has been shown to be effective in atopic eczema [530, 599]. Prior to using azathioprine, one should measure the enzyme thiopurine methyltransferase (TPMT) since, when there are defects, rapid development of myelodepression can occur [504].

The therapeutic effect of azathioprine treatment only becomes visible after weeks or months. Regular controls of blood count and liver values are recommended. Side effects include nausea, leukopenia, and very rarely allergic reactions.

7.8.1.4 Methotrexate

Methotrexate is an antimetabolite of folic acid and used as antineoplastic substance in the treatment of rheumatoid arthritis and psoriasis. It can also be used in severe cases of atopic eczema [475]. In a randomized trial comparing methotrexate with azathioprine, it was found that methotrexate is equally effective as azathioprine [718].

Methotrexate can be given orally or parenterally. It is usually given once a week, either starting with doses of 7.5 mg per week and increasing to 15 mg per week or directly starting with 15 mg per week, each time followed by the application of folate (5 mg 1 day after the methotrexate application). We prefer the subcutaneous application which can be performed by the patient himself. Side effects include myelosuppression and hepatotoxicity, which has to be checked regularly. Methotrexate is contraindicated in pregnancy and during lactation [355, 475, 739, 823]. For children, it should only be given with careful indication [785].

7.8.1.5 Mycophenolate Mofetil

Mycophenolate mofetil is regularly used in organ transplantation but also more and more in inflammatory skin diseases such as autoimmune bullous disease and psoriasis. It also has been found effective in atopic eczema [544, 593]. It is given in patients where cyclosporin A is contraindicated. Mycophenolate mofetil inhibits the inosine monophosphate dehydrogenase and thus the purine synthesis [52, 286, 308]. Under mycophenolate mofetil, blood count and liver, renal, and electrolyte values have to be controlled in 2-week intervals. In a controlled observer-blinded randomized trial, mycophenolate was compared to cyclosporin in patients with severe atopic dermatitis, showing that mycophenolate mofetil was as effective as cyclosporin A in maintenance therapy in patients with atopic dermatitis. However, the clinical improvement after mycophenolate took a longer time in comparison to cyclosporin A [297].

7.8.1.6 Cyclophosphamide

Cyclophosphamide, which is widely used in hematological and collagen disease, should not be given in atopic dermatitis. It is an alkylating agent with a special action on a subgroup of T cells, mainly regulatory T cells. It has been shown that several autoimmune diseases may be increased as is allergic contact dermatitis [352].

7.8.1.7 Summary

Severe cases of atopic eczema have to be treated with systemic therapies. Before the era of biologics or JAK inhibitors, conventional immunosuppressives were the only choice. Apart from cyclosporin A, azathioprine, mycophenolate mofetil, and methotrexate were in use and might still be used occasionally. Cyclosporin A is approved and still has a place for short-term usage. Several side effects have to be considered. The side effects of cyclosporin A include gastrointestinal complaints, headache, and severe disturbance of renal function with resulting hypertension. A new era has been opened with the introduction of several small molecules and biologics.

7.8.2 Modern Small Molecules

7.8.2.1 Janus Kinase (JAK) Inhibitors

Mode of Action

Janus Kinase (JAK) inhibitors are among the most promising newly developed mode-of-actions utilized for atopic dermatitis treatment. In principle, members of the JAK family—namely JAK1, JAK2, JAK3, and Tyrosine Kinase (Tyk)2—form heterodimers or multimers at the inner part of the cell membrane. These dimers mediate intracellular signaling of multiple cytokines, including type 2 cytokines IL-4 and IL-13 (Jak1/Tyk2) as well as IL-31 and TSLP (Jak1/Jak2), IL-10 family members including IL-22 (Jak1/Tyk2), acute phase cytokines such as IL-6 (Jak1/Jak2), type 1 cytokine IFN-g (Jak1/Jak2), IFN-a/b (Jak1/Tyk2), and type 3 cytokines such as IL-23 (Jak2/Tyk2) [562, 829] (Fig. 7.13).

JAK activation leads to activation of transcription factors of the Signal transducer and activation of transcription (STAT) family. Collectively, the JAK/STAT molecules are a very efficient and most likely evolutionary conserved intracellular signaling cascade of many inflammatory stimuli.

This central pro-inflammatory signaling cascade can be inhibited by small molecules. These are oral medications that have to be given once or twice daily. Early JAK inhibitors such as tofacitinib or delgocitinib were not followed as a systemic therapy because of side effects and are currently tried as topical therapies, e.g., psoriasis or atopic dermatitis [68, 537]. Recently delgocitinib was approved as a topical treatment of atopic dermatitis in Japan. Ruxolitinib, a JAK1/2 inhibitor, is also in clinical development as a topical treatment for vitiligo and atopic dermatitis [395].

Clinical Efficacy

Subsequently, more selective JAK inhibitors were either approved (baricitinib, a JAK1/JAK2 inhibitor) or entered late-stage clinical development

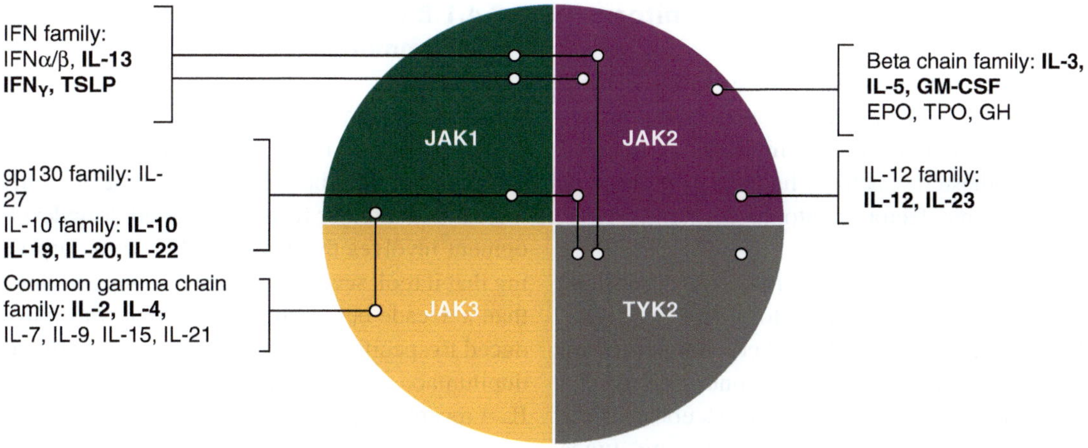

Fig. 7.13 JAK molecules form heterodimers to mediate intracellular signaling of many cytokines. Obtained from Ref. [561]

(upadacitinib and abrocitinib, both JAK1 inhibitors) for systemic treatment of atopic dermatitis [545].

Baricitinib showed efficacy above placebo in so far eight phase III trials either in combination with topical steroids or alone. 2 mg and 4 mg baricitiniab are available, both given once daily. Around 30% of the patients with moderate to severe atopic dermatitis reached an Investigator Global Assessment (IGA) score of 0 or 1 after 16 weeks of 4 mg baricitinib treatment in combination with topical steroids. Given as a monotherapy, around 15% achieve this endpoint after 16 weeks. This corresponds to a mean reduction of the EASI score of close to 60% [618, 752].

Upadactinib is a more selective JAK1 inhibitor that was tested in six phase III trials either as monotherapy, in combination with topical steroids, or head-to-head versus dupilumab. It is available in 15 mg and 30 mg tablets, both given once daily. Around 50% of the patients achieved the primary endpoint (IGA 0/1) after 16 weeks in all trials. Also, around 50% achieved at least a 90% improvement of the EASI score (EASI90) at week 16 of the treatment with 30 mg upadacitinib. At week 16, these upadacitinib was more effective than dupilumab [291].

Abrocitinib was tested in 100 mg and 200 mg tablets in seven phase III clinical trials, also including monotherapy, combination with topical corticosteroids, or a head-to-head comparison with dupilumab. The primary endpoint in abrocitinib trials was week 12 and thus 4 weeks earlier than in baricitinib or upadacitinib trials. Around 40% (200 mg) and 25% (100 mg) achieved the primary endpoint of IGA 0/1. At least 75% improvement of the EASI score (EASI75) was achieved in 60% (200 mg) or 45% (100 mg) of all patients, respectively [754].

Side Effects and Monitoring

Side effects of special interest observed in the large clinical trial program of selective JAK inhibitors in atopic dermatitis are the development of acne/folliculitis (in up to 15% of the patients depending on study drug and study), nausea, infections with viruses of the herpes group (eczema herpeticum or herpes simplex, zoster), elevation of blood lipids, reduction of platelet counts, and neutropenia. In the large study program of these inhibitors in the population of rheumatoid arthritis patients, signals for thromboembolism or major cardiovascular events (MACE) were identified [730]; it seems this risk is low in atopic dermatitis patients, but real-world evidence is needed here. Thus, it is recommended that patients are screened for infections (hepatitis, tuberculosis) prior to drug initiation and then subsequently get monitored with blood cell count, lipid state, and liver and kidney status assessed [545].

7.8.3 Phosphodiesterase Inhibitors

On the basis of studies showing a weakened reactivity of cyclic AMP and a decreased responsiveness to beta-adrenergic stimuli, an augmented phosphodiesterase activity has been postulated as a pathogenic factor in atopic dermatitis [131, 737].

The phosphodiesterase inhibitor apremilast is approved for moderate to severe psoriasis. Several clinical trials have been conducted on atopic dermatitis. The latest one compared a dose of 40 mg twice daily to placebo and the dose approved for psoriasis (30 mg twice daily). While the 30 mg dose was not more effective than placebo, the 40 mg dose reached moderate efficacy; however, the study was discontinued due to side effects [751]. Thus, PDE4 inhibitors seem unlikely to become available as systemic treatment options at the moment.

In contrast, a topical formulation of crisaborole is approved for the treatment of atopic dermatitis in the US. It is a safe treatment with good antipruritic effect, but overall weaker efficacy than mid-potent topical steroids. It is approved, but not marketed in Europe [367].

7.8.4 Biologics

Biologics have been introduced in medicine 30 years ago, using the production of recombinant proteins with modern gene technology thus allowing very specific actions on well-defined target structures. They comprise monoclonal antibodies against cytokines, monoclonal antibodies against specific receptors, soluble cytokines, and soluble receptors.

In a broader definition, also intravenous immunoglobulins or interferons may be called "biologics."

In the following, the most important biologics of possible relevance for atopic dermatitis will be discussed.

7.8.4.1 Biologics Targeting Type 2 Immunity

Anti-Interleukin-4/-Interleukin-13

Given the central role of type 2 immunity in the pathogenesis of atopic dermatitis, it seems only logical that a major focus of targeted drug development involves this pathway. It is thus surprising that it took several drug generations and more than a decade before the first biologic was introduced to specifically target this pathway—that is dupilumab, a monoclonal antibody against the IL-4 receptor alpha (IL-4Ra).

Both IL-4 and IL-13 bind to receptor dimers—IL-4 to a dimer of IL-4Ra and the common gamma chain, IL-13 to IL-14Ra and IL-13R1 [22]. Thus, by blocking the IL-4Ra effects of both IL-4 and IL-13 are neutralized.

Clinical Efficacy of Dupilumab

Dupilumab is approved for adult patients with atopic dermatitis in need of systemic therapy since 2017 in Europe in a dose regimen of 600 mg s.c. as starting dose and then 300 mg s.c. every 2 weeks. It was tested in multiple phase III clinical trials and also real-world evidence data. Overall, between 30% and 40% of patients achieve a response of almost clear or clear on an Investigator global assessment (IGA) scale after 16 weeks when combined with topical corticosteroids (TCS). This corresponds to around two-thirds of the patients achieving a 75% improvement in their EASI score from baseline. Response rates as a monotherapy are somewhat lower and in real-world dupilumab is most frequently combined with TCS. The response to dupilumab seems to be quite stable over at least 1 year [8, 71, 748]. Studies in adolescents and children are currently ongoing and point to a similar efficacy and safety as in adults [753].

Side Effects of Dupilumab

Overall, dupilumab is a safe treatment option. The rate of severe infections is not increased, vaccination seems to be effective under treatment

[72], and although long-term treatment data is missing, there are no signals of increased cancer development or severe cardiovascular events. Nevertheless, there are side effects of special interest, namely conjunctivitis and injection-side reactions. While the latter rarely causes real problems in daily clinical routine, conjunctivitis can occur in up to 15–20% of all patients treated with dupilumab. In exceptional cases, conjunctivitis might be a reason to discontinue the therapy; however, in the vast majority lid hygiene, referral to an ophthalmologist and eventually treatment with topical steroids or calcineurin inhibitors are effective measurements [31, 796]. Interestingly, conjunctivitis is not observed in patients treated with dupilumab for allergic asthma. The underlying pathogenesis is not yet clear and this phenomenon cannot be explained.

Anti-Interleukin-13

Two monoclonal antibodies against the cytokine IL-13 itself are close to approval for atopic dermatitis, namely tralokinumab and lebrikizumab. The efficacy of tralokinumab has been proven in three clinical phase III trials so far, the ECTZRA program [744, 881]. Around 30% of the patients included reached an EASI75 response across the three trials at week 16, which was superior to placebo. For lebrikizumab, two phase II trials are published. At the primary endpoints at week 12, EASI50 response was reached in 82% versus 62% in the placebo group [750]. Side effects of both tralokinumab and lebrikizumab are similar to the ones of dupilumab with a tendency for lower rates of conjunctivitis. They are administered subcutaneously every 4 weeks.

Anti-Interleukin-31

The role of IL-31 in neuro-immunology is described in Chap. 5. Nemolizumab is a monoclonal antibody targeting the IL-31 receptor alpha (IL-31Ra). In phase II and phase III clinical trials, the expected high efficacy regarding itch reduction was confirmed with around 40% itch reduction at 16 weeks. Effects on the skin were somewhat lower at this early time point, with EASI75 reached in 46% of all patients versus 33% in the placebo group [377, 673]. Nemolizumab was well tolerated, with the most common side effect of injection-site reactions in up to 10% of the patients.

Anti-Interleukin-5

Interleukin-5 is the crucial cytokine in the recruitment, production, and activation of eosinophil granulocytes which represent a major characteristic of tissue inflammation both in asthma and in atopic dermatitis.

First clinical trials with a monoclonal antibody against IL-5 in asthma showed disappointing clinical results, although there was a clear-cut effect in the reduction of peripheral eosinophil counts. On the contrary, mepolizumab was highly effective in the rare group of patients with hypereosinophilic syndrome (HES) [598, 670].

In a placebo-controlled study with only two injections of mepolizumab in atopic dermatitis, there was a significant but only moderate clinical effect [568].

While mepolizumab was approved for several eosinophilic diseases in 2021, it will not be further pursued for the indication of atopic dermatitis.

Anti-IgE

Since, almost 20 years, the monoclonal antibody against human IgE (omalizumab) is available for the treatment of severe asthma [114, 509]. It is a humanized IgG1 molecule and also has effects in allergic rhinitis, IgE-mediated food allergy [456], and it is approved for the treatment of chronic urticaria [7]. Omalizumab induces a marked and rapid decrease of serum-free IgE levels and has to be given in a dose according to the actual serum IgE concentration with good safety profile [149, 334].

There have been a variety of case reports and case series with successful omalizumab treatment in atopic dermatitis [244, 828]. We performed a pilot study on a total of 11 patients with severe atopic eczema and concomitant asthma who had been treated with systemic immunosuppressives and phototherapy without good effect before. In 6 of 11 patients, there was a marked improvement [51]. These patients had serum IgE concentrations sometimes reaching 15,000 kU/L; therefore, it was not possible to adjust the dose according to the recommendation of the producer, but we just use the typical dose used in asthma patients with 150 mg every 2 weeks.

A controlled study by Stingl et al. showed no significant effect [318]. Recently, Wollenberg showed in a systematic review some effects, especially in patients with lower IgE levels [885].

In summary, omalizumab treatment may be effective in a small subgroup of patient with atopic dermatitis.

Combination approaches with prior plasmapheresis removing excessively increased IgE values resulted in slightly better results [910]. However, immune-apheresis is an invasive procedure that does not result in long-term clinical improvement and should thus be preserved for very therapy-resistant patients as the last treatment option [617, 794]. Finally, contradicting results are reported regarding the efficacy of rituximab [731, 745], a monoclonal antibody targeting CD20 and thus removing all B cells from the periphery, add to the conclusion that targeting humoral immunity may not be the primary treatment choice in atopic dermatitis—or that specific endotypes of atopic dermatitis need to be identified for these treatment options.

Biologics Targeting Type 3 Immunity or Innate Immunity

Biologics targeting type 3 (Th17) immunity are a success story since the 1990s in the field of psoriasis treatment [77]. Antibodies specifically neutralizing TNF, IL-23, or IL-17 molecules are highly efficient to treat psoriasis and show an overall good safety profile. Thus, it is logical that over time almost all of these options have also been tried to treat atopic dermatitis. Overall, efficacy levels are much less in atopic dermatitis than in psoriasis. This is in line with the mutually antagonistic immune response patterns of atopic dermatitis and psoriasis. However, as stated in Chap. 5, especially chronic atopic dermatitis also shows some influx of Th17 cells. It cannot be excluded that these therapies are efficient in a subtype of atopic dermatitis patients at this time.

Beyond therapies approved for psoriasis, several biologics neutralizing innate immunity have been or currently are investigated for their efficacy in atopic dermatitis—among them IL-6 or IL-1a.

Anti-TNF Strategies

Tumor necrosis factor (TNF) is a central cytokine of delayed-type hypersensitivity which plays a major role in Th1-mediated immune reactions. Anti-TNF has shown remarkable effects in rheumatic diseases such as Crohn's disease, rheumatoid arthritis, and psoriasis.

There are several products available such as monoclonal antibodies against TNF (infliximab, golimumab, adalimumab, certolizumab) but also soluble receptor antagonists of the TNF receptor (etanercept).

There are some case reports describing mild to moderate effects of atopic dermatitis [124]. However, this is opposed by numerous case series describing worsening of atopic dermatitis with induced eosinophilia, dry skin, and increased pruritus [224, 361, 482]. Furthermore, a variety of serious side effects including allergic reactions, eosinophilia, and dry skin as well as the development of sepsis might occasionally be observed [482].

We therefore feel that anti-TNF strategies are not overall recommendable to treat atopic dermatitis—even if we cannot exclude that there might be a subset of atopic dermatitis patients that benefit from this strategy.

Anti-Interleukin-17 and Interleukin-22

The monoclonal antibody against IL-17 secukinumab was tested without any efficacy regarding clinical or molecular improvement in a placebo-controlled pahse II trial at week 16 [815]. This also included sub-analysis of a small cohort of Asian patients that was previously reported to have a certain Th17 component in their pathogenesis (see Chap. 5). Thus, neutralization of IL-17 is not promising as a global approach in atopic dermatitis. It is unknown whether distinct atopic dermatitis endotypes might respond better.

This seems to be the case for the neutralization of IL-22. Fezakinumab, a monoclonal antibody directed against IL-22, showed an overall moderate efficacy in atopic dermatitis. Patients with higher baseline levels of IL-22 seemed to respond better to a post hoc analysis [109, 290]. If this holds true, it could be a way to stratify atopic dermatitis patients and tailor the therapeutic decision to distinct endotypes. IL-22 receptor antagonization is a strategy currently in very early clinical trials.

Anti-Interleukin-12/23

IL-12/23 inhibition with the monoclonal antibody ustekinumab impacts both type 3 (Th17) immunity and type 1 (Th1) immunity. There are several case reports on the successful treatment of atopic dermatitis using ustekinumab, but solid controlled clinical trials are missing. The best evidence is made from a cross-over trial including 33 patients that started on a placebo arm or ustekinumab arm and then switched at week 16. Here, numerical efficacy did not achieve statistical significance [392]. In summary, all psoriasis biologics do not show convincing efficacy from a global point of view. Relevant endotypes of atopic dermatitis patients that might benefit from this treatment strategy are not (yet) identified.

Intravenous Immunoglobulins

The intravenous application of high doses of immunoglobulins has proven helpful in a variety of autoimmune diseases such as dermatomyositis and idiopathic thrombocytopenic purpura.

There are some case reports regarding the use of IVIg in atopic dermatitis [584] showing a transitory effect. Due to the high costs, this therapeutic option remains only for a limited number of patients.

7.9 Pre- and Probiotics and Polyunsaturated Fatty Acids

Probiotics such as lactobacillus mixtures have been used in atopic dermatitis and shown to lead to an improvement [359, 379]. This group also described a preventive effect of probiotics given during pregnancy. Other studies [240, 667] however showed no significant effects. This coincides with our own experiences.

In a study on 800 infants, the effect of a prebiotic mixture of immunoactive oligosaccharides has been studied. There was a significant effect in a decreased occurrence of atopic dermatitis [280].

Whether the alteration of the intestinal or cutaneous microbiome will play a role in clinical practice is still controversial and might require personalized approaches.

There is a long tradition of hypothetical considerations that polyunsaturated fatty acids (PUFA) such as gamma-linolenic acid and eicosapentaenoic acid may have beneficial effects on atopic inflammation and atopic eczema [59]. A prospective randomized trial performed by our group showed no significant effects over placebo (Fig. 7.14). Maybe this therapeutic option could have a place in allergy prevention.

7.9.1 Summary

The progress through the introduction of biologics into medicine, which has been achieved in other diseases such as psoriasis, rheumatoid arthritis or Crohn's disease, or asthma, has now reached atopic dermatitis. Antibodies targeting type 2 immunity are either approved (dupilumab, tralokinumab) or close to approval (leb-

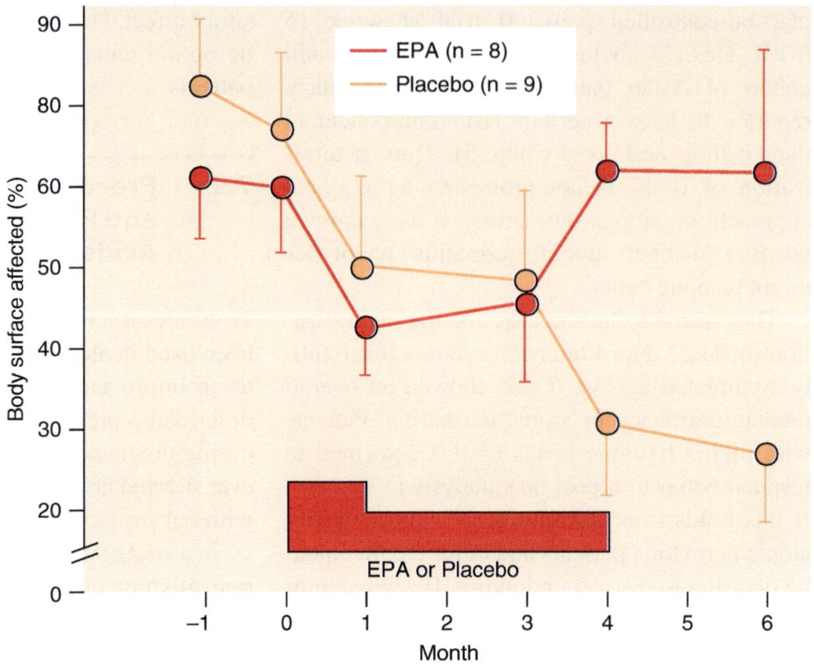

Fig. 7.14 Clinical improvement in patients with atopic eczema under oral eicosapentaenoic acid (EPA) and placebo; in the long-term observation over 6 months, placebo was better than verum

rikizumab), with further substances in early clinical development. However, the complex pathogenesis and high heterogeneity of atopic dermatitis make it seem unlikely that neutralization of only one cytokine or cytokine receptor will be as efficient as seen in, e.g., psoriasis, where neutralization of the type 3 immunity results in improvement rates of at least 90% in more than 80% of all patients. Thus, endotyping and precision medicine are most likely important components of therapeutic algorithms in the future.

7.10 Psychosomatic Strategies

The skin as an expression organ of the soul has an eminent esthetic function. Therefore, it is not surprising that skin diseases not only become manifest in somatic complaints but often also lead to psychological problems (see also Chap. 3 "Burden"). The intensity of this psychosomatic interaction varies individually. One has always consider that skin conditions have to be regarded both in a psychosomatic and in a somatopsychic way [204].

7.10.1 Exploration and Evaluation of Psychosomatic Involvement in the Disease

It is extremely important first to detect and evaluate together with the patient how far psychological factors influence the skin disease toward exacerbation or eventually improvement. This requires an open conversation and motivation for self-perception. It is crucial not to give the impression that atopic dermatitis is a "psychological" disease. It has always to be stated that atopic dermatitis primarily is a skin disease which can be modulated through neural irritation and psychological influences but does not have per se a psychiatric cause! (see Chap. 5).

This is especially important in the treatment of infants or small children where organic causes obviously are central; the induction of "feelings of guilt" in the mother or the father has to be absolutely avoided!

With increasing age, it is natural that the more severe the eczematous skin lesions are and the more often the frustrating experience of therapeutic failure has been observed, psychological alterations begin which have to be analyzed and discussed in a patient-doctor relationship carried by mutual trust.

Note: There are many patients with very severe atopic eczema who are psychologically absolutely normal and benefit only little from psychosomatic or psychotherapeutic interventions.

Every human being has his/her everyday problems, stress, and emotional conflicts. It is a normal and "human" basis of patient-doctor interaction to also cover these aspects in the exploration of the history. This would need no special training. However—this cannot be denied—modern medicine is moving toward a direction of utmost specialization in a way that residents in a university hospital call for a psychosomatic consultant with the note: "The patient is crying" [630]. From our experience, we advise the parents of children with atopic dermatitis to know about psychosomatic interactions and try to realize and observe these psychodynamics of family situations with their impact on the skin disease of the offspring themselves [203].

The treatment of skin diseases always needs patience; good effects can never be forced. Especially the basic therapy of the disturbed skin barrier function should not develop into a compulsory behavior in the form of a "skin hygiene ritual" which naturally will build-up aversion in the child against parental authority.

7.10.2 Therapeutic Modalities

As soon as psychological components are recognized as relevant for the individual disease of a patient, the best possible therapeutic option has to be selected. This always has to be done on the basis of somatic general skin treatment. Cooperation between a dermatologist and psychologist or psychosomatic physician is absolutely essential [204]!

In Table 7.6, various opportunities for psychosomatic therapeutic options are enlisted, reaching from placebo treatment to psychoanalysis [773].

Through the introduction of short-time analytic procedures with less time- and cost-associated sessions, also psychoanalytically oriented therapeutic options can make sense. However, it has to be mentioned that in the exploration of emotions, eczema flares may be triggered.

Rarely psychopharmaceuticals should be used, preferably those with also antihistaminergic components thus having concomitant antipruritic effects (see Sect. 5.4). The well-known placebo effect is particularly notable in allergies and especially atopic dermatitis and may help to explain why so many anecdotal reports of effective "complementary" or "alternative" methods are reported (see Sect. 7.10).

From our own experience with placebo-controlled clinical trials using new therapeutics, we know that it is the pure personal impact ("doctor's devotion to patients") of a physician which can have surprising effects on the treatment of atopic dermatitis. After many years, JR still is receiving Christmas postcards "Thank you Doctor, you have cured me!" from patients with severe atopic dermatitis who had been in the placebo group and experienced long-lasting significant improvement (Fig. 7.13).

The logical consequence of this is not the recommendation to prescribe placebos but to inten-

Table 7.6 Therapeutic options in atopic dermatitis with psychosomatic involvement (in addition to classical dermatologic treatment)

Placebo treatment
Psychopharmaceuticals (sedatives, antihistamines, antidepressants)
Psychosomatic counseling
Behavioral therapy (cognitive behavioral stress management)
Family therapy
Relaxation techniques
Autogenic training
Biofeedback
Hypnosis
Psychotherapy/group psychotherapy
Psychoanalysis

sify the personal involvement of a reassuring physician-patient interaction.

7.10.3 Behavioral Therapy

In atopic dermatitis, several behavioral therapeutical techniques have been used; they all comprise the classical stages [904]:

- Detection and characterization of problematic behavior.
- Selection of relevant stimuli and consequences.
- Intervention.
- Evaluation of success.

In the beginning, mostly relaxation techniques are used like the large muscle relaxation. However, other methods like autogenic training and biofeedback are widely used [204].

Recently a new technique of "mindfulness" in coping with stress has also been used for atopic dermatitis [564].

These techniques have to be practiced with the patient; they cannot be learned on theoretical recommendation. Therefore, this is a central part of educational programs in atopic dermatitis (Chap. 8).

Autogenic training as well as imagination techniques (e.g., cold imagination or the imagination of "healthy" environmental influences) may help in calming down the inflamed skin [204].

Changes in behavior can be achieved via conditioning based on general principles of learning which have to be learned and practiced by the patient, leading to improvement (Table 7.7).

Practical techniques comprise recommendations for certain behaviors [505] focusing especially on scratching and the concomitant damage to the skin and maintenance of inflammation. This can be done by "distraction" techniques like using instruments for scratching (scratch cube) instead of the skin in respective situations. Sometimes already the recommendation to keep an "itch diary," where the patient makes a written note regarding the intensity of his itch sensations, can be helpful by the pure act of handwriting and distraction from scratching.

Table 7.7 Techniques of behavioral therapy and conditioning

Classical	"Desensitization" (e.g., reciprocal inhibition with relaxation techniques after classification of a hierarchy of irritants) Flooding (exposure to an overwhelming dose of the stimulus) Assertiveness training (practicing the competence to express own feelings and wishes without hurting other individuals) Communication therapy of couples
Operant	Positive reinforcement Negative reinforcement Punishment Ignorance (e.g., "time-out") Oversatiation
Observational	Model learning from comparable situations
Cognitive	Development of a new understanding of interactions Bibliotherapy Paradoxical communication

In coping with the many burdens associated with this disease, many patients have lost hope and are additionally desperate when they often hear the term "incurable." This is where cognitive behavioral therapy starts which also acts against the peculiar "perfectionism" observed in many patients with atopic dermatitis.

Furthermore, the social competence which often is compromised in many patients with facial eczema has to be promoted. Always it has to be mentioned that patients with atopic dermatitis are not "neurotic" and do not have a psychiatric disease!

The understanding and practicing of cooperative communication improve the self-confidence of the patient. In this context, so-called role plays are helpful like they are used in programs for "eczema school." Wrong ways of thinking ("I am ugly"; "everybody is looking at me") can be overcome. Studies with volunteers wearing eyeglasses through which one could measure the direction of the gaze of the observer show clearly that patients suffering from facial dermatoses always believe that they are more and more intensively observed than is actually true with regard to the observing environment.

In a randomized controlled trial, a cognitive behavioral stress management program has been studied in 28 patients with severe atopic dermatitis. A "public speaking" effort was the stimulus for acute stress. After undergoing cognitive behavioral stress management programs, the experimental group showed lower salivary cortisol levels under acute stress and remained calmer as measured by the cortisol-awakening response [723, 724].

The same group showed that relaxation techniques were able to induce a significant reduction in scratch response after showing a video with scratching people [722].

Hypnosis may be used in selected cases in order to relax fixed behavioral patterns and reflexes [736].

A general experience that should be emphasized: It is so much easier to detect emotional conflicts and difficulties than to clear them.

7.10.4 Summary

Atopic dermatitis is primarily a skin disease however modulated via neural stimuli and reaction patterns and psychological influences. An intense exploration with regard to the influence of conflict situations or stress is helpful in many patients. On the basis of this, specific psychosomatic counseling can be recommended. The therapeutic options include behavioral therapy with different procedures, e.g., relaxation techniques, which also can be included in eczema school programs.

7.11 Unconventional Methods

There are few fields in medicine where "alternative," "complementary," or "unconventional" methods have such a degree of popularity as in the management of atopic dermatitis (Fig. 7.15). Reports from the lay press about presumptuous "new miracle ointments or tablets" or "cures through bioscientific methods" (anonymous "cream from the other world," 1992) support this trend [28, 248, 538, 671].

The increasing budgetary restraints in many countries give rise to a trend that "normal," scientifically oriented physicians also are tempted to use unconventional methods if they are desired by the patient, in order to earn easy money, and thus support the routine office. Some people repeat the old—but wrong—argument "who cures is right"; this sentence is not logical since it compares different categories similar to "who wins is beautiful"; correctly the sentence should be "Who cures does good; but whether he is right is another question."

The increasing specialization and introduction of technology into medicine, together with the acceleration and dwindling time physicians have for the individual patient and a deep longing for a harmonic world where illness and health of the whole human being are seen together, is growing in a romantic imagination of the unity of body and soul; man is part of nature and religion. Especially in Germany, this romanticism on the basis of the philosophical school of German idealism (Kant, Fichte, Schelling, Hegel) has strong roots in all levels of the population. The hunt for the "blue flower" in idealized nature is still very

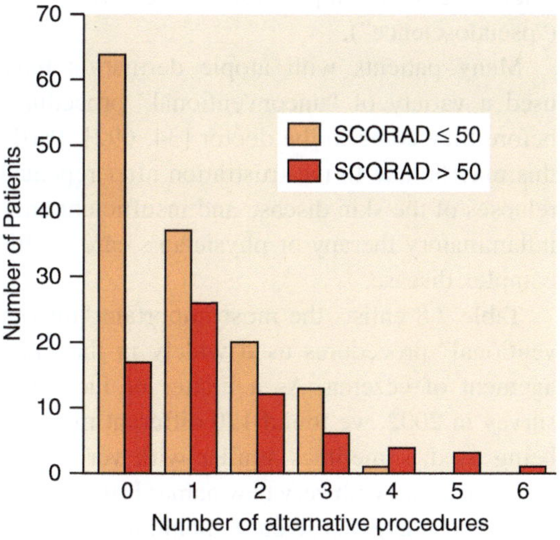

Fig. 7.15 Number of various "alternative"/"complementary" methods used in a 3-month period by patients with atopic dermatitis ($N = 204$) [692]

Table 7.8 Most commonly used "alternative"/"unconventional" procedures in allergy (alphabetical order!)

Acupuncture
Autologous blood injection
Autohomologous immunotherapy
Bach flower therapy
Bioresonance
Diet/curative fasting
Electroacupuncture
Hair mineral analyses
Homeopathy
Kinesiology
Neural therapy
Pendulum
Phytotherapy
Traditional Chinese medicine

According to Dorsch and Ring [191]

Table 7.9 Unconventional procedures: categories of plausibility

New scientific procedures in the phase of clinical trials
Plausible concept founded on case reports; however, no exact studies are available
Procedure with little plausibility and lacking convincing case reports
Procedure lacking evidence of efficacy in spite of scientific studies
Procedure with such low plausibility or potential hazard that it is not advised to perform scientific studies
True quackery like fraud in mixing cortisone in presumptuous "cortisone-free" preparations

attractive. Disease is seen as a disturbance of the originally harmonic world, and biological processes are interpreted philosophically or with religious content. There is an old experience: The "unconventional"/"alternative" medicine of today is the scientific medicine of the past century. Some of the thoughts are justified and interesting, but they are combined with often quite outdated or obsolete methods.

When these diffuse irrational sentiments are combined with most modern technology (e.g., bioresonance), they become tricky and give the patient the wrong impression of a scientific basis ("pseudoscience").

Many patients with atopic dermatitis have used a variety of "unconventional" procedures before they come to the doctor [34, 692]. Partly this may be due to the frustration after repeated relapses of the skin disease and insufficient anti-inflammatory therapy or physician's care in this complex disease.

Table 7.8 enlists the most important "unconventional" procedures used widely in the management of eczema. As a matter of fact, in a survey in 2002, we found 120 different methods being used, sometimes similar with very small differences but with very new names [191]. When people postulate that science should have no hesitance to study these procedures, this is a difficult task.

Therefore, we need plausibility criteria in sorting out various categories among the spectrum of "unconventional" procedures which may make sense or may be justified in certain patients (Table 7.9). It is noteworthy that sometimes so-called unconventional methods have interesting and plausible concepts and may lead to new therapeutic procedures which should be investigated with scientific methods, e.g., general health promotion according to Kneipp [406].

Many authors use the term "unconventional" or "complementary" for certain procedures which in fact present a meaningful addendum to classical dermatology therapy like:

- Psychosomatic counseling and relaxation techniques.
- Dietary recommendations.
- Climate therapy.
- Phytotherapeutic procedures.
- Physical therapy.
- Sports therapy and ergotherapy.
- Acupuncture (see below) (cum grano salis).

Contrary to these procedures, one can find a wide spectrum of methods which, according to current evidence, cannot be recommended since there is no evidence of efficacy or the diagnostic reliability in controlled studies can be compared to throwing a dice (Table 7.10) [309, 692]. In the following, some procedures will be briefly discussed and evaluated. The practicing physician should at least know what his patients have read or even tried themselves. It makes no good

Table 7.10 Unconventional procedures which cannot be recommended according to current evidence

Autohomologous immunotherapy
Bach flower therapy
Bioresonance
Electroacupuncture
Kinesiology
Pendulum diagnostics
Hair mineral analysis
Food-specific IgG for diagnostics and dietary recommendations

Table 7.11 Phytotherapeutic approaches in atopic dermatitis (selection)

Chamomile (*Matricariae flos*)
Marigold (*Calendulae flos*)
Hamamelis leaves and bark (*Hamamelidis folium et cortex*)
Oak bark (*Quercus cortex*)
Pansy herbs (*Violae tricoloris herba*)
Sage leaves (*Salvia folium*)
Bittersweet stalks (*Dulcamarae stipites*)
St. John's wort flowers (*Hyperici flos*)
Mahonia (*Mahonia aquifolium*)
Balloon vine (*Cardiospermum halicacabum*)
Evening primrose (*Oenothera biennis*)
Rockrose (*Cistus incanus*)

According to Reuter et al. [626]

impression when the doctor has to look up on the Internet what the patient is telling him; I help myself in these situations with the question "Well, how did this doctor actually do this?" Then the patient tells the story, and one can make at least a guess.

7.11.1 Evaluation of Some "Unconventional" Procedures

7.11.1.1 Acupuncture

Acupuncture comes from Chinese medicine and uses alterations of "energy streams" on the body surface and their alteration in illness through needle puncture. The needles have to be applied very precisely on certain classical "acupuncture points" and left there for several minutes. This is connected with pain; however, there should be no or minimal bleeding.

Acupuncture is used in school medicine in the therapy of pain. Regarding allergic reactions, acupuncture has been tried in experimental studies in hay fever with significant effects: skin test reactions and itch could be influenced by acupuncture [590]. In this context, further studies are necessary; however, in single cases, acupuncture may be tried in atopic dermatitis [123, 900]. It has been found that in placebo-controlled clinical trials, under acupuncture, certain central nervous areas in the brain involved in the processing of the itch sensation may be downregulated [591]. Both placebo and nocebo responses can be documented in brain activation patterns [540].

7.11.1.2 Phytotherapy and Traditional Chinese Medicine

Plant extracts have been used in medicine since early history, and many of today's pharmacological evidence-based drugs have been developed from plants. In dermatology, numerous plants are used against inflammation and for wound healing, but there is also a vast literature on phytotherapy in atopic dermatitis (Table 7.11).

In the last decades, the interest in East Asian medical concepts has increased considerably. Especially traditional Chinese medicine (TCM) has become very fashionable in the USA and Europe; these procedures have a strong connection with philosophical and religious concepts but use a variety of herbal extracts with considerable effects [45]. Significant improvements of eczema have been reported after the application of a mixture of ten different Chinese herbs in atopic eczema [26, 734, 735]. Often it is impossible to select single substances in these mixtures and study them for their evidence. Recently, a prospective randomized placebo-controlled trial reported significant effects of oral Xiaox-Iao-feng-sun (XFS), a mixture of 12 Chinese herbal preparations in atopic dermatitis [137] from Taiwan.

It should be mentioned that these herbal extracts cannot be regarded generally as "safe": severe side reactions have been reported [466] with hepatotoxicity and fatal consequences as well as reversible dilated cardiomyopathy [230]. In some herbal mixtures, potent glucocorticosteroids have been detected [560]. These herbal mixtures should only be used under medical control and with knowledge of the content. Furthermore, plants can have very strong allergenic properties inducing allergic contact dermatitis also after systemic use. A similar degree of evidence can be found for Japanese phytotherapeutic measures (Campo medicine).

7.11.1.3 Homeopathy

Homeopathy was introduced into medicine by the German physician Samuel Hahnemann (1775–1843) who—in his time at the level of actual science—tried to understand and use pharmacological properties of a variety of substances. Unfortunately, the contact to scientific medicine with critical analysis and continuous methodological improvement has been lost over time in favor of a general characterization of "philosophy" (Weltanschauung). Like industry supporters of homeopathy have a strong lobby activity with health care providers and politicians.

The basis of the homeopathy concept is the rule of "similarity" (similia similibus): Droplets, little balls (globuli), tablets, or injections are prepared with extreme dilutions of substances which are regarded to play a causal role in the disease. There is an inverse measurement of "potency" in that the higher the dilution, the more potent the preparation is believed to be. In some cases, even dilutions of 10^{23} are used, which means that, according to Loschmidt's number, there is no single molecule left in the solution [863].

The concept of diluting effective substances is also used in allergen-specific immunotherapy (hyposensitization); however, in this case, a clear-cut dose-response effect with increasing efficacy with increasing concentrations is applied.

There was marked publicity some years ago when a group of a well-renowned scientists published in "Nature" that these extreme dilutions of allergens indeed were able to inhibit allergen-induced histamine release from peripheral basophil leukocytes [53]. Also, a clinical trial was performed with significant effects and published in "The Lancet" [495]. The authors explained the effects of these dilutions by molecular vibrations thus leading to a "memory of water." As expected, these results could not be reproduced in any other lab. The editor of "Nature" ordered an external independent evaluation (the group consisted of a physicist, a statistician, and a magician) and found that the laboratory data were faked—without the boss knowing—by a close coworker trying to please the master!

It is extremely difficult to perform controlled studies with homeopathic regimens [401]; however, some studies showing positive effects in hay fever have been published; however, negative results are more common [218].

We performed a randomized, placebo-controlled, double-blind clinical trial studying the effect of classic homeopathic therapy in atopic eczema and found no significant effect of homeopathy compared to placebo. However, both verum and placebo therapy led to a marked improvement over the observational period of almost 1 year [738].

7.11.1.4 Cell Extracts and Thymus Factors

On the basis of good experiences with "fresh cell therapy" in the 50s of the twentieth century, also cellular extracts have been used in eczema as well as soluble supernatants of cell cultures, especially so-called thymus preparations. The best-known extracts are called thymosin or thymostimulin from calf thymus as well as thymopentin as a synthetic pentapeptide [455]. The so-called transfer factor gained from stimulated leukocyte suspensions also has immunomodulating effects. All these procedures were more or less disappearing after the outbreak of bovine spongiform encephalitis (BSE).

7.11.1.5 Bach Flower Therapy

The English physician Dr. Edward Bach introduced a therapeutical concept using leaves of flowers of different colors which are supposed to influence the psychic conditions of humans by their vibrations. The concept has a strong resemblance to romantic medicine and philosophy and is very difficult to study under scientific conditions.

7.11.1.6 Anthroposophic Medicine

The concept of anthroposophic medicine is very complex and does not describe the effects of single substances or procedures, but rather represents a religious holistic concept with a specific emphasis on "natural" procedures and lifestyle. Antibiotics or vaccinations are avoided, the children should experience the natural course of infectious diseases.

However, it has to be mentioned that epidemiological trials studying children from anthroposophic families have shown that they develop less allergies than the normal population [20, 21]. Similar findings have been observed when studying farmers' children in alpine regions of Bavaria, Austria, and Switzerland where it was shown that farmers' children growing up on a farm and whose mother had worked in the stable during pregnancy develop less allergies [632] (see Chap. 2).

7.11.1.7 Bioresonance

Bioresonance describes somatic electromagnetic vibrations which can be measured and which are disturbed in certain diseases; these can be diagnosed and corrected by the introduction of allergens both in diagnostic and therapeutic use. Bioresonance can be regarded as a mixture of magic guru and modern high-tech medicine. There is no physical basis for this concept; there has been no effect in placebo-controlled double-blind studies [692, 716, 891].

Recently a double-blind study was performed showing that a new bioresonance technique was not able to differentiate between the skin of healthy or atopic individuals or a meatball or cadaver skin [191].

7.11.1.8 Electroacupuncture According to Voll

This procedure combines Chinese acupuncture with Western technology and uses energy streams of the patient altered through allergens. Again, in control studies, no diagnostic effect could be proven [99].

7.11.1.9 Kinesiology

The American physician Diamond developed the method of kinesiology ("touch for health"), assuming that muscular tension is an expression of the holistic energy field of a human individual and allows diagnostic information about possible disease elicitors. The examiner stands in front of the patient who has elevated his upper arm horizontally and tries to press the arm down against resistance. As soon as he puts a vial with relevant allergen in front of the sternum, acute relaxation of the muscle occurs, and the arm drops down. We have tried this procedure in a double-blind placebo-controlled clinical trial; first of all, we had to include a coworker under a "hidden name" in the course of the master in order to learn the methodology and gain the "apostolic blessings" so that nobody could say we did not perform the method properly. Although there were single patients where surprisingly some effect could be observed, in the randomized clinical trial, the diagnostic reliability however was even below that of throwing a dice (below 50%) [435].

7.11.2 General Recommendations for Dealing with "Alternative" Methods

When a patient asks for "alternative" therapies, we can safely state that scientific medicine always has a choice of several alternatives of scientifically well-based treatments. Also, new plausible therapeutic options may be used in a pilot study and then evaluated in a controlled trial. However, what is already investigated and rejected or absolutely not plausible should be avoided in the interest of the patient. As physicians, we are obliged to tell our patients the truth and treat them according to our knowledge and conscience. At the same time, we should never be arrogant or emotionally involved in quarreling with the patients or induce feelings of guilt. Physicians treating atopic dermatitis have to have a composure of utmost tolerance; however, tolerance is an attitude toward individual subjects, not against philosophical ideologies!

It is very helpful when patients are informed in a group as we do this in our eczema school program (see below) and discuss the controversies among themselves; there is always a patient who already has made a very negative experience with some alternative methods and thus has a much higher authority than the doctor, who is regarded to be a "narrow-minded" supporter of "school medicine."

The physician can act as a moderator and does not appear to be the super teacher. In our contact with patients, we avoid academic debates; we say, "Lady (Sir)—this is a matter of religion, and we do not discuss religion with our patients."

7.11.3 Summary

There is almost no field in medicine where "alternative," "complementary," or "unconventional" methods are so popular as in the management of atopic dermatitis. Therefore, it is important for the physician at least to know the name and the principle of the most commonly used procedures. When trying to categorize unconventional methods according to plausibility, there are a variety of procedures which may be recommended as a useful supplement to classical dermatologic therapy such as psychosomatic counseling, relaxation techniques, certain dietary recommendations, climate therapy, certain forms of phytotherapy, physical therapy, sports therapy, and—maybe to be better studied—acupuncture. On the contrary, there are procedures which, according to current knowledge, cannot be recommended. Double-blind trials with homeopathy have not shown significant improvements; similarly, negative results have been published from controlled trials to bioresonance and kinesiology. When talking to the patient about unconventional methods, the atmosphere should be calm and never lead to the induction of "feelings of guilt" in the patient. It will be an interesting field experiment to observe the number of treatments from this field in the context of growing opportunities regarding topical and systemic specific agents.

8 Prevention

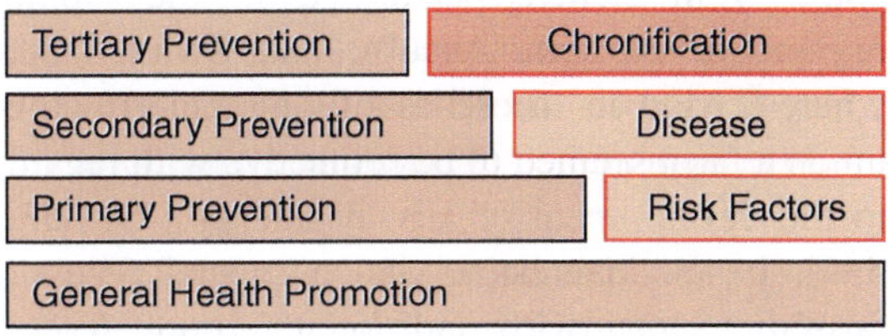

Fig. 8.1 Various levels of health promotion and prevention of disease

In addition to general activities to promote health the term "prevention" includes recommendations at three levels called

- Primary,
- Secondary and
- Tertiary prevention (Fig. 8.1).

8.1 Primary Prevention

The basis of rational recommendations for primary prevention of allergy or eczema is precise knowledge about causes and mechanisms of the development of these conditions as well as methods for the definition of possible risk groups (see Chap. 2).

8.1.1 Risk Groups

In all recommendations for primary prevention, it has to be distinguished between strategies involving the whole population and those which are only recommended for risk families.

While identifying risk groups beyond family history among atopic dermatitis patients, the most simple way to define allergy risk is family history, i.e., children whose parents are suffering or have suffered from an atopic disease (one or both parents) are at greater risk. Measurable laboratory biomarkers from cord blood have been investigated, but—in spite of progress in molecular genetics and experimental immunology—are not yet available for routine purposes such as T cell subpopulations, phosphodiesterase concentrations in mononuclear cells, IgE or IgE receptor expression, and filaggrin mutation.

8.1.2 Allergy Development

Our knowledge regarding causal factors in allergy development is limited and comprises, apart from allergen exposure, anthropogenic and biogenic

K. Eyerich, J. Ring, *Atopic Dermatitis - Eczema*, https://doi.org/10.1007/978-3-031-12499-0_8

Table 8.1 General avoidance of irritant factors

• Skin-irritative clothing, wool, nylon, too vehement skin cleaning, too early use of potentially sensitizing jewelry, e.g., nickel ear piercing
• Airways (dust, fog, air pollutants such as tobacco smoke, traffic exhaust, and volatile organic compounds VOCs)
• Nutrition (irritative or directly pharmacologically active compounds such as too hot spices and alcohol)
• Psychosocial (avoidance of unpleasant mental or emotional stress)

influences from the environment, which can act as modulators either in a protective or an enhancing sense (see Sect. 2.5 "Risk Factors"). The avoidance of allergy-enhancing factors might make sense in primary prevention.

Current recommendations comprise avoidance strategies, preferably regarding nutrition, but also other environmental factors from indoor and outdoor air (Table 8.1). An S3 guideline in Germany for primary allergy prevention is available and will be actualized [687].

Prevention strategies regarding nutrition and diet are covered under "hypoallergenic infant formula" and "nutrition."

8.1.3 Avoidance Strategies and General Recommendations

8.1.3.1 Pet Keeping

While over decades the classical recommendation was to strictly avoid fur- and feather-bearing animals in the house, a variety of recent studies have brought new evidence in a more differentiated way. It has been shown that persons with extremely high contact to pets (maximal cat allergen exposure in indoor air corresponding to keeping several cats) may develop protecting antibodies (quoted in [596, 597]).

Still, the recommendation to avoid cats is actual. This may be different with regard to dogs. There are studies which show a decreased allergy prevalence in families where dogs are kept. Therefore, the strict recommendation to avoid dogs is no longer relevant. With regard to the mechanisms, it may be speculated that dogs with their natural "coprophilic" behavior can alter the microbiome in the family environment!

For the general population there is no reason to restrict pet keeping with regard to primary allergy prevention. In this context, these strategies comprise allergies in general and are not specific to atopic dermatitis. There is however also no reason to keep pets for allergy prevention!

8.1.3.2 Farming Environment

One of the most exciting findings in the past has come from studies performed in the alpine regions of Bavaria, Austria, and Switzerland, where it has been found that living and growing up on a farm seemed to be protective with regard to the development of airway allergy [19, 353, 534]. It was interesting that a special type of farming culture with traditional farming (cows and cultivation) was protective, as well as the number of different species kept on a farm seemed to be important in the sense of "diversity" as a protective element.

Particularly pronounced were the effects when the mother of a child had worked in the stable during pregnancy [201, 662].

Regarding nutrition on the farm, see below.

8.1.3.3 Use of Parasites "Worms" in Atopy Prevention

According to the "jungle" or "hygiene" hypothesis, immunodeviation towards Th2 reaction pattern occurs when the natural stimulation of the immune system by parasitic infestation is lacking due to improved hygiene [237, 238, 601, 780].

Therefore, people have tried to induce similar immune-modulating effects by applying worms or helminth substances in order to decrease Th2 reactions.

There are clinical trials with parasites of the species Trichuris as well as Necator americanus. Most of the studies are still experimental however first clinical trials have not shown convincing effects [37].

One study described a good therapeutic effect of a compound named IPBD WB1001 as a small molecule having shown to inhibit proinflammatory cytokines and T cell migration. This compound was extracted from bacteria living in entomopathogenic nematodes (2-isopropyl-5-(E)-2-phenylethenyl) benzene-1,3-diol).

8.1.3.4 Aeroallergens

In the indoor air, where human beings spend most of their lifetime, it is advisable to produce a climate which does not favor mold growth; i.e., too high humidity and poor ventilation.

Exposure against house dust mites, especially in the bedroom, may play a role for allergic individuals; however, for primary prevention, reduction of mite exposure has not shown effective evidence.

8.1.3.5 Air Pollutants

The major air pollutant in the indoor air is derived from environmental tobacco smoke. Many studies have shown increased allergy and eczema prevalence rates in children passively exposed to tobacco smoke [690, 837]. Therefore, avoidance of smoking not only for the mother and during pregnancy, but also generally for the family is one of the most important recommendations for primary allergy prevention.

In the outdoor air, pollutants derived from car traffic exhaust are most relevant, especially fine and ultrafine particles, which has been shown in children living close to heavy traffic roads [449, 522]. Therefore, it is recommended to keep exposure against traffic exhaust as low as possible.

Apart from the alpine farmer's story, there is evidence from other studies that the Western lifestyle is associated with increased allergy and eczema prevalence according to the hygiene hypothesis [47, 769] (see Chap. 2).

8.1.3.6 Vaccination and Immunomodulatory Strategies

One of the questions most often asked by mothers in daily practice is whether their children can be vaccinated. There are rumors that "natural infection," e.g., with measles virus, may be more protective and more "healthy" than the vaccination. There is a great deal of philosophical involvement in these debates. Once, a very nice and intelligent father of such a religious community told me (JR) that "there must be some reason for these childhood infectious diseases in evolution and some benefit for mankind." Not very politely, I answered "Yes, you are right, there is indeed a reason, these infections are effective against overpopulation."

Adequately performed vaccinations do not increase the allergy risk, neither for airway nor for skin atopy. Of course, vaccination should not be performed during an acute flare of the disease. Therefore, all children with atopic dermatitis can receive normal vaccinations like other children! The second most asked question regarding egg allergy and vaccinations produced on eggs also can be answered clearly: "There is no contraindication for these vaccinations; in children with severe egg anaphylaxis it is recommended to test the vaccine prior to application."

The effect of immunomodulatory strategies such as application of pre- and probiotics will be covered below.

There are hints that the use of antibiotics in early life may be associated with the development of atopic dermatitis and other atopic diseases; however, the risk-benefit ratio is clearly positive, so there is no need to avoid antibiotics when they are necessary [625].

8.1.3.7 General Recommendations

General recommendations for primary prevention—also for secondary and tertiary prevention—comprise avoidance of irritants of all categories (see Table 6.1). This includes clothing, skin hygiene, jewelry, etc. [440]. A recent study found that nylon clothing, dust, and shampoos may play a role as triggers of eczema flares in children.

An epidemiological trial had found an association between increased water hardness and eczema prevalence in the United Kingdom [499]. However, the use of ion-coupled water softeners does not seem to have enough evidence to be recommended as a primary preventive strategy [254].

8.1.3.8 Pharmacological Primary Prevention

Attempts to induce primary prevention with pharmacological substances such as histamine antagonists have not shown the desired effect as was found in the ETAC (early treatment of atopic child) study when the infants were treated with cetirizine at first signs of atopic dermatitis over 2 years.

8.1.4 Nutrition and Dietary Recommendations

8.1.4.1 Breastfeeding

The longest-known and scientifically best-investigated recommendation for primary allergy prevention starts at birth and includes strict breastfeeding from day 1. From epidemiological investigations as well as animal experimental studies it is known that, in the first month of life, there is a special "window of opportunity" during which an organism can develop tolerance against environmental substances [12, 117, 339].

Breastfeeding thus is the only "general antiallergic diet" which can be recommended; however, the effect is limited and does not last very long. Therefore, the recommendations comprise only the first 4 months of life. Whether the positive effect of breast milk corresponds only to allergen avoidance, namely of cow proteins, or whether there may be active protective factors in breast milk is a matter of speculation.

The fact that in breast milk also small amounts of allergenic proteins depending upon the maternal diet may be detected implies dietary recommendations for lactating mothers. In Scandinavian studies, a certain effect of oligoallergenic diet during lactation has been observed [315].

In the last years, the evidence regarding breastfeeding and prevention of eczema has been more and more controversially discussed. There are also studies which show increased rates of eczema in breastfed children and meta-analyses have concluded that there was no convincing evidence of a protective effect of exclusive breastfeeding in eczema [238].

8.1.4.2 Solid Food in the First Year of Life

With regard to the introduction of solid food, the recommendations have changed slightly: While previously introduction of solid food was recommended only after the sixth month, this has now been shortened to the fourth month of life. There is no evidence of a definite preventive effect of delayed introduction of solid food. Also a certain diversity of food groups—with special emphasis on yoghurt—seems to be helpful [662].

8.1.4.3 General Recommendations

There is no general antiallergic diet. There have been studies showing that regular consumption of fish already in the first year of life may have a protective effect. Generally, Mediterranean diet with a high amount of polyunsaturated fatty acids may have beneficial effects. This also holds true for dietary recommendations during pregnancy. Generally, also obesity seems to be a risk factor for asthma. Therefore, normal diet and avoidance of obesity is also recommended.

It is important that the diet in the first year of life contains all the necessary elements and vitamins and a certain degree of diversity according to general nutrition recommendations (Fig. 8.2).

8.1.4.4 Nutrition During Pregnancy

For the time during pregnancy, recommendations are difficult and generally controversially discussed (see probiotics); there is limited evidence from prospective clinical trials.

Mostly nutrition for a pregnant woman is not easy and connected with a lot of problems. Therefore, it is important not to make it more difficult. Most important is avoidance of smoking (see above) and too much calories (control of body weight), since obese pregnant women tend to give birth to overweight children. New studies have shown that increased body mass index is associated with higher prevalence of asthma [839]. There are no good studies with regard to atopic dermatitis.

Avoidance of overweight has therefore been included in current dietary recommendations for allergy prevention.

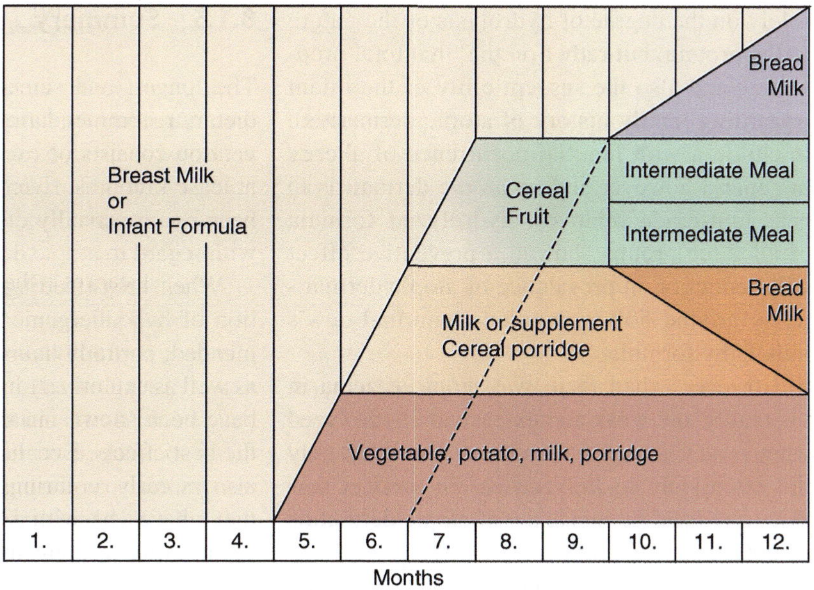

Fig. 8.2 Dietary schedule for healthy nutrition in the first year of life (with friendly permission of C. Kugler)

Possible regular intake of fish—probably because of high amounts of polyunsaturated fatty acids—during pregnancy and lactation may have beneficial effects [196].

8.1.4.5 Hypoallergenic Formula

Whenever breastfeeding is not possible for one or another reason, there are a variety of "hypoallergenic" infant formulas which can be used as a supplement to cow's milk [818].

The term "hypoallergenic" can only be used when certain requirements are fulfilled by law, i.e., among others a concentration of allergenic protein of less than 1% in the original product in Germany. From the point of view of food technology, mostly hydrolysis is used to achieve these levels by either enzymatic digestion, ultra-high temperature, or ultrafiltration. Therefore, also the term "hydrolysate formula" is used. Apart from the chemical nature of the major ingredients of the original material, namely casein or whey molecules, the intensity of the hydrolysis, which can lead to either partially or extensively hydrolyzed food, is crucial. Earlier mostly weak hydrolysates had been used for prevention, while now extensively hydrolyzed formula are only given when there is already existing cow's milk allergy.

Among many studies with regard to the efficacy of hypoallergenic infant nutrition in allergy prevention, the GINI study (German Infant Nutritional Intervention) has yielded quite reliable results. More than 2000 newborns were investigated in a prospective randomized and double-blind study. Apart from a control group, one group was exclusively breastfed, and three groups received hydrolysate formula of different degrees. As parameters of outcome, the occurrence of atopic dermatitis, food allergy, or urticaria was observed [54, 55]. The group with exclusive breastfeeding was not included in the final evaluation since for ethical reasons neither randomization nor blinding could be performed here. However, it is interesting that some of the extensively hydrolyzed formula had a similar allergy-preventive or even better effect than exclusive breastfeeding. The formula groups received

- Partially hydrolyzed whey,
- Extensively hydrolyzed whey,
- Extensively hydrolyzed casein.

In a careful analysis of the results, the authors came to the conclusion that there is a preventive effect of hypoallergenic infant formula which however does not seem to depend solely on the degree of hydrolysis or the nature of the protein, but rather on the final total preparation and also the susceptibility of the infant (regarding family history of atopic dermatitis). In children with familial occurrence of allergy in general however and no atopic dermatitis in near first-grade relatives, hydrolyzed formula of all three groups showed a preventive effect with reduction in prevalence of atopic dermatitis by around 50% compared to normal cow's milk baby formula.

However, when there was atopic eczema in the family, the weak and extensively hydrolyzed whey products were no longer effective, but only the extensively hydrolyzed casein product was able to reduce the incidence of atopic dermatitis by 50%.

Apart from hypoallergenic products, there are allergen-free amino acid mixtures (e.g., Neocate) which can also be given as therapeutic nutrition.

8.1.4.6 Pre- and Probiotics

Preventive effects of probiotics are discussed controversially (see Chap. 2). Possible effects of prebiotic oligosaccharides have been reported in a controlled study [282].

There have been attempts to reduce allergy development by prophylactic intake of probiotics during pregnancy [379] which however have not found enough evidence for general recommendation.

8.1.4.7 Barrier Restoration

While initial results suggested it could be possible to prevent initial development of atopic dermatitis in high-risk infants by applying emollients (Simpson et al. [337, 749]; Horimukai et al.) larger trials could not confirm this [128]. Whether this might be promising in a subtype of atopic dermatitis or could depend on the emollient used is currently unknown. New studies with better emollients are on the way, since the rationale of the concept is quite attractive. Introduction of an allergen-poor food diet did not result in primary prevention [141], neither as a single intervention nor in combination with emollients.

8.1.5 Summary

The longest and scientifically best investigated dietary recommendation for primary allergy prevention consists of exclusive breastfeeding over at least 4 months. Even this recommendation has been controversially discussed in the recent past with regard to atopic dermatitis.

When breastfeeding is not possible, application of hypoallergenic infant formula is recommended; partially hydrolyzed whey preparations as well as extensively hydrolyzed casein products have been shown in large clinical trials to yield the best effects. Eventually, regular intake of fish also as early as during pregnancy and lactation may have beneficial effects as well as a Mediterranean diet. The role of introduction of solid food seems to be less important, it can be started after the fourth month of life. Recent studies have shown that overweight is associated with a higher risk of asthma; therefore, avoidance of high-calorie diets have also been included in recommendations for allergy prevention.

Recommendations for primary prevention also comprise avoidance strategies and general considerations. In the last years, these recommendations have been less rigid with regard to pet keeping: While cats should still be avoided, dog keeping does not seem to go along with an increased risk of allergy, but may even have protective effects. However, there is no indication for the general population to keep pets for allergy prevention.

Indoors, climate conditions of too high humidity allowing mold growth should be avoided. The most important recommendation with regard to air pollutants is avoidance of tobacco smoke in the indoor air, traffic exhaust in the outdoor air. There is no reason why atopic individuals should not be vaccinated like normal children. Interesting results from epidemiological trials such as in remote islands or alpine farm environments are very important for research, but cannot be translated easily into practical prevention recommendations.

8.2 Secondary Prevention

Secondary prevention describes the detection of risk groups by early screening programs and the prevention or reduction of developing symptoms or disease. In the case of allergy, this means screening for atopic sensitization and application of preventive measures only in these individuals. The general measures correspond to the above-discussed recommendations for primary prevention.

8.3 Tertiary Prevention: Rehabilitation

Tertiary prevention, also called rehabilitation, is one of the most important strategies in the long-term management of allergic patients; it describes all activities after the first diagnosis and treatment in the acute phase in order to achieve as long as possible remission intervals thus allowing participation in normal active life in society and occupation. Among the total of rehabilitation costs of most insurance or government agencies, approx. 1–2% regard allergic skin and airway diseases.

In many countries, there are legal conditions for outpatient or inpatient rehabilitation measures which also contain rules for standardization and quality control in the general management of patients with atopic dermatitis. In Central Europe, inpatient facilities specialized in allergic airway and skin diseases are available. In quality control and management programs, studies with regard to the quality of life and patient satisfaction as well as days of work loss have been performed. For the indication "atopic dermatitis," similar to "allergic airway disease," there was an estimated reduction of costs of around 1000 € already in the first 6 months after an inpatient rehabilitation.

For adolescents, the question with regard to the choice of occupation is often a great problem in atopic individuals, especially when they suffer from hand eczema. An individual and adequate occupational counseling play an important role for these adolescents. It needs to be evaluated and the patient informed, but there should be no prohibited occupations. There are occupations with a high risk due to intensive contact with potent allergens such as baker, cook, or animal caretaker, or strongly irritative substances for the skin, such as a hairdresser or car mechanic. In individuals with severe atopic dermatitis, one generally would advise to avoid occupations with great skin strain.

Also counseling with regard to pet keeping, hobbies and vacation should be given. What is important is the individual and independent interaction with the informed patient with regard to basic therapeutic measures both in avoidance strategies of specific and nonspecific irritants and in active protection.

8.3.1 Socioeconomic Impact

There is a high degree of variability with regard to the yearly costs of atopic dermatitis when only doctor's visits or drug prescriptions are counted or when also indirect costs for the patient are included.

In the outpatient sector, the introduction of an "office fee" for outpatients in Germany in January 2004 led to a marked reduction in visits of patients with atopic dermatitis in the dermatologist's office. At the same time there was a steep increase of "alternative," "unconventional" treatments as well as no evidence-based treatment of eczema with systemic glucocorticosteroids, especially in patients with rare doctor visits [709].

8.3.2 Summary

Rehabilitation is the most important aspect of tertiary prevention in atopic eczema where inpatient treatments are most successful. By adequate tertiary prevention already in the first year after an inpatient stay, direct and indirect illness costs can be reduced markedly.

8.4 Climate Therapy in Secondary and Tertiary Prevention

The term "climate therapy" describes a complex medical treatment which includes beneficial effects of certain climatic regions, but not exclusively these effects.

Already early sources of medical history in scriptures of Hippocrates and his disciples or from ancient China and Rome reveal that humans were seeking cure from chronic diseases in special places with climate characteristics. In the nineteenth century, these aspects were studied by scientific medicine especially for airway diseases. A special date is the year 1852 when the young physician from Southwest Germany who had to take refuge in Switzerland after the revolution of 1848, Alexander Spengler, came to Davos to take care of the population and later opened a sanatorium for lung diseases. Later the Dutch physician Holsboer intensified these treatments which became very popular all over the world and found their literary description in Thomas Mann's "The Magic Mountain" ("Der Zauberberg"). In 1953, climate therapy was started at the North Sea island of Norderney under Jo Hartung. The first German patient orgainzaiton the "Hay Fever Association" (Heufieberbund), today "Deutscher Allergie- und Asthmabund" (daab) was founded in 1898 on the island of Helgoland, and this was not a coincidence!

Also in 1898, the German Hermann Burchard founded a special hospital for lung diseases in Davos-Wolfgang which was guided after the Second World War by Christian Virchow, a great-nephew of Rudolf Virchow as "high-altitude clinic for asthma patients." In 1960, Siegfried Borelli discovered, after early work with Alfred Marchionini (in 1956), that the climate of Davos also had beneficial effects on certain skin diseases, especially atopic dermatitis [83].

In modern meteorology, climate describes the characteristic interplay and composure of atmospheric factors over a certain area together with the specific meteorological conditions of weather.

Table 8.2 Factors influencing or determining a characteristic climate (according to Vocks et al. [830, 831])

Geographic factors	Meteorologic factors (weather)
• Altitude above sea level • Distance to sea • Connection to high mountains and valleys • Composition of soil • Type of vegetation • Most frequent wind directions	• Solar irradiation • Precipitation (fog, rain, snow) • Air humidity • Air temperature • Air pressure • Air movement (wind) • Aerosol composition (natural, anthropogenic)

From this definition it becomes clear that specific climates can only be found under very specific geographic and meteorologic conditions. These are areas on the seashore or the Dead Sea on the one hand and high altitude on the other hand. In between, daily weather changes contribute much more to the actual climate than a specific geographic characteristic [755].

Table 8.2 describes relevant geographic and meteorologic factors for determining a "climate." Apart from photoactinic factors with thermic-hygric effects, there is a complex interaction also with regard to oxygen concentrations as well as the ionization of the air and the composure of aerosol particles.

8.4.1 High Altitude, North Sea, and Dead Sea

Climate therapy tries to treat patients by using the exposure to physicochemical effects of the atmosphere with the aim to avoid noxious substances and, on the other hand, adapt to natural environmental irritants.

In various scientific investigations, influences of the Davos high-altitude climate on autonomic nervous system, immunologic reactivity as well as general clinical parameters important for asthma or atopic dermatitis have been found [346] (Table 8.3).

In the healthy climate of Davos, the low allergen content of air, especially the absence of house dust mites has special importance for asthma and atopic dermatitis [721] (see Chap. 6).

Table 8.3 Climate characteristics of the high mountain valley in Davos (Switzerland) important for asthma and atopic eczema (Vocks et al. [84, 831])

Protective effects
Clean air (pollutants)
Clean air (microbes)
Improved tolerance to cold ("dry cold")
Reduced number of allergens
• Pollen
• Mites
• Molds
Absence of gusty winds
Relaxation in the ambient alpine landscape
Possibly stimulating ("irritating") effects on immune system
Lower average temperature over the year compared to low lands (ca 3 centigrade)
Lower air humidity
Effect on suprarenal glands with an increase in endogenous cortisol production
Increase of endogenous erythrocyte production (oxygen carrier)

Similar climate effects have been described on North Sea islands (except for house dust mites) and to a lesser extent on other seashores. Experiences with the climate therapy on the Dead Sea in Israel report beneficial effects in psoriasis and to a minor extent on eczema, mostly due to the increased long-wave UV radiation and the high salt content of the water [310].

The protected high-altitude situation in Davos also is characterized by a relatively low occurrence of wind, which is accepted well by most patients. Too strong gusty winds may irritate the skin and the airways.

Climate therapy can either be performed as an inpatient model for acute exacerbation of eczema or as rehabilitation in specialized clinics [101, 232, 755].

Scientific investigations with regard to the itch sensation showed an interesting dependence of itch intensity on meteorologic changes; Especially when the weather changed, and before a change of air humidity, many patients suffer from more intense itch sensations.

Of practical importance is the fact that under climate therapy conditions, a significant steroid-sparing effect can be observed. After a short phase of adaptation with occasional and reversible flares in the first days, most patients experience improvement and long-lasting stabilization without strong systemic or topical therapeutics [217].

In many patients, adequate allergy diagnostics (see Chap. 6) are only possible under the conditions of climate therapy, since under normal conditions at home they either suffer from generalized eczema, and the skin cannot be tested, or they have to be treated with systemic or topical anti-inflammatory substances not allowing allergy testing.

A randomized comparative study of rehabilitation measures in the Netherlands compared the high-altitude situation in Davos with similar treatment in the Netherlands in asthma and showed significant improvement by high-altitude climate therapy [279].

Of course, climate never can act alone, but always in connection with classic dermatologic as well as general treatment, including psychosomatic counseling, dietary recommendations, sports and ergotherapy, etc., in a complex intervention. For severe patients, it is easier when they have adequate time and the right ambience to learn and accept the conditions of their disease and gain motivation to change certain factors in their lifestyle. Therefore, also educational programs are often easier and more effective under these conditions than in the normal, often stressful, life at home.

A climate-therapeutical intervention should cover a period of 4 weeks, better 6 weeks. It is sad that in our more and more hectic times, with the acceleration of daily life, many patients cannot afford this period.

8.4.2 Summary

Climate therapy describes a complex treatment schedule in areas with specific characteristic geographic and meteorologic conditions for allergy, asthma, or atopic dermatitis, in Central Europe particularly North Sea islands as well as high altitudes, in Israel the Dead Sea. Numerous investigations described influences, especially of the Davos high-altitude climate on autonomic nervous system, immune reactions as well as allergologic parameters in atopic dermatitis. Acute inpatients stays as well as inpatient rehabilitation measures under climate therapy conditions lead to improvement in many patients with severe atopic dermatitis, often lasting over years and sometimes decisively changing the progression of the disease towards improvement. In some patients, adequate allergy diagnostics is only possible under allergen-poor climate-therapeutical conditions.

8.5 Educational Programs ("Eczema School")

From the manifold illustrations and texts with regard to clinical symptomatology and multiple causes and trigger factors as well as diagnostic therapeutic and preventive recommendations, it becomes clear that it is not possible to give all this information in the average daily routine office [259].

8.5.1 Development of "Eczema School"

Therefore, at the end of the 80s, several groups started to develop educational programs for certain diseases which started as group sessions mostly devoted to giving information. In 1993, the German Minister of Health started a project to improve the care and prevention of atopic eczema in children. On the basis of this expertise, the development of an educational program was started in a national consensus and in an interdisciplinary setting including psychological, pedagogic, and also nutritional aspects. From this project, the "working group eczema school" ("Arbeitsgemeinschaft Neurodermitisschulung" AGNES) developed an educational program as an institution to guarantee permanent quality control and standardization of this program [185, 269, 758]. Later this was followed by an initiative also for adults [322]. Similar programs have been developed and are in use in many countries [760, 908].

8.5.2 Contents

The contents of this "eczema school" comprise not only information on structure and function of the skin, disturbances in skin barrier, and immune mechanisms in atopic dermatitis, but also knowledge on individual provocation factors and their avoidance. In addition, psychologic aspects of symptom perception, together with relaxation techniques and role plays for coping with emotional aspects, are trained. Furthermore, family dynamic aspects and psychosocial aspects are covered [259, 840]. Special emphasis is given to psychosomatic aspects and relaxation techniques. Recently new programs for stress reduction via "mindfulness" have shown promising results [564] Finally, the various therapeutic options including discussion on unconventional procedures are covered.

8.5.3 Evaluation

This complex intervention program "Eczema School" has been studied in a prospective randomized trial with a control group in a waiting loop. In over 1000 patients, the program was found to be significantly effective [758]. It was of particular interest that not only the parameters of quality of life and psychologic well-being or coping with illness-induced stress showed improvement, but also the very simple real intensity of eczematous skin lesion as measured in the scoring system SCORAD.

8.5.4 Practical Performance

The eczema school is offered in six consequent 2-h sessions (e.g., every Wednesday evening from 7.00 to 9.00 pm) for maximum 6–12 parents of 6 children. It is essential that there is an interdisciplinary approach: At least one physician—dermatologist, pediatrician, or allergist—a psychologist or psychosomatic physician and a nutrition expert have to work together in order to guarantee the quality and get reimbursement from insurances. The inclusion of a specially trained nurse is optional.

8.5.5 Qualification of Trainers

In order to guarantee the quality of the program, only individuals with a certificate as "eczema trainer" are allowed to do the school. It has to be learned that not every physician is also a good teacher. In Germany, there are specialized "eczema academies" which are entitled to offer "train-the-trainer seminars" for physicians, psychologists, and nutritional experts. In a program of 40 h, including practical exercises, a hospitation in an already existing eczema school and final supervision (personal or video) of an own session has to be documented before the individual is accepted as an "eczema trainer." This model of eczema school is now spread all over Germany and has become so successful that it has been copied by many other countries.

New target groups for educational programs include nurses, nursery nurses, but also special emphasis should be given to reaching difficult groups in society.

8.5.6 Music Therapy

In the context of educational programs, also music therapy has been used; together with melodies and rhythms—depending on the life events and the actual situation—with improvisation, singing and instrumental performance, emotions of the patients are registered and evaluated in the group session. This interpersonal perception, together with the physical expression, allows the patient a very special and facilitated communication—often without words.

In music therapy, one can differentiate between

- Receptive music therapy for relaxation and calming down.
- Active music therapy with the aim of musical improvisation in order to facilitate communication and own musical activities which help the patient to cope with difficult life situations.

8.5.7 Summary

In the 90s, in a national consensus supported by the German Ministry of Health, an interdisciplinary educational program for atopic eczema was developed which comprises six consequent 2-h sessions for maximally 6–12 parents of 6 children. The educational program is interdisciplinary in nature with a physician (dermatologist, pediatrician, or allergist), a psychologist, and a nutritionist, optionally together with a specialized nurse. This educational program "eczema school" was studied in a prospective controlled randomized trial and found to be significantly effective both for improving quality of life, but also for improving actual eczematous skin lesions. In Germany, this program is reimbursed by the insurances. In order to guarantee the standardization and quality control, train-the-trainer seminars in order to get the qualification "eczema trainer" are offered in various "eczema academies" in Germany in a standardized fashion. Music therapy may be of additional help in these programs.

9 Outlook into the Future

The last century brought us enormous insights into the pathogenesis, the clinical course, comorbidities, the stigmatization, and loss of quality of life of patients suffering from atopic dermatitis as well as their surroundings. Today, we know how prevalent atopic dermatitis is all over the world and which consequences this disease has on our socioeconomic environment. We know about the pathogenesis mosaics that range from genetic predisposition, epigenetic contribution, innate and specific immunity, an impaired epidermal barrier, and disturbed microbial colonization of the skin. Bigger epidemiological trials, registries, and improved methods will help us to get an even more granular picture. This holds also true for advancing research methods such as single-cell techniques and artificial intelligence.

What is missing is to project all this knowledge to an individual patient. It is more than just speculation that atopic dermatitis comprises several clinically relevant endotypes—but we are just at the beginning to understand how to define these. Clinically relevant questions such as the prediction of the natural clinical course of the disease, the risk to develop comorbidities, or the prediction of a therapeutic response are still impossible to answer. This becomes more and more relevant, as we have an increasing number of possibilities on the therapeutics side—we might think about primary or at least secondary prevention in some patients using emollients, food diet, or immunotherapy; we have more and more developments of innovative topical therapies, conventional and smart immunomodulators, and biological therapies. The biggest unmet need is now to develop precise diagnostics that tailors this therapeutic toolbox to an individual patient. So far, this diagnostic toolbox consists of the clinical view (which will always be the most important aspect), family and personal history of the patient, a small portfolio of laboratory tools such as IgE levels or S. aureus detection from smear test cultures, as well as the description of the skin architecture. In the future, image-based artificial intelligence algorithms, as well as molecular diagnostics, is needed to improve the tailored care for each individual atopic dermatitis patient (Fig. 9.1).

With increasing help on the diagnostic side, the role for us as physicians will drastically change—from a diagnostistian to an interpreter of given suggestions. We will need to understand and integrate automated diagnostic findings—and translate them to the individual patient with all empathy and logical reasoning at the same time. It is a very interesting time to be a doctor treating atopic dermatitis!

K. Eyerich, J. Ring, *Atopic Dermatitis - Eczema*, https://doi.org/10.1007/978-3-031-12499-0_9

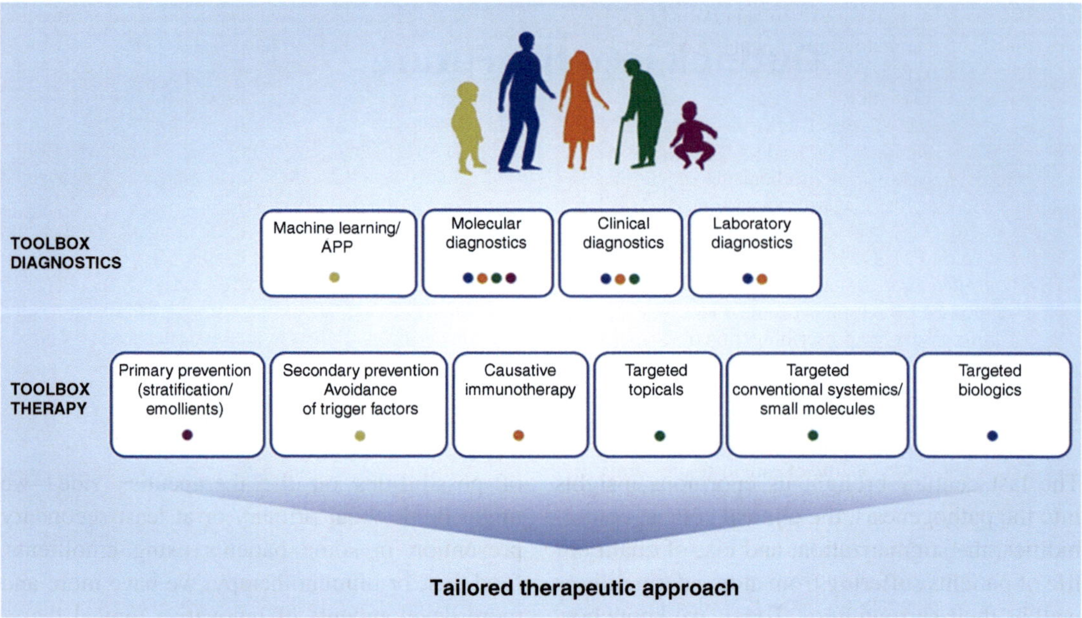

Fig. 9.1 Outlook into the future of atopic dermatitis. From Ref. [223]

10 Concluding Remarks: How To Live With Eczema/Atopic Dermatitis

The many informations and commentaries in this book, starting from the clinical morphology and epidemiology via pathophysiology, diagnostics, therapy, and prevention, make clear that atopic dermatitis is a very complex disease which cannot be treated well in a quick physician-patient contact and by writing a simple prescription for a cream, pill, or an injection.

In spite of clear-cut psychosomatic interactions with deteriorations of skin lesions in specific stress situations, it has to be stated that atopic dermatitis is neither a "psychiatric" nor a "mental" disease, but a skin disease which can be modulated by psychological influences—negatively and positively! The development of atopic eczema never is the product of "guilt"—neither of the patient nor of the mother or father—rather it is the result of a complex interplay of genetic predisposition and environmental factors.

Although patients may be very severely affected, it is possible in most cases to improve the disease in a way that a normal and enjoyable life is possible. To achieve this, the efforts not only of the patient, but also of his/her social environment, in family and occupation, and continuous activity and observation of various aspects are necessary. These include strategies for daily skincare and avoidance of noxious influences. Psychological influences never should be overestimated; however, also not be neglected. It may happen that a short eczema flare can start in a period of extreme happiness.

It should be stressed that patients with atopic dermatitis—similar to those with atopic airway disease—are not helpless victims of their destiny. Even if the genetic predisposition cannot be changed at this time, and the patients will have the tendency to hypersensitivity and dryness of the skin and possible development of eczema, we try to avoid the term "incurable" for this disease. The excruciating eczematous skin lesions can be very well treated—and our therapeutic possibilities increase more and more, now ranging from potential prevention over causative approaches to symptomatic treatments with topical agents, oral treatments, or biologics interacting with Th2 immunity. The big challenge in AD is currently to translate the growing knowledge about the molecular basis of AD into tailored clinical decisions—the basis of precision medicine. We can state that most likely there are relevant endotypes of AD, and numerous biomarkers are proposed to stratify AD patients, but none of them has truly arrived in daily clinical practice.

Thus, still the basis of a good prognosis for a relatively normal life is the confidential cooperation in mutual trust between patient and physician, who should have special experience in this

K. Eyerich, J. Ring, *Atopic Dermatitis - Eczema*, https://doi.org/10.1007/978-3-031-12499-0_10

disease and who knows the problems and can give advice to the patient, even in difficult times. This approach will restore the joy of life and the capability to work by offering adequate therapeutic strategies.

We try to awake in the patients the drive to take responsibility for their skin disease and its management, what we like to call "patient empowerment."

We tell our patients:

"You will be your own skin doctor; you will know what cream to apply at which time of the day to which area of your body and in which concentration and what you should take systemically in order to be symptom-free. For possible catastrophes, we still feel responsible and you can come back to us whenever you like, we will deal with your problem!"

References

1. Aaboud M, Aad G, Abbott B, Abdallah J, Abdinov O, Abeloos B, et al. Measurement of detector-corrected observables sensitive to the anomalous production of events with jets and large missing transverse momentum in p p collisions at s = 13 TeV using the ATLAS detector. Eur Phys J C Part Fields. 2017;77(11):765.
2. Abeck D, Mempel M. Staphylococcus aureus colonization in atopic dermatitis and its therapeutic implications. Br J Dermatol. 1998;139(Suppl 53):13–6.
3. Abels C, Proksch E. Therapy of atopic dermatitis. Hautarzt. 2006;57(8):711–23; quiz 24-5
4. Abuabara K, van Zuuren EJ, Flohr C. Why does the BJD require registration of systematic reviews and meta-analyses? Br J Dermatol. 2019;180(2):249–50.
5. Adachi J, Endo K, Fukuzumi T, Tanigawa N, Aoki T. Increasing incidence of streptococcal impetigo in atopic dermatitis. J Dermatol Sci. 1998;17(1):45–53.
6. Agache I, Akdis C. Global atlas of allergy; 2017. https://medialibrary.eaaci.org/mediatheque/media.aspx?mediaId=60228&channel=8518.
7. Agache I, Rocha C, Pereira A, Song Y, Alonso-Coello P, Sola I, et al. Efficacy and safety of treatment with omalizumab for chronic spontaneous urticaria: a systematic review for the EAACI Biologicals Guidelines. Allergy. 2021;76(1):59–70.
8. Agache I, Song Y, Posso M, Alonso-Coello P, Rocha C, Sola I, et al. Efficacy and safety of dupilumab for moderate-to-severe atopic dermatitis: a systematic review for the EAACI Biologicals Guidelines. Allergy. 2020;76(1):45–58.
9. Aguilar-Pimentel JA, Cho YL, Gerlini R, Calzada-Wack J, Wimmer M, Mayer-Kuckuk P, et al. Increased estrogen to androgen ratio enhances immunoglobulin levels and impairs B cell function in male mice. Sci Rep. 2020;10(1):18334.
10. Ahmad-Nejad P, Mrabet-Dahbi S, Breuer K, Klotz M, Werfel T, Herz U, et al. The toll-like receptor 2 R753Q polymorphism defines a subgroup of patients with atopic dermatitis having severe phenotype. J Allergy Clin Immunol. 2004;113(3):565–7.
11. Akdis CA, Akdis M, Bieber T, Bindslev-Jensen C, Boguniewicz M, Eigenmann P, et al. Diagnosis and treatment of atopic dermatitis in children and adults: European Academy of Allergology and Clinical Immunology/American Academy of Allergy, Asthma and Immunology/PRACTALL Consensus Report. Allergy. 2006;61(8):969–87.
12. Akdis CA, Akdis M, Trautmann A, Blaser K. Immune regulation in atopic dermatitis. Curr Opin Immunol. 2000;12(6):641–6.
13. Akdis CA, Blaser K, Akdis M. Mechanisms of allergen-specific immunotherapy. Chem Immunol Allergy. 2006;91:195–203.
14. Akerstrom U, Reitamo S, Langeland T, Berg M, Rustad L, Korhonen L, et al. Comparison of moisturizing creams for the prevention of atopic dermatitis relapse: a randomized double-blind controlled multicentre clinical trial. Acta Derm Venereol. 2015;95(5):587–92.
15. Akhavan A, Rudikoff D. The treatment of atopic dermatitis with systemic immunosuppressive agents. Clin Dermatol. 2003;21(3):225–40.
16. Akira S, Uematsu S, Takeuchi O. Pathogen recognition and innate immunity. Cell. 2006;124(4):783–801.
17. Alessandrini F, Schulz H, Takenaka S, Lentner B, Karg E, Behrendt H, et al. Effects of ultrafine carbon particle inhalation on allergic inflammation of the lung. J Allergy Clin Immunol. 2006;117(4):824–30.
18. Alexander H, Paller AS, Traidl-Hoffmann C, Beck LA, De Benedetto A, Dhar S, et al. The role of bacterial skin infections in atopic dermatitis: expert statement and review from the International Eczema Council Skin Infection Group. Br J Dermatol. 2020;182(6):1331–42.
19. Alfven T, Braun-Fahrlander C, Brunekreef B, von Mutius E, Riedler J, Scheynius A, et al. Allergic diseases and atopic sensitization in children related to farming and anthroposophic lifestyle—The PARSIFAL study. Allergy. 2006;61(4):414–21.
20. Alm JS, Swartz J, Bjorksten B, Engstrand L, Engstrom J, Kuhn I, et al. An anthroposophic lifestyle and intestinal microflora in infancy. Pediatr Allergy Immunol. 2002;13(6):402–11.
21. Alm JS, Swartz J, Lilja G, Scheynius A, Pershagen G. Atopy in children of families with an anthroposophic lifestyle. Lancet. 1999;353(9163):1485–8.
22. Andrews AL, Holloway JW, Holgate ST, Davies DE. IL-4 receptor alpha is an important modulator

K. Eyerich, J. Ring, *Atopic Dermatitis - Eczema*, https://doi.org/10.1007/978-3-031-12499-0

of IL-4 and IL-13 receptor binding: implications for the development of therapeutic targets. J Immunol. 2006;176(12):7456–61.
23. Anzai A, Wang EHC, Lee EY, Aoki V, Christiano AM. Pathomechanisms of immune-mediated alopecia. Int Immunol. 2019;31(7):439–47.
24. Apfelbacher CJ, Ofenloch RF, Weisshaar E, Molin S, Bauer A, Mahler V, et al. Chronic hand eczema in Germany: 5-year follow-up data from the CARPE registry. Contact Dermatitis. 2019;80(1):45–53.
25. Arellano FM, Wentworth CE, Arana A, Fernandez C, Paul CF. Risk of lymphoma following exposure to calcineurin inhibitors and topical steroids in patients with atopic dermatitis. J Invest Dermatol. 2007;127(4):808–16.
26. Armstrong NC, Ernst E. The treatment of eczema with Chinese herbs: a systematic review of randomized clinical trials. Br J Clin Pharmacol. 1999;48(2):262–4.
27. Arshad SH, Bateman B, Matthews SM. Primary prevention of asthma and atopy during childhood by allergen avoidance in infancy: a randomised controlled study. Thorax. 2003;58(6):489–93.
28. Artik S, Ruzicka T. Complementary therapy for atopic eczema and other allergic skin diseases. Dermatol Ther. 2003;16(2):150–63.
29. Asgari MM, Tsai AL, Avalos L, Sokil M, Quesenberry CP Jr. Association between topical calcineurin inhibitor use and keratinocyte carcinoma risk among adults with atopic dermatitis. JAMA Dermatol. 2020;156(10):1066–73.
30. Asher MI, Montefort S, Bjorksten B, Lai CK, Strachan DP, Weiland SK, et al. Worldwide time trends in the prevalence of symptoms of asthma, allergic rhinoconjunctivitis, and eczema in childhood: ISAAC Phases One and Three repeat multicountry cross-sectional surveys. Lancet. 2006;368(9537):733–43.
31. Aszodi N, Thurau S, Seegraber M, de Bruin-Weller M, Wollenberg A. Management of dupilumab-associated conjunctivitis in atopic dermatitis. J Dtsch Dermatol Ges. 2019;17(5):488–91.
32. Atherton DJ, Sewell M, Soothill JF, Wells RS, Chilvers CE. A double-blind controlled crossover trial of an antigen-avoidance diet in atopic eczema. Lancet. 1978;1(8061):401–3.
33. Augustin M, Misery L, von Kobyletzki L, et al. Unveiling the true costs and societal impacts of moderate-to-severe atopic dermatitis in Europe. J Eur Acad Dermatol Venereol. 2022;36(Suppl. 7):3–16.
34. Augustin M, Zschocke I, Buhrke U. Attitudes and prior experience with respect to alternative medicine among dermatological patients: the Freiburg questionnaire on attitudes to naturopathy (FAN). Forsch Komplementarmed. 1999;6(Suppl 2):26–9.
35. Augustin M, Zschocke I, Lange S, Seidenglanz K, Amon U. Quality of life in skin diseases: methodological and practical comparison of different quality of life questionnaires in psoriasis and atopic dermatitis. Hautarzt. 1999;50(10):715–22.
36. Bae JM, Choi YY, Park CO, Chung KY, Lee KH. Efficacy of allergen-specific immunotherapy for atopic dermatitis: a systematic review and meta-analysis of randomized controlled trials. J Allergy Clin Immunol. 2013;132(1):110–7.
37. Bager P, Arnved J, Ronborg S, Wohlfahrt J, Poulsen LK, Westergaard T, et al. Trichuris suis ova therapy for allergic rhinitis: a randomized, double-blind, placebo-controlled clinical trial. J Allergy Clin Immunol. 2010;125(1):123–30. e1-3
38. Bair B, Dodd J, Heidelberg K, Krach K. Cataracts in atopic dermatitis: a case presentation and review of the literature. Arch Dermatol. 2011;147(5):585–8.
39. Balaji H, Heratizadeh A, Wichmann K, Niebuhr M, Crameri R, Scheynius A, et al. Malassezia sympodialis thioredoxin-specific T cells are highly cross-reactive to human thioredoxin in atopic dermatitis. J Allergy Clin Immunol. 2011;128(1):92–9 e4.
40. Bandmann HJ. In: Miescher G, Storck H, editors. Ekzem und ekzematoide Dermatitiden im Kindesalter. Berlin: Springer; 1962.
41. Bannister MJ, Freeman S. Adult-onset atopic dermatitis. Australasian J Dermatol. 2000;41(4):225–8.
42. Bard S, Paravisini A, Aviles-Izquierdo JA, Fernandez-Cruz E, Sanchez-Ramon S. Eczematous dermatitis in the setting of hyper-IgE syndrome successfully treated with omalizumab. Arch Dermatol. 2008;144(12):1662–3.
43. Baur X, Dewair M, Fruhmann G, Aschauer H, Pfletschinger J, Braunitzer G. Hypersensitivity to chironomids (non-biting midges): localization of the antigenic determinants within certain polypeptide sequences of hemoglobins (erythrocruorins) of Chironomus thummi thummi (Diptera). J Allergy Clin Immunol. 1982;69(1 Pt 1):66–76.
44. Becker D, Langer E, Seemann M, Seemann G, Fell I, Saloga J, et al. Clinical efficacy of blue light full body irradiation as treatment option for severe atopic dermatitis. PLoS One. 2011;6(6):e20566.
45. Bedi MK, Shenefelt PD. Herbal therapy in dermatology. Arch Dermatol. 2002;138(2):232–42.
46. Behrendt H, Ring J. In: Heppt W, Bachert C, editors. Genetik und Umwelteinflüsse in der Epidemiologie von Allergien. Stuttgart: Thieme; 2011.
47. Behrendt H, Ring J. In: Wilderer PA, Grambow M, Molls M, Oexle K, editors. Allergy - a disease of civilization. Berlin: Springer; 2022.
48. Behrendt H, Tomczok J, Sliwa-Tomczok W, Kasche A, Ebner von Eschenbach C, Becker WM, et al. Timothy grass (Phleum pratense L.) pollen as allergen carriers and initiators of an allergic response. Int Arch Allergy Immunol. 1999;118(2-4):414–8.
49. Behrens T, Taeger D, Maziak W, Duhme H, Rzehak P, Weiland SK, et al. Self-reported traffic density and atopic disease in children. Results of the ISAAC Phase III survey in Muenster, Germany. Pediatr Allergy Immunol. 2004;15(4):331–9.
50. Behrens S, von Kobyletzki G, Gruss C, Reuther T, Altmeyer P, Kerscher M. PUVA-bath photochemotherapy (PUVA-soak therapy) of recalcitrant

dermatoses of the palms and soles. Photodermatol Photoimmunol Photomed. 1999;15(2):47–51.
51. Belloni B, Ziai M, Lim A, Lemercier B, Sbornik M, Weidinger S, et al. Low-dose anti-IgE therapy in patients with atopic eczema with high serum IgE levels. J Allergy Clin Immunol. 2007;120(5):1223–5.
52. Benez A, Fierlbeck G. Successful long-term treatment of severe atopic dermatitis with mycophenolate mofetil. Br J Dermatol. 2001;144(3):638–9.
53. Benveniste J, Ducot B, Spira A. Memory of water revisited. Nature. 1994;370(6488):322.
54. von Berg A, Filipiak-Pittroff B, Kramer U, Link E, Bollrath C, Brockow I, et al. Preventive effect of hydrolyzed infant formulas persists until age 6 years: long-term results from the German Infant Nutritional Intervention Study (GINI). J Allergy Clin Immunol. 2008;121(6):1442–7.
55. von Berg A, Koletzko S, Grubl A, Filipiak-Pittroff B, Wichmann HE, Bauer CP, et al. The effect of hydrolyzed cow's milk formula for allergy prevention in the first year of life: the German Infant Nutritional Intervention Study, a randomized double-blind trial. J Allergy Clin Immunol. 2003;111(3):533–40.
56. Bergmann RL, Bergmann KE, Lau-Schadensdorf S, Luck W, Dannemann A, Bauer CP, et al. Atopic diseases in infancy. The German multicenter atopy study (MAS-90). Pediatr Allergy Immunol. 1994;5(6 Suppl):19–25.
57. Bergmann KC, Ring J. History of allergy. Basel: Karger; 2014.
58. Berth-Jones J, Damstra RJ, Golsch S, Livden JK, Van Hooteghem O, Allegra F, et al. Twice weekly fluticasone propionate added to emollient maintenance treatment to reduce risk of relapse in atopic dermatitis: randomised, double blind, parallel group study. BMJ. 2003;326(7403):1367.
59. Berth-Jones J, Graham-Brown RA. Placebo-controlled trial of essential fatty acid supplementation in atopic dermatitis. Lancet. 1993;341(8860):1557–60.
60. Besnier E. La Practique Dermatologique. 1901;II:3.
61. Beyer K, Wahn U. Is atopic dermatitis predictable? Pediatr Allergy Immunol. 1999;10(12 Suppl):7–10.
62. Bharati A, Yesudian PD. Positivity of iron studies in pruritus of unknown origin. J Eur Acad Dermatol Venereol. 2008;22(5):617–8.
63. Bieber T. Fc epsilon RII/CD23 on epidermal Langerhans' cells. Res Immunol. 1992;143(4):445–7.
64. Bieber T. Atopic dermatitis. N Engl J Med. 2008;358(14):1483–94.
65. Bieber T, Ring J. Terfenadine and automobile driving. A placebo controlled double-blind study of the effect of different antihistamines on driving behavior. Med Klin (Munich). 1987;82(20):683–6.
66. Biedermann T. Dissecting the role of infections in atopic dermatitis. Acta Derm Venereol. 2006;86(2):99–109.
67. Bindslev-Jensen C, Ballmer-Weber BK, Bengtsson U, Blanco C, Ebner C, Hourihane J, et al. Standardization of food challenges in patients with immediate reactions to foods—Position paper from the European Academy of Allergology and Clinical Immunology. Allergy. 2004;59(7):690–7.
68. Bissonnette R, Papp KA, Poulin Y, Gooderham M, Raman M, Mallbris L, et al. Topical tofacitinib for atopic dermatitis: a phase IIa randomized trial. Br J Dermatol. 2016;175(5):902–11.
69. Bjorksten B. Environment and infant immunity. Proc Nutr Soc. 1999;58(3):729–32.
70. Bjorksten B, Sepp E, Julge K, Voor T, Mikelsaar M. Allergy development and the intestinal microflora during the first year of life. J Allergy Clin Immunol. 2001;108(4):516–20.
71. Blauvelt A, de Bruin-Weller M, Gooderham M, Cather JC, Weisman J, Pariser D, et al. Long-term management of moderate-to-severe atopic dermatitis with dupilumab and concomitant topical corticosteroids (LIBERTY AD CHRONOS): a 1-year, randomised, double-blinded, placebo-controlled, phase 3 trial. Lancet. 2017;389(10086):2287–303.
72. Blauvelt A, Simpson EL, Tyring SK, Purcell LA, Shumel B, Petro CD, et al. Dupilumab does not affect correlates of vaccine-induced immunity: A randomized, placebo-controlled trial in adults with moderate-to-severe atopic dermatitis. J Am Acad Dermatol. 2019;80(1):158–67 e1.
73. Blennerhassett MG. Nerve and mast cell interaction: cell conflict or information exchange? Prog Clin Biol Res. 1994;390:225–41.
74. Blume-Peytavi U, Cork MJ, Faergemann J, Szczapa J, Vanaclocha F, Gelmetti C. Bathing and cleansing in newborns from day 1 to first year of life: recommendations from a European round table meeting. J Eur Acad Dermatol Venereol. 2009;23(7):751–9.
75. Bockelbrink A, Heinrich J, Schafer I, Zutavern A, Borte M, Herbarth O, et al. Atopic eczema in children: another harmful sequel of divorce. Allergy. 2006;61(12):1397–402.
76. Bode HH. Dwarfism following long-term topical corticosteroid therapy. JAMA. 1980;244(8):813–4.
77. Boehncke WH, Schon MP. Psoriasis. Lancet. 2015;386(9997):983–94.
78. Boehner A, Todorova A, Ring J. Nummular eczema. In: Katsambas A, et al., editors. Handbook of dermatological treatment. 3rd ed. Berlin New York: Springer; in press.
79. Boettger MK, Bar KJ, Dohrmann A, Muller H, Mertins L, Brockmeyer NH, et al. Increased vagal modulation in atopic dermatitis. J Dermatol Sci. 2009;53(1):55–9.
80. van den Bogaard EH, Bergboer JG, Vonk-Bergers M, van Vlijmen-Willems IM, Hato SV, van der Valk PG, et al. Coal tar induces AHR-dependent skin barrier repair in atopic dermatitis. J Clin Invest. 2013;123(2):917–27.
81. Boguniewicz M, Sampson H, Leung SB, Harbeck R, Leung DY. Effects of cefuroxime axetil on Staphylococcus aureus colonization and superantigen production in atopic dermatitis. J Allergy Clin Immunol. 2001;108(4):651–2.

82. Boos AC, Hagl B, Schlesinger A, Halm BE, Ballenberger N, Pinarci M, et al. Atopic dermatitis, STAT3- and DOCK8-hyper-IgE syndromes differ in IgE-based sensitization pattern. Allergy. 2014;69(7):943–53.
83. Borelli S. Die dermatologische Klinik und Poliklinik am Biederstein der Technischen Universitat Munchen und die Deutsche Klinik Alexanderhaus Davos. Lindner: Munich; 1995.
84. Borelli S, Michailov P, Ene-Popescu C. Changes in the environment dependent allergic reactivity in patients with neurodermatitis constitutionalis following high-altitude climate therapy. Hautarzt. 1967;18(10):456–8.
85. Borelli S, Schnyder UW. In: Miescher G, Storck H, editors. Neurodermitis constitutionalis sive atopica. II. Ätiologie, pathophysiologie, pathogenese, therapie. Berlin: Springer; 1962.
86. Bork K, Hoede N. Juvenile papulous dermatitis. Hautarzt. 1978;29(4):216–8.
87. Bornhovd EC, Schuller E, Bieber T, Wollenberg A. Immunosuppressive macrolides and their use in dermatology. Hautarzt. 2000;51(9):646–54.
88. Bos JD. Atopiform dermatitis. Br J Dermatol. 2002;147(3):426–9.
89. Bos JD, Van Leent EJ, Sillevis Smitt JH. The millennium criteria for the diagnosis of atopic dermatitis. Exp Dermatol. 1998;7(4):132–8.
90. Bovet D, Staub AM. Action protectrice des éthers-phénoliques au cours de l'intoxication histaminique. CR Soc Biol Paris. 1934;124:547–9.
91. Bozek A, Fisher A, Filipowska B, Mazur B, Jarzab J. Clinical features and immunological markers of atopic dermatitis in elderly patients. Int Arch Allergy Immunol. 2012;157(4):372–8.
92. Bozek A, Jarzab J, Mielnik M, Bogacz A, Kozlowska R, Mangold D. Can atopy have a protective effect against cancer? PLoS One. 2020;15(2):e0226950.
93. Bradley M, Soderhall C, Wahlgren CF, Luthman H, Nordenskjold M, Kockum I. The Wiskott-Aldrich syndrome gene as a candidate gene for atopic dermatitis. Acta Derm Venereol. 2001;81(5):340–2.
94. Braun-Fahrlander C, Gassner M, Grize L, Takken-Sahli K, Neu U, Stricker T, et al. No further increase in asthma, hay fever and atopic sensitisation in adolescents living in Switzerland. Eur Respir J. 2004;23(3):407–13.
95. Braun-Falco O, Korting HC. In: Ruzicka T, Ring J, Przybilla B, editors. Syndets in the treatment of atopic eczema. Springer; 1991.
96. Braun-Falco O, Ring J. Therapy of atopic eczema. Hautarzt. 1984;35(9):447–54.
97. Braun-Falco O, Ryckmanns F, Heilgemeir GP, Ring J. A syndrome: uncombable hair. Observation of 6 members of a family with pili canaliculi, associated with pili torti, progressive alopecia, atopic eczema and hamartomas. Hautarzt. 1982;33(7):366–72.
98. Brenninkmeijer EE, Schram ME, Leeflang MM, Bos JD, Spuls PI. Diagnostic criteria for atopic dermatitis: a systematic review. Br J Dermatol. 2008;158(4):754–65.
99. Bresser H. "Allergy testing" with "Dr. Voll electroacupuncture". Hautarzt. 1993;44(6):408–9.
100. Breuer K, Heratizadeh A, Wulf A, Baumann U, Constien A, Tetau D, et al. Late eczematous reactions to food in children with atopic dermatitis. Clin Exp Allergy. 2004;34(5):817–24.
101. Breuer K, Kapp A. Inpatient rehabilitation of adults with atopic dermatitis. Hautarzt. 2006;57(7):592, 4-602
102. Broberg A, Augustsson A. Atopic dermatitis and melanocytic naevi. Br J Dermatol. 2000;142(2):306–9.
103. Broberg A, Faergemann J. Topical antimycotic treatment of atopic dermatitis in the head/neck area. A double-blind randomised study. Acta Derm Venereol. 1995;75(1):46–9.
104. Brockow K, Abeck D, Ring J. Systemic therapy in the treatment concept of atopic eczema. Reliable treatment methods and experimental developments. Hautarzt. 1999;50(5):323–9.
105. Brockow K, Grabenhorst P, Abeck D, Traupe B, Ring J, Hoppe U, et al. Effect of gentian violet, corticosteroid and tar preparations in Staphylococcus-aureus-colonized atopic eczema. Dermatology. 1999;199(3):231–6.
106. Brocq L. L'eczéma considéré comme une réaction cutaneé. Ann Dermatol Syphiligr (Paris). 1903;4:172.
107. de Bruin-Weller M, Gadkari A, Auziere S, Simpson EL, Puig L, Barbarot S, et al. The patient-reported disease burden in adults with atopic dermatitis: a cross-sectional study in Europe and Canada. J Eur Acad Dermatol Venereol. 2020;34(5):1026–36.
108. Brune A, Metze D, Luger TA, Stander S. Antipruritic therapy with the oral opioid receptor antagonist naltrexone. Open, non-placebo controlled administration in 133 patients. Hautarzt. 2004;55(12):1130–6.
109. Brunner PM, Pavel AB, Khattri S, Leonard A, Malik K, Rose S, et al. Baseline IL-22 expression in patients with atopic dermatitis stratifies tissue responses to fezakinumab. J Allergy Clin Immunol. 2019;143(1):142–54.
110. Brunner PM, Silverberg JI, Guttman-Yassky E, Paller AS, Kabashima K, Amagai M, et al. Increasing comorbidities suggest that atopic dermatitis is a systemic disorder. J Invest Dermatol. 2017;137(1):18–25.
111. Bruynzeel-Koomen CA, Van Wichen DF, Spry CJ, Venge P, Bruynzeel PL. Active participation of eosinophils in patch test reactions to inhalant allergens in patients with atopic dermatitis. Br J Dermatol. 1988;118(2):229–38.
112. Buckley RH, Becker WG. Abnormalities in the regulation of human IgE synthesis. Immunol Rev. 1978;41:288–314.
113. Buddenkotte J, Steinhoff M. Pathophysiology and therapy of pruritus in allergic and atopic diseases. Allergy. 2010;65(7):805–21. https://doi.org/10.1111/j.1398-9995.2010.01995.x.
114. Buhl R, Soler M, Matz J, Townley R, O'Brien J, Noga O, et al. Omalizumab provides long-term

control in patients with moderate-to-severe allergic asthma. Eur Respir J. 2002;20(1):73–8.
115. Bunikowski R, Staab D, Kussebi F, Brautigam M, Weidinger G, Renz H, et al. Low-dose cyclosporin A microemulsion in children with severe atopic dermatitis: clinical and immunological effects. Pediatr Allergy Immunol. 2001;12(4):216–23.
116. Burbank AJ, Peden DB. Assessing the impact of air pollution on childhood asthma morbidity: how, when and what to do. Curr Opin Allergy Clin Immunol. 2019;18:124–31.
117. Burks AW, Laubach S, Jones SM. Oral tolerance, food allergy, and immunotherapy: implications for future treatment. J Allergy Clin Immunol. 2008;121(6):1344–50.
118. Buske-Kirschbaum A, Schmitt J, Plessow F, Romanos M, Weidinger S, Roessner V. Psychoendocrine and psychoneuroimmunological mechanisms in the comorbidity of atopic eczema and attention deficit/hyperactivity disorder. Psychoneuroendocrinology. 2013;38(1):12–23.
119. Bussmann C, Bockenhoff A, Henke H, Werfel T, Novak N. Does allergen-specific immunotherapy represent a therapeutic option for patients with atopic dermatitis? J Allergy Clin Immunol. 2006;118(6):1292–8.
120. Butler JM, Marks R, Sutherland R. Cutaneous and cardiac valvular pigmentation with minocycline. Clin Exp Dermatol. 1985;10(5):432–7.
121. Bylund S, Kobyletzki LB, Svalstedt M, Svensson A. Prevalence and incidence of atopic dermatitis: a systematic review. Acta Derm Venereol. 2020;100(12):adv00160.
122. Campione E, Lanna C, Diluvio L, Cannizzaro MV, Grelli S, Galluzzo M, et al. Skin immunity and its dysregulation in atopic dermatitis, hidradenitis suppurativa and vitiligo. Cell Cycle. 2020;19(3):257–67.
123. Carlsson CP, Wallengren J. Therapeutic and experimental therapeutic studies on acupuncture and itch: review of the literature. J Eur Acad Dermatol Venereol. 2010;24(9):1013–6.
124. Cassano N, Loconsole F, Coviello C, Vena GA. Infliximab in recalcitrant severe atopic eczema associated with contact allergy. Int J Immunopathol Pharmacol. 2006;19(1):237–40.
125. Castellsague J, Kuiper JG, Pottegard A, Anveden Berglind I, Dedman D, Gutierrez L, et al. A cohort study on the risk of lymphoma and skin cancer in users of topical tacrolimus, pimecrolimus, and corticosteroids (Joint European Longitudinal Lymphoma and Skin Cancer Evaluation - JOELLE study). Clin Epidemiol. 2018;10:299–310.
126. Catala A, Munoz-Santos C, Galvan-Casas C, Roncero Riesco M, Revilla Nebreda D, Sola-Truyols A, et al. Cutaneous reactions after SARS-CoV-2 vaccination: a cross-sectional Spanish nationwide study of 405 cases. Br J Dermatol. 2021;186(1):142–52.
127. Cevikbas F, Wang X, Akiyama T, Kempkes C, Savinko T, Antal A, et al. A sensory neuron-expressed IL-31 receptor mediates T helper cell-dependent itch: Involvement of TRPV1 and TRPA1. J Allergy Clin Immunol. 2014;133(2):448–60.
128. Chalmers JR, Haines RH, Bradshaw LE, Montgomery AA, Thomas KS, Brown SJ, et al. Daily emollient during infancy for prevention of eczema: the BEEP randomised controlled trial. Lancet. 2020;395(10228):962–72.
129. Chamlin SL, Lai JS, Cella D, Frieden IJ, Williams ML, Mancini AJ, et al. Childhood atopic dermatitis impact scale: reliability, discriminative and concurrent validity, and responsiveness. Arch Dermatol. 2007;143(6):768–72.
130. Chan SC, Hanifin JM. Differential inhibitor effects on cyclic adenosine monophosphate-phosphodiesterase isoforms in atopic and normal leukocytes. J Lab Clin Med. 1993;121(1):44–51.
131. Chan SC, Kim JW, Henderson WR Jr, Hanifin JM. Altered prostaglandin E2 regulation of cytokine production in atopic dermatitis. J Immunol. 1993;151(6):3345–52.
132. Chan AR, Sandhu VK, Drucker AM, Fleming P, Lynde CW. Adult-onset atopic dermatitis: presentations and progress. J Cutan Med Surg. 2020;24(3):267–72.
133. Chaoimh CN, Lad D, Nico C, Puppels GJ, Wong XFCC, Common JE, Murray DM, Irvine AD, Hourihane JO. Early initiation of short-term emollient use for the prevention of atopic dermatitis in high-risk infants-The STOP-AD randomised controlled trial. Allergy. 2022.
134. Charman CR, Venn AJ, Ravenscroft JC, Williams HC. Translating patient-oriented eczema measure (POEM) scores into clinical practice by suggesting severity strata derived using anchor-based methods. Br J Dermatol. 2013;169(6):1326–32.
135. Charman CR, Venn AJ, Williams HC. The patient-oriented eczema measure: development and initial validation of a new tool for measuring atopic eczema severity from the patients' perspective. Arch Dermatol. 2004;140(12):1513–9.
136. Chen W, Mempel M, Schober W, Behrendt H, Ring J. Gender difference, sex hormones, and immediate type hypersensitivity reactions. Allergy. 2008;63(11):1418–27.
137. Cheng HM, Chiang LC, Jan YM, Chen GW, Li TC. The efficacy and safety of a Chinese herbal product (Xiao-Feng-San) for the treatment of refractory atopic dermatitis: a randomized, double-blind, placebo-controlled trial. Int Arch Allergy Immunol. 2011;155(2):141–8.
138. Cheng R, Zhang H, Zong W, Tang J, Han X, Zhang L, et al. Development and validation of new diagnostic criteria for atopic dermatitis in children of China. J Eur Acad Dermatol Venereol. 2020;34(3):542–8.
139. Chida Y, Hamer M, Steptoe A. A bidirectional relationship between psychosocial factors and atopic disorders: a systematic review and meta-analysis. Psychosom Med. 2008;70(1):102–16.
140. Christiansen JV, Gadborg E, Kleiter I, Ludvigsen K, Meier CH, Norholm A, et al. Efficacy of bufexamac

(NFN) cream in skin diseases. A double-blind multicentre trial. Dermatologica. 1977;154(3):177–84.
141. Cipriani F, Dondi A, Ricci G. Recent advances in epidemiology and prevention of atopic eczema. Pediatr Allergy Immunol. 2014;25(7):630–8.
142. Coca AF, Cooke RA. On the classification of the phenomena of hypersensitiveness. J Immunol. 1923;8:163–82.
143. Coca AF, Grove E. Studies in hypersensitiveness. XIII. A study of the atopic reagins. J Immunol. 1925;10:445.
144. Colver GB, Mortimer PS, Millard PR, Dawber RP, Ryan TJ. The 'dirty neck'—A reticulate pigmentation in atopics. Clin Exp Dermatol. 1987;12(1):1–4.
145. Cookson WO, Moffatt MF. The genetics of atopic dermatitis. Curr Opin Allergy Clin Immunol. 2002;2(5):383–7.
146. Coombs RRA, Gell PGH. Classification of allergic reactions responsible for drug hypersensitivity reactions. Philadelphia, PA: Davis; 1968.
147. Corbo GM, Ferrante E, Macciocchi B, Foresi A, De Angelis V, Fabrizi G, et al. Bronchial hyperresponsiveness in atopic dermatitis. Allergy. 1989;44(8):595–8.
148. Cork MJ, Robinson D, Vasilopoulos Y, Ferguson A, Moustafa M, Mac Gowan A, et al. Predisposition to sensitive skin and atopic eczema. Community Pract. 2005;78(12):440–2.
149. Cox L, Platts-Mills TA, Finegold I, Schwartz LB, Simons FE, Wallace DV, et al. American Academy of Allergy, Asthma & Immunology/American College of Allergy, Asthma and Immunology Joint Task Force Report on omalizumab-associated anaphylaxis. J Allergy Clin Immunol. 2007;120(6):1373–7.
150. Cramer C, Ranft U, Ring J, Mohrenschlager M, Behrendt H, Oppermann H, et al. Allergic sensitization and disease in mother-child pairs from Germany: role of early childhood environment. Int Arch Allergy Immunol. 2007;143(4):282–9.
151. Crumrine D, Khnykin D, Krieg P, Man MQ, Celli A, Mauro TM, et al. Mutations in recessive congenital ichthyoses illuminate the origin and functions of the corneocyte lipid envelope. J Invest Dermatol. 2019;139(4):760–8.
152. Czarnecka-Operacz M, Jenerowicz D. Topical calcineurin inhibitors in the treatment of atopic dermatitis - an update on safety issues. J Dtsch Dermatol Ges. 2012;10(3):167–72.
153. Czarnecka-Operacz M, Silny W. Specific immunotherapy in atopic dermatitis—Four-year treatment in different age and airborne allergy type subgroups. Acta Dermatovenerol Croat. 2006;14(4):230–40.
154. Czarnowicki T, He H, Krueger JG, Guttman-Yassky E. Atopic dermatitis endotypes and implications for targeted therapeutics. J Allergy Clin Immunol. 2019;143(1):1–11.
155. Czerny A. Die exsudative diathese. Jb. Kinderheilk. Jb Kinderheilk. 1905;61(3):199.
156. Dale HH, Laidlaw BP. The physiological action of β-Imidazolylethylamine. J Physiol. 1910;41:318.
157. Darsow U. Desensitization—at home and without pricks. How effective is sublingual immunotherapy? Interview by Erik Heintz. MMW Fortschr Med. 2005;147(33-34):15.
158. Darsow U, Laifaoui J, Kerschenlohr K, Wollenberg A, Przybilla B, Wuthrich B, et al. The prevalence of positive reactions in the atopy patch test with aeroallergens and food allergens in subjects with atopic eczema: a European multicenter study. Allergy. 2004;59(12):1318–25.
159. Darsow U, Mautner VF, Bromm B, Scharein E, Ring J. The Eppendorf Pruritus Questionnaire. Hautarzt. 1997;48(10):730–3.
160. Darsow U, Ring J. Significance of pollen and animal hair for the outcome of atopic eczema. Hautarzt. 1995;46(7):505–6.
161. Darsow U, Ring J. Airborne and dietary allergens in atopic eczema: a comprehensive review of diagnostic tests. Clin Exp Dermatol. 2000;25(7):544–51.
162. Darsow U, Ring J. Atopy patch testing with aeroallergens and food. Hautarzt. 2005;56(12):1133–40.
163. Darsow U, Sbornik M, Rombold S, Katzer K, von Sonnenburg F, Behrendt H, et al. Long-term safety of replication-defective smallpox vaccine (MVA-BN) in atopic eczema and allergic rhinitis. J Eur Acad Dermatol Venereol. 2016;30(11):1971–7.
164. Darsow U, Scharein E, Bromm B, Ring J. Skin testing of the pruritogenic activity of histamine and cytokines (interleukin-2 and tumour necrosis factor-alpha) at the dermal-epidermal junction. Br J Dermatol. 1997;137(3):415–7.
165. Darsow U, Scharein E, Simon D, Walter G, Bromm B, Ring J. New aspects of itch pathophysiology: component analysis of atopic itch using the 'Eppendorf Itch Questionnaire'. Int Arch Allergy Immunol. 2001;124(1-3):326–31.
166. Darsow U, Vieluf D, Ring J. Atopy patch test with different vehicles and allergen concentrations: an approach to standardization. J Allergy Clin Immunol. 1995;95(3):677–84.
167. Darsow U, Vieluf D, Ring J. The atopy patch test: an increased rate of reactivity in patients who have an air-exposed pattern of atopic eczema. Br J Dermatol. 1996;135(2):182–6.
168. Darsow U, Vieluf D, Ring J. Evaluating the relevance of aeroallergen sensitization in atopic eczema with the atopy patch test: a randomized, double-blind multicenter study. J Am Ass Dermatol. 1999;40:187–93.
169. Darsow U, Wollenberg A, Simon D, Taieb A, Werfel T, Oranje A, et al. ETFAD/EADV eczema task force 2009 position paper on diagnosis and treatment of atopic dermatitis. J Eur Acad Dermatol Venereol. 2010;24(3):317–28.
170. Davallow Ghajar L, Wood Heickman LK, Conaway M, Rogol AD. Low risk of adrenal insufficiency after use of low- to moderate-potency topical corticosteroids for children with atopic dermatitis. Clin Pediatr (Phila). 2019;58(4):406–12.

171. David TJ. Dietary treatment of atopic eczema. Arch Dis Child. 1989;64(10):1506–9.
172. David TJ, Cambridge GC. Bacterial infection and atopic eczema. Arch Dis Child. 1986;61(1):20–3.
173. David TJ, Waddington E, Stanton RH. Nutritional hazards of elimination diets in children with atopic eczema. Arch Dis Child. 1984;59(4):323–5.
174. De Benedetto A, Agnihothri R, McGirt LY, Bankova LG, Beck LA. Atopic dermatitis: a disease caused by innate immune defects? J Invest Dermatol. 2009;129(1):14–30.
175. Degos R. Dermatologie. Collection Médico-chirurgicale à Révision Annuelle. Paris: Flammarion; 1953.
176. Deleuran M, Ellingsen AR, Paludan K, Schou C, Thestrup-Pedersen K. Purified Der p1 and p2 patch tests in patients with atopic dermatitis: evidence for both allergenicity and proteolytic irritancy. Acta Derm Venereol. 1998;78(4):241–3.
177. Desai NS, Poindexter GB, Monthrope YM, Bendeck SE, Swerlick RA, Chen SC. A pilot quality-of-life instrument for pruritus. J Am Acad Dermatol. 2008;59(2):234–44.
178. Devillers AC, de Waard-van der Spek FB, Mulder PG, Oranje AP. Treatment of refractory atopic dermatitis using 'wet-wrap' dressings and diluted corticosteroids: results of standardized treatment in both children and adults. Dermatology. 2002;204(1):50–5.
179. Devlin J, David TJ. Intolerance to oral and intravenous calcium supplements in atopic eczema. J R Soc Med. 1990;83(8):497–8.
180. Di Pascuale MA, Elizondo A, Gao YY, Raju VK, Tseng SC. Gigantic waves in the tear film generated by bubbles from a large glaucoma bleb. Arch Ophthalmol. 2007;125(4):573–4.
181. Diebschlag W, Diebschlag, B. Hausstauballergien. Gesundheitliche und hygienische Aspekte. Herbert Utz Verlag; 2000.
182. Diepgen TL. Atopic dermatitis: the role of environmental and social factors, the European experience. J Am Acad Dermatol. 2001;45(1 Suppl):S44–8.
183. Diepgen TL, Elsner P, Schliemann S, Fartasch M, Kollner A, Skudlik C, et al. Guideline on the management of hand eczema ICD-10 Code: L20. L23. L24. L25. L30. J Dtsch Dermatol Ges. 2009;7(Suppl 3):S1–16.
184. Diepgen T, Fartasch M, Hornstein OP. Kriterien zur Beurteilung der atopischen Hautdiathese. Dermatosen. 1991;39:79–83.
185. Diepgen TL, Fartasch M, Ring J, Scheewe S, Staab D, Szczepanski R, et al. Education programs on atopic eczema. Design and first results of the German Randomized Intervention Multicenter Study. Hautarzt. 2003;54(10):946–51.
186. Dieris-Hirche J, Gieler U, Kupfer JP, Milch WE. Suicidal ideation, anxiety and depression in adult patients with atopic dermatitis. Hautarzt. 2009;60(8):641–6.
187. Diezel W, Schewe T, Rohde E, Rosenbach T, Czarnetzki BM. Ammonium bituminosulfonate (Ichthyol). Anti-inflammatory effect and inhibition of the 5-lipoxygenase enzyme. Hautarzt. 1992;43(12):772–4.
188. Dinkloh A, Worm M, Geier J, Schnuch A, Wollenberg A. Contact sensitization in patients with suspected cosmetic intolerance: results of the IVDK 2006-2011. J Eur Acad Dermatol Venereol. 2015;29(6):1071–81.
189. Dirven-Meijer PC, Glazenburg EJ, Mulder PG, Oranje AP. Prevalence of atopic dermatitis in children younger than 4 years in a demarcated area in central Netherlands: the West Veluwe Study Group. Br J Dermatol. 2008;158(4):846–7.
190. Dittmar HC, Pflieger D, Schempp CM, Schopf E, Simon JC. Comparison of balneophototherapy and UVA/B mono-phototherapy in patients with subacute atopic dermatitis. Hautarzt. 1999;50(9):649–53.
191. Dorsch W, Ring J. Komplementärverfahren oder sogenannte alternativmethoden in der Allergologie. Allergo J. 2002;11:163–70.
192. Dorsch W, Ring J, Reimann HJ, Geiger R. Mediator studies in skin blister fluid from patients with dual skin reactions after intradermal allergen injection. J Allergy Clin Immunol. 1982;70(4):236–42.
193. Dubowitz V. Familial low birthweight dwarfism with an unusual facies and a skin eruption. J Med Genet. 1965;2(1):12–7.
194. Dufresne H, Bataille P, Bellon N, Compain S, Deladriere E, Bekel L, et al. Risk factors for corticophobia in atopic dermatitis. J Eur Acad Dermatol Venereol. 2020;34(12):e846–9.
195. Dunstan JA, Mori TA, Barden A, Beilin LJ, Holt PG, Calder PC, et al. Effects of n-3 polyunsaturated fatty acid supplementation in pregnancy on maternal and fetal erythrocyte fatty acid composition. Eur J Clin Nutr. 2004;58(3):429–37.
196. Dunstan JA, Roper J, Mitoulas L, Hartmann PE, Simmer K, Prescott SL. The effect of supplementation with fish oil during pregnancy on breast milk immunoglobulin A, soluble CD14, cytokine levels and fatty acid composition. Clin Exp Allergy. 2004;34(8):1237–42.
197. Dupre A, Christol B, Bonafe JL, Lassere J. Orf and atopic dermatitis. Br J Dermatol. 1981;105(1):103–4.
198. Eberlein B, Huss-Marp J, Pfab F, Fischer R, Franz R, Schlich M, et al. Influence of alpine mountain climate of Bavaria on patients with atopic diseases: studies at the Environmental Research Station Schneefernerhaus (UFS - Zugspitze) - a pilot study. Clin Transl Allergy. 2014;4:17.
199. Eberlein-Konig B, Przybilla B, Kuhnl P, Pechak J, Gebefugi I, Kleinschmidt J, et al. Influence of airborne nitrogen dioxide or formaldehyde on parameters of skin function and cellular activation in patients with atopic eczema and control subjects. J Allergy Clin Immunol. 1998;101(1 Pt 1):141–3.
200. Edgren G. Prognose und Erblichkeitsmomente bei Eczema infantum. Eine klinisch-statistische Untersuchung von Allergieerscheinungen. Acta Paediatr Scand. 1943;30(Suppl 2):1–204.

201. Ege MJ, Herzum I, Buchele G, Krauss-Etschmann S, Lauener RP, Roponen M, et al. Prenatal exposure to a farm environment modifies atopic sensitization at birth. J Allergy Clin Immunol. 2008;122(2):407–12, 12 e1-4
202. Egelrud T, Regnier M, Sondell B, Shroot B, Schmidt R. Expression of stratum corneum chymotryptic enzyme in reconstructed human epidermis and its suppression by retinoic acid. Acta Derm Venereol. 1993;73(3):181–4.
203. Egle UT, Hardt J, Nickel R, Kappis B, Hoffmann SO. Long-term effects of adverse childhood experiences - actual evidence and needs for research1/2. Z Psychosom Med Psychother. 2002;48(4):411–34.
204. Ehlers A, Stangier U, Gieler U. Treatment of atopic dermatitis: a comparison of psychological and dermatological approaches to relapse prevention. J Consult Clin Psychol. 1995;63(4):624–35.
205. Ehlken B, Mohrenschlager M, Kugland B, Berger K, Quednau K, Ring J. Cost-of-illness study in patients suffering from atopic eczema in Germany. Hautarzt. 2005;56(12):1144–51.
206. Eichenfield LF, Lucky AW, Boguniewicz M, Langley RG, Cherill R, Marshall K, et al. Safety and efficacy of pimecrolimus (ASM 981) cream 1% in the treatment of mild and moderate atopic dermatitis in children and adolescents. J Am Acad Dermatol. 2002;46(4):495–504.
207. von Eiff AW. Psychologie und Klinikstress. Therapiewoche. 1984;S7(34):192–6.
208. Eigenmann PA, Sicherer SH, Borkowski TA, Cohen BA, Sampson HA. Prevalence of IgE-mediated food allergy among children with atopic dermatitis. Pediatrics. 1998;101(3):E8.
209. Elias PM, Menon GK. Structural and lipid biochemical correlates of the epidermal permeability barrier. Adv Lipid Res. 1991;24:1–26.
210. Ellis CN, Drake LA, Prendergast MM, Abramovits W, Boguniewicz M, Daniel CR, et al. Cost of atopic dermatitis and eczema in the United States. J Am Acad Dermatol. 2002;46(3):361–70.
211. Ellis C, Luger T, Abeck D, Allen R, Graham-Brown RA, De Prost Y, et al. International consensus conference on atopic dermatitis II (ICCAD II): clinical update and current treatment strategies. Br J Dermatol. 2003;148(Suppl 63):3–10.
212. Elman S, Hynan LS, Gabriel V, Mayo MJ. The 5-D itch scale: a new measure of pruritus. Br J Dermatol. 2010;162(3):587–93.
213. Emerson RM, Charman CR, Williams HC. The Nottingham Eczema Severity Score: preliminary refinement of the Rajka and Langeland grading. Br J Dermatol. 2000;142(2):288–97.
214. Enders F, Przybilla B, Ring J, Burg G, Braun-Falco O. Epicutaneous testing with a standard series. Results in 12,026 patients. Hautarzt. 1988;39(12):779–86.
215. Enders F, Przybilla B, Ring J, Gollhausen R. Patch test results in 1987 compared to trends from the period 1977-1983. Contact Dermatitis. 1989;20(3):230–2.
216. Engman MF, Weiss RS, Engman ME. Eczema and environment. Med Clin North Am. 1936;20:651–63.
217. Engst R, Vocks E. High-mountain climate therapy for skin diseases and allergies—Mode of action, therapeutic results, and immunologic effects. Rehabilitation (Stuttg). 2000;39(4):215–22.
218. Ernst E, Barnes J. Meta-analysis of homoeopathy trials. Lancet. 1998;351(9099):366. author reply 7-8
219. Ewing CI, Ashcroft C, Gibbs AC, Jones GA, Connor PJ, David TJ. Flucloxacillin in the treatment of atopic dermatitis. Br J Dermatol. 1998;138(6):1022–9.
220. Exl BM, Deland U, Secretin MC, Preysch U, Wall M, Shmerling DH. Improved general health status in an unselected infant population following an allergen-reduced dietary intervention programme: the ZUFF-STUDY-PROGRAMME. Part II: infant growth and health status to age 6 months. ZUg-FrauenFeld. Eur J Nutr. 2000;39(4):145–56.
221. Eyerich K, Eyerich S. Immune response patterns in non-communicable inflammatory skin diseases. J Eur Acad Dermatol Venereol. 2018;32(5):692–703.
222. Eyerich S, Eyerich K, Traidl-Hoffmann C, Biedermann T. Cutaneous barriers and skin immunity: differentiating a connected network. Trends Immunol. 2018;39(4):315–27.
223. Eyerich S, Metz M, Bossios A, Eyerich K. New biological treatments for asthma and skin allergies. Allergy. 2020;75(3):546–60.
224. Eyerich S, Onken AT, Weidinger S, Franke A, Nasorri F, Pennino D, et al. Mutual antagonism of T cells causing psoriasis and atopic eczema. N Engl J Med. 2011;365(3):231–8.
225. Falk ES. Ketotifen in the treatment of atopic dermatitis. Results of a double blind study. Riv Eur Sci Med Farmacol. 1993;15(2):63–6.
226. Falth-Magnusson K, Oman H, Kjellman NI. Maternal abstention from cow milk and egg in allergy risk pregnancies. Effect on antibody production in the mother and the newborn. Allergy. 1987;42(1):64–73.
227. Faye O, Meledie N'Djong AP, Diadie S, Coniquet S, Niamba PA, Atadokpede F, et al. Validation of the patient-oriented SCORing for atopic dermatitis tool for black skin. J Eur Acad Dermatol Venereol. 2020;34(4):795–9.
228. Felix R, Shuster S. A new method for the measurement of itch and the response to treatment. Br J Dermatol. 1975;93(3):303–12.
229. Feng J, Yang P, Mack MR, Dryn D, Luo J, Gong X, et al. Sensory TRP channels contribute differentially to skin inflammation and persistent itch. Nat commun. 2017;8(1):980.
230. Ferguson JE, Chalmers RJ, Rowlands DJ. Reversible dilated cardiomyopathy following treatment of atopic eczema with Chinese herbal medicine. Br J Dermatol. 1997;136(4):592–3.
231. Ferie J, Dinkela A, Mbata M, Idindili B, Schmid-Grendelmeier P, Hatz C. Skin disorders among

school children in rural Tanzania and an assessment of therapeutic needs. Trop Doct. 2006;36(4):219–21.
232. Fieten KB, Weststrate AC, van Zuuren EJ, Bruijnzeel-Koomen CA, Pasmans SG. Alpine climate treatment of atopic dermatitis: a systematic review. Allergy. 2015;70(1):12–25.
233. Finlay AY. Quality of life measurement in dermatology: a practical guide. Br J Dermatol. 1997;136(3):305–14.
234. Finlay AY, Khan GK. Dermatology life quality index (DLQI)—A simple practical measure for routine clinical use. Clin Exp Dermatol. 1994;19(3):210–6.
235. Fishbein AB, Mueller K, Lor J, Smith P, Paller AS, Kaat A. Systematic review and meta-analysis comparing topical corticosteroids with vehicle/moisturizer in childhood atopic dermatitis. J Pediatr Nurs. 2019;47:36–43.
236. Fisher MS, Kripke ML. Systemic alteration induced in mice by ultraviolet light irradiation and its relationship to ultraviolet carcinogenesis. Proc Natl Acad Sci U S A. 1977;74(4):1688–92.
237. Flohr C, Pascoe D, Williams HC. Atopic dermatitis and the 'hygiene hypothesis': too clean to be true? Br J Dermatol. 2005;152(2):202–16.
238. Flohr C, Yeo L. Atopic dermatitis and the hygiene hypothesis revisited. Curr Probl Dermatol. 2011;41:1–34.
239. Folster-Holst R, Kiene P, Brodersen JP, Christophers E. Dermatitis papulosa juvenilis. Hautarzt. 1996;47(2):129–31.
240. Folster-Holst R, Muller F, Schnopp N, Abeck D, Kreiselmaier I, Lenz T, et al. Prospective, randomized controlled trial on Lactobacillus rhamnosus in infants with moderate to severe atopic dermatitis. Br J Dermatol. 2006;155(6):1256–61.
241. Folster-Holst R, Pape M, Buss YL, Christophers E, Weichenthal M. Low prevalence of the intrinsic form of atopic dermatitis among adult patients. Allergy. 2006;61(5):629–32.
242. Folster-Holst R, Weichenthal M, Steinsland K, Polzhofer G, Christophers E. Eczema infantum and its prognosis. Acta Derm Venereol. 2004;84(5):410–2.
243. Fonacier LS, Aquino MR. The role of contact allergy in atopic dermatitis. Immunol Allergy Clin North Am. 2010;30(3):337–50.
244. Forman SB, Garrett AB. Success of omalizumab as monotherapy in adult atopic dermatitis: case report and discussion of the high-affinity immunoglobulin E receptor. FcepsilonRI. Cutis. 2007;80(1): 38–40.
245. Frei R, Lauener RP, Crameri R, O'Mahony L. Microbiota and dietary interactions: an update to the hygiene hypothesis? Allergy. 2012;67(4):451–61.
246. Freitag G, Hoppner T. Results of a postmarketing drug monitoring survey with a polidocanol-urea preparation for dry, itching skin. Curr Med Res Opin. 1997;13(9):529–37.
247. Frosch PJ, Schwanitz HJ, Macher E. A double blind trial of H1 and H2 receptor antagonists in the treatment of atopic dermatitis. Arch Dermatol Res. 1984;276(1):36–40.
248. Fuhrmann T, Smith N, Tausk F. Use of complementary and alternative medicine among adults with skin disease: updated results from a national survey. J Am Acad Dermatol. 2010;63(6):1000–5.
249. Furue M, Terao H, Rikihisa W, Urabe K, Kinukawa N, Nose Y, et al. Clinical dose and adverse effects of topical steroids in daily management of atopic dermatitis. Br J Dermatol. 2003;148(1):128–33.
250. Fyhrquist N, Muirhead G, Prast-Nielsen S, Jeanmougin M, Olah P, Skoog T, et al. Microbe-host interplay in atopic dermatitis and psoriasis. Nat Commun. 2019;10(1):4703.
251. Gabes M, Chamlin SL, Lai JS, Cella D, Mancini AJ, Apfelbacher CJ. Development of a validated short-form of the childhood atopic dermatitis impact scale, the CADIS-SF15. J Eur Acad Dermatol Venereol. 2020;34(8):1773–8.
252. Galli SJ. The mast cell-IgE paradox: from homeostasis to anaphylaxis. Am J Pathol. 2016;186(2):212–24.
253. Gambichler T, Boms S, Susok L, Dickel H, Finis C, Abu Rached N, Barras M, Stucker M, Kasakovski D. Cutaneous findings following COVID-19 vaccination: review of world literature and own experience. J Eur Acad Dermatol Venereol. 2022;36:172–80.
254. Gamble RG, Dellavalle RP. Ion-exchange water softener use and eczema. Arch Dermatol. 2011;147(10):1208–10.
255. Garzorz N, Alsisi M, Todorova A, Atenhan A, Thomas J, Lauffer F, et al. Dissecting susceptibility from exogenous triggers: the model of alopecia areata and associated inflammatory skin diseases. J Eur Acad Dermatol Venereol. 2015;29(12):2429–35.
256. Gauger A, Fischer S, Mempel M, Schaefer T, Foelster-Holst R, Abeck D, et al. Efficacy and functionality of silver-coated textiles in patients with atopic eczema. J Eur Acad Dermatol Venereol. 2006;20(5):534–41.
257. Gauger A, Mempel M, Schekatz A, Schafer T, Ring J, Abeck D. Silver-coated textiles reduce Staphylococcus aureus colonization in patients with atopic eczema. Dermatology. 2003;207(1):15–21.
258. Gdalevich M, Mimouni D, David M, Mimouni M. Breast-feeding and the onset of atopic dermatitis in childhood: a systematic review and meta-analysis of prospective studies. J Am Acad Dermatol. 2001;45(4):520–7.
259. Gebert N, Hummelink R, Konning J, Staab D, Schmidt S, Szczepanski R, et al. Efficacy of a self-management program for childhood asthma—A prospective controlled study. Patient Educ Couns. 1998;35(3):213–20.
260. Gehring W, Wenz J, Gloor M. Influence of topically applied ceramide/phospholipid mixture on the barrier function of intact skin, atopic skin and experimentally induced barrier damage. Int J Cosmet Sci. 1997;19(4):143–56.
261. Gelfand HH, Cinder JC, Grant SF, Soiffer M. Evaluation of histamine-gamma globulin (hista-

globin) in the treatment of various allergic conditions. Ann Allergy. 1963;21:150–5.
262. Gelmetti C. Skin cleansing in children. J Eur Acad Dermatol Venereol. 2001;15(Suppl 1):12–5.
263. George SM, Karanovic S, Harrison DA, Rani A, Birnie AJ, Bath-Hextall FJ, et al. Interventions to reduce Staphylococcus aureus in the management of eczema. Cochrane Database Syst Rev. 2019;2019(10):CD003871.
264. Giannetti A, Fantini F, Cimitan A, Pincelli C. Vasoactive intestinal polypeptide and substance P in the pathogenesis of atopic dermatitis. Acta Derm Venereol Suppl (Stockh). 1992;176:90–2.
265. Gibbs NK, Norval M. Photoimmunosuppression: a brief overview. Photodermatol Photoimmunol Photomed. 2013;29(2):57–64.
266. Gieler U, Ehlers A, Hohler T, Burkard G. The psychosocial status of patients with endogenous eczema. A study using cluster analysis for the correlation of psychological factors with somatic findings. Hautarzt. 1990;41(8):416–23.
267. Gieler U, Harth W. Psychodermatology. Hautarzt. 2008;59(4):287–8.
268. Gieler U, Niemeier V, Kupfer J, Harth W. Psychosomatic dermatology. Hautarzt. 2008;59(5):415–32. quiz 33
269. Gieler U, Scheewe S, Niemeier V, Kupfer J, Diepgen T, Staab D. Interdisciplinary model project neurodermatitis—Education for children and adolescents. Kinderkrankenschwester. 2003;22(4):152–8.
270. Girolomoni G, Luger T, Nosbaum A, Gruben D, Romero W, Llamado LJ, et al. The economic and psychosocial comorbidity burden among adults with moderate-to-severe atopic dermatitis in europe: analysis of a cross-sectional survey. Dermatol Ther (Heidelb). 2021;11(1):117–30.
271. Glaser R, Navid F, Schuller W, Jantschitsch C, Harder J, Schroder JM, et al. UV-B radiation induces the expression of antimicrobial peptides in human keratinocytes in vitro and in vivo. J Allergy Clin Immunol. 2009;123(5):1117–23.
272. Gloor M, Gehring W. Effects of emulsions on the stratum corneum barrier and hydration. Hautarzt. 2003;54(4):324–30.
273. Goldblum RW, Piper WN. Artificial lichenification produced by a scratching machine. J Invest Dermatol. 1954;22(5):405–15.
274. Goldminz AM, Scheinman PL. A case series of dupilumab-treated allergic contact dermatitis patients. Dermatol Ther. 2018;31(6):e12701.
275. Gondo A, Saeki N, Tokuda Y. Challenge reactions in atopic dermatitis after percutaneous entry of mite antigen. Br J Dermatol. 1986;115(4):485–93.
276. Grewe M, Vogelsang K, Ruzicka T, Stege H, Krutmann J. Neurotrophin-4 production by human epidermal keratinocytes: increased expression in atopic dermatitis. J Invest Dermatol. 2000;114(6):1108–12.
277. Grimbacher B, Holland SM, Gallin JI, Greenberg F, Hill SC, Malech HL, et al. Hyper-IgE syndrome with recurrent infections—An autosomal dominant multisystem disorder. N Engl J Med. 1999;340(9):692–702.
278. Grimbacher B, Schaffer AA, Holland SM, Davis J, Gallin JI, Malech HL, et al. Genetic linkage of hyper-IgE syndrome to chromosome 4. Am J Hum Genet. 1999;65(3):735–44.
279. Grootendorst DC, Dahlen SE, Van Den Bos JW, Duiverman EJ, Veselic-Charvat M, Vrijlandt EJ, et al. Benefits of high altitude allergen avoidance in atopic adolescents with moderate to severe asthma, over and above treatment with high dose inhaled steroids. Clin Exp Allergy. 2001;31(3):400–8.
280. Gruber C. Probiotics and prebiotics in allergy prevention and treatment: future prospects. Expert review of clinical immunology. 2012;8(1):17–9.
281. Gruber C, Illi S, Lau S, Nickel R, Forster J, Kamin W, et al. Transient suppression of atopy in early childhood is associated with high vaccination coverage. Pediatrics. 2003;111(3):e282–8.
282. Gruber C, van Stuijvenberg M, Mosca F, Moro G, Chirico G, Braegger CP, et al. Reduced occurrence of early atopic dermatitis because of immunoactive prebiotics among low-atopy-risk infants. J Allergy Clin Immunol. 2010;126(4):791–7.
283. Grundmann-Kollmann M, Behrens S, Krahn G, Leiter U, Ochsendorf F, Kaufmann R, et al. Treatment of psoriasis with calcipotriene plus psoralen-UV-A-bath therapy. Arch Dermatol. 1999;135(7):861–2.
284. Grundmann-Kollmann M, Behrens S, Peter RU, Kerscher M. Treatment of severe recalcitrant dermatoses of the palms and soles with PUVA-bath versus PUVA-cream therapy. Photodermatol Photoimmunol Photomed. 1999;15(2):87–9.
285. Grundmann-Kollmann M, Behrens S, Podda M, Peter RU, Kaufmann R, Kerscher M. Phototherapy for atopic eczema with narrow-band UVB. J Am Acad Dermatol. 1999;40(6 Pt 1):995–7.
286. Grundmann-Kollmann M, Korting HC, Behrens S, Leiter U, Krahn G, Kaufmann R, et al. Successful treatment of severe refractory atopic dermatitis with mycophenolate mofetil. Br J Dermatol. 1999;141(1):175–6.
287. Gudjonsson JE, Kabashima K, Eyerich K. Mechanisms of skin autoimmunity: cellular and soluble immune components of the skin. J Allergy Clin Immunol. 2020;146(1):8–16.
288. Gueniche A, Knaudt B, Schuck E, Volz T, Bastien P, Martin R, et al. Effects of nonpathogenic gram-negative bacterium Vitreoscilla filiformis lysate on atopic dermatitis: a prospective, randomized, double-blind, placebo-controlled clinical study. Br J Dermatol. 2008;159(6):1357–63.
289. Gustafsson D, Sjoberg O, Foucard T. Development of allergies and asthma in infants and young children with atopic dermatitis—A prospective follow-up to 7 years of age. Allergy. 2000;55(3):240–5.
290. Guttman-Yassky E, Brunner PM, Neumann AU, Khattri S, Pavel AB, Malik K, et al. Efficacy and safety of fezakinumab (an IL-22 monoclonal anti-

body) in adults with moderate-to-severe atopic dermatitis inadequately controlled by conventional treatments: A randomized, double-blind, phase 2a trial. J Am Acad Dermatol. 2018;78(5):872–81 e6.
291. Guttman-Yassky E, Thaci D, Pangan AL, Hong HC, Papp KA, Reich K, et al. Upadacitinib in adults with moderate to severe atopic dermatitis: 16-week results from a randomized, placebo-controlled trial. J Allergy Clin Immunol. 2020;145(3):877–84.
292. Gutzmer R, Langer K, Lisewski M, Mommert S, Rieckborn D, Kapp A, et al. Expression and function of histamine receptors 1 and 2 on human monocyte-derived dendritic cells. J Allergy Clin Immunol. 2002;109(3):524–31.
293. Gutzmer R, Mommert S, Gschwandtner M, Zwingmann K, Stark H, Werfel T. The histamine H4 receptor is functionally expressed on T(H)2 cells. J Allergy Clin Immunol. 2009;123(3):619–25.
294. Hafenreffer S. Nosodochium, in quo cutis, eique adaerentium partium, affectus omnes, singulari methodo, et cognoscendi e curandi fidelissime traduntur. Ulm: Kuhnen; 1660. p. 98–102.
295. Haapakoski R, Karisola P, Fyhrquist N, Savinko T, Lehtimaki S, Wolff H, et al. Toll-like receptor activation during cutaneous allergen sensitization blocks development of asthma through IFN-gamma-dependent mechanisms. J Invest Dermatol. 2013;133(4):964–72.
296. Hachem JP, Wagberg F, Schmuth M, Crumrine D, Lissens W, Jayakumar A, et al. Serine protease activity and residual LEKTI expression determine phenotype in Netherton syndrome. J Invest Dermatol. 2006;126(7):1609–21.
297. Haeck IM, Knol MJ, Ten Berge O, van Velsen SG, de Bruin-Weller MS, Bruijnzeel-Koomen CA. Enteric-coated mycophenolate sodium versus cyclosporin A as long-term treatment in adult patients with severe atopic dermatitis: a randomized controlled trial. J Am Acad Dermatol. 2011;64(6):1074–84.
298. Haeck IM, Rouwen TJ, Timmer-de Mik L, de Bruin-Weller MS, Bruijnzeel-Koomen CA. Topical corticosteroids in atopic dermatitis and the risk of glaucoma and cataracts. J Am Acad Dermatol. 2011;64(2):275–81.
299. Hajar T, Leshem YA, Hanifin JM, Nedorost ST, Lio PA, Paller AS, et al. A systematic review of topical corticosteroid withdrawal ("steroid addiction") in patients with atopic dermatitis and other dermatoses. J Am Acad Dermatol. 2015;72(3):541–9 e2.
300. Hajdarbegovic E, Thio B, Nijsten T. Lower lifetime prevalence of atopy in rheumatoid arthritis. Rheumatol Int. 2014;34(6):847–8.
301. Hajdu K, Kapitany A, Dajnoki Z, Soltesz L, Barath S, Hendrik Z, et al. Improvement of clinical and immunological parameters after allergen-specific immunotherapy in atopic dermatitis. J Eur Acad Dermatol Venereol. 2021;35(6):1357–61.
302. Halken S, Hansen KS, Jacobsen HP, Estmann A, Faelling AE, Hansen LG, et al. Comparison of a partially hydrolyzed infant formula with two extensively hydrolyzed formulas for allergy prevention: a prospective, randomized study. Pediatr Allergy Immunol. 2000;11(3):149–61.
303. Hanifin J, Gupta AK, Rajagopalan R. Intermittent dosing of fluticasone propionate cream for reducing the risk of relapse in atopic dermatitis patients. Br J Dermatol. 2002;147(3):528–37.
304. Hanifin JM, Lobitz WC Jr. Newer concepts of atopic dermatitis. Arch Dermatol. 1977;113(5):663–70.
305. Hanifin JM, Rajka G. Diagnostic features of atopic dermatitis. Acta Derm Venereol. 1980;60(92):44–7.
306. Hannuksela M, Kalimo K, Lammintausta K, Mattila T, Turjanmaa K, Varjonen E, et al. Dose ranging study: cetirizine in the treatment of atopic dermatitis in adults. Ann Allergy. 1993;70(2):127–33.
307. Hannuksela-Svahn A, Pukkala E, Laara E, Poikolainen K, Karvonen J. Psoriasis, its treatment, and cancer in a cohort of Finnish patients. J Invest Dermatol. 2000;114(3):587–90.
308. Hansen ER, Buus S, Deleuran M, Andersen KE. Treatment of atopic dermatitis with mycophenolate mofetil. Br J Dermatol. 2000;143(6):1324–6.
309. Happle R. The essence of alternative medicine. A dermatologist's view from Germany. Arch Dermatol. 1998;134(11):1455–60.
310. Harari M, Shani J, Seidl V, Hristakieva E. Climatotherapy of atopic dermatitis at the Dead Sea: demographic evaluation and cost-effectiveness. Int J Dermatol. 2000;39(1):59–69.
311. Harding NJ, Birch JM, Hepworth SJ, McKinney PA. Atopic dysfunction and risk of central nervous system tumours in children. Eur J Cancer. 2008;44(1):92–9.
312. Harper JI, Ahmed I, Barclay G, Lacour M, Hoeger P, Cork MJ, et al. Cyclosporin for severe childhood atopic dermatitis: short course versus continuous therapy. Br J Dermatol. 2000;142(1):52–8.
313. Harper JI, Berth-Jones J, Camp RD, Dillon MJ, Finlay AY, Holden CA, et al. Cyclosporin for atopic dermatitis in children. Dermatology. 2001;203(1):3–6.
314. Harrop J, Chinn S, Verlato G, Olivieri M, Norback D, Wjst M, et al. Eczema, atopy and allergen exposure in adults: a population-based study. Clin Exp Allergy. 2007;37(4):526–35.
315. Hattevig G, Sigurs N, Kjellman B. Effects of maternal dietary avoidance during lactation on allergy in children at 10 years of age. Acta Paediatr. 1999;88(1):7–12.
316. Hatz HJ. Glucocorticoide. Immunologische Grundlagen, Pharmakologie und Therapierichtlinien. Stuttgart: Wissenschaftliche Verlagsgesellschaft mbH; 1998.
317. Hayashida S, Furusho N, Uchi H, Miyazaki S, Eiraku K, Gondo C, et al. Are lifetime prevalence of impetigo, molluscum and herpes infection really increased in children having atopic dermatitis? J Dermatol Sci. 2010;60(3):173–8.
318. Heil PM, Maurer D, Klein B, Hultsch T, Stingl G. Omalizumab therapy in atopic dermatitis: deple-

tion of IgE does not improve the clinical course - a randomized, placebo-controlled and double blind pilot study. J Dtsch Dermatol Ges. 2010;8(12):990–8.
319. Hemels HG. The effect of propranolol on the acetylcholine-induced sweat gland response in atopic and non-atopic subjects. Br J Dermatol. 1970;83(2):312–4.
320. Henseler T, Christophers E. Disease concomitance in psoriasis. J Am Acad Dermatol. 1995;32(6):982–6.
321. Heratizadeh A, Breuer K, Kapp A, Werfel T. Systemic therapy of atopic dermatitis. Hautarzt. 2003;54(10):937–45.
322. Heratizadeh A, Werfel T, Wollenberg A, Abraham S, Plank-Habibi S, Schnopp C, et al. Effects of structured patient education in adults with atopic dermatitis: Multicenter randomized controlled trial. J Allergy Clin Immunol. 2017;140(3):845–53 e3.
323. Herbert O, Barnetson RS, Weninger W, Kramer U, Behrendt H, Ring J. Western lifestyle and increased prevalence of atopic diseases: an example from a small papua new guinean island. World Allergy Organ J. 2009;2(7):130–7.
324. Herz U, Ahrens B, Scheffold A, Joachim R, Radbruch A, Renz H. Impact of in utero Th2 immunity on T cell deviation and subsequent immediate-type hypersensitivity in the neonate. Eur J Immunol. 2000;30(2):714–8.
325. Herzberg J. Little known forms of neurodermitis. Hautarzt. 1973;24(2):47–51.
326. Heymann WR. "Tar smarts" may have a new meaning for atopic dermatitis and psoriasis. J Am Acad Dermatol. 2019;80(1):56–7.
327. Hide DW, Matthews S, Matthews L, Stevens M, Ridout S, Twiselton R, et al. Effect of allergen avoidance in infancy on allergic manifestations at age two years. J Allergy Clin Immunol. 1994;93(5):842–6.
328. Hilliquin P, Allanore Y, Coste J, Renoux M, Kahan A, Menkes CJ. Reduced incidence and prevalence of atopy in rheumatoid arthritis. Results of a case-control study. Rheumatology (Oxford). 2000;39(9):1020–6.
329. Hindley D, Galloway G, Murray J, Gardener L. A randomised study of "wet wraps" versus conventional treatment for atopic eczema. Arch Dis Child. 2006;91(2):164–8.
330. Hjorth N, Schmidt H, Thomsen K. Fusidic acid plus betamethasone in infected or potentially infected eczema. Pharmatherapeutica. 1985;4(2):126–31.
331. Hlela C, Lunjani N, Gumedze F, Kakande B, Khumalo NP. Affordable moisturisers are effective in atopic eczema: a randomised controlled trial. S Afr Med J. 2015;105(9):780–4.
332. Ho RC, Giam YC, Ng TP, Mak A, Goh D, Zhang MW, et al. The influence of childhood atopic dermatitis on health of mothers, and its impact on Asian families. Pediatr Allergy Immunol. 2010;21(3):501–7.
333. Hoare C, Li Wan Po A, Williams H. Systematic review of treatments for atopic eczema. Health Technol Assess. 2000;4(37):1–191.
334. Holgate S, Casale T, Wenzel S, Bousquet J, Deniz Y, Reisner C. The anti-inflammatory effects of omalizumab confirm the central role of IgE in allergic inflammation. J Allergy Clin Immunol. 2005;115(3):459–65.
335. Honigsmann H. History of phototherapy in dermatology. Photochem Photobiol Sci. 2013a;12(1):16–21.
336. Honigsmann H. Phototherapy. J Invest Dermatol. 2013b;133(E1):E18–20.
337. Horimukai K, Morita K, Narita M, Kondo M, Kitazawa H, Nozaki M, Shigematsu Y, Yoshida K, Niizeki H, Motomura K, Sago H, Takimoto T, Inoue E, Kamemura N, Kido H, Hisatsune J, Sugai M, Murota H, Katayama I, Sasaki T, Amagai M, Morita H, Matsuda A, Matsumoto K, Saito H, Ohya Y. Application of moisturizer to neonates prevents development of atopic dermatitis. J Allergy Clin Immunol. 2014;134:824–30.
338. Host A, Andrae S, Charkin S, Diaz-Vazquez C, Dreborg S, Eigenmann PA, et al. Allergy testing in children: why, who, when and how? Allergy. 2003;58(7):559–69.
339. Host A, Halken S, Muraro A, Dreborg S, Niggemann B, Aalberse R, et al. Dietary prevention of allergic diseases in infants and small children. Pediatr Allergy Immunol. 2008;19(1):1–4.
340. Howell MD, Kim BE, Gao P, Grant AV, Boguniewicz M, DeBenedetto A, et al. Cytokine modulation of atopic dermatitis filaggrin skin expression. J Allergy Clin Immunol. 2009;124(3 Suppl 2):R7–R12.
341. Hradetzky S, Werfel T, Rosner LM. Autoallergy in atopic dermatitis. Allergo J Int. 2015;24(1):16–22.
342. Hua T, Yousaf M, Gwillim E, Yew YW, Lee B, Hua K, et al. Does daily bathing or showering worsen atopic dermatitis severity? A systematic review and meta-analysis. Arch Dermatol Res. 2021;313(9):729–35.
343. Huang JT, Abrams M, Tlougan B, Rademaker A, Paller AS. Treatment of Staphylococcus aureus colonization in atopic dermatitis decreases disease severity. Pediatrics. 2009;123(5):e808–14.
344. Huang YH, Huang LH, Kuo CF, Yu KH. Familial aggregation of atopic dermatitis and co-aggregation of allergic diseases in affected families in Taiwan. J Dermatol Sci. 2020;100(1):15–22.
345. Hubiche T, Ged C, Benard A, Leaute-Labreze C, McElreavey K, de Verneuil H, et al. Analysis of SPINK 5, KLK 7 and FLG genotypes in a French atopic dermatitis cohort. Acta Derm Venereol. 2007;87(6):499–505.
346. Humpeler E, Skrabal F, Bartsch G. Influence of exposure to moderate altitude on the plasma concentraton of cortisol, aldosterone, renin, testosterone, and gonadotropins. Eur J Appl Physiol Occup Physiol. 1980;45(2-3):167–76.
347. Hundley JL, Yosipovitch G. Mirtazapine for reducing nocturnal itch in patients with chronic pruritus: a pilot study. J Am Acad Dermatol. 2004;50(6):889–91.
348. Huss-Marp J, Darsow U, Brockow K, Pfab F, Weichenmeier I, Schober W, et al. Can immunoglobulin E-measurement replace challenge tests in

allergic rhinoconjunctivits to grass pollen? Clin Exp Allergy. 2011;41(8):1116–24.
349. Huss-Marp J, Eberlein-Konig B, Breuer K, Mair S, Ansel A, Darsow U, et al. Influence of short-term exposure to airborne Der p 1 and volatile organic compounds on skin barrier function and dermal blood flow in patients with atopic eczema and healthy individuals. Clin Exp Allergy. 2006;36(3):338–45.
350. Huss-Marp J, Kramer U, Eberlein B, Pfab F, Ring J, Behrendt H, et al. Reduced exhaled nitric oxide values in children with asthma after inpatient rehabilitation at high altitude. J Allergy Clin Immunol. 2007;120(2):471–2.
351. Iikura Y, Naspitz CK, Mikawa H, Talaricoficho S, Baba M, Sole D, et al. Prevention of asthma by ketotifen in infants with atopic dermatitis. Ann Allergy. 1992;68(3):233–6.
352. Ikezawa Y, Nakazawa M, Tamura C, Takahashi K, Minami M, Ikezawa Z. Cyclophosphamide decreases the number, percentage and the function of CD25+ CD4+ regulatory T cells, which suppress induction of contact hypersensitivity. J Dermatol Sci. 2005;39(2):105–12.
353. Illi S, Depner M, Genuneit J, Horak E, Loss G, Strunz-Lehner C, et al. Protection from childhood asthma and allergy in Alpine farm environments-the GABRIEL Advanced Studies. J Allergy Clin Immunol. 2012;129(6):1470–7 e6.
354. Incorvaia C, Al-Ahmad M, Ansotegui IJ, Arasi S, Bachert C, Bos C, et al. Personalized medicine for allergy treatment: allergen immunotherapy still a unique and unmatched model. Allergy. 2021;76(4):1041–52.
355. Irvine AD, Jones AP, Beattie P, Baron S, Browne F, Ashoor F, et al. A randomized controlled trial protocol assessing the effectiveness, safety and cost-effectiveness of methotrexate vs. ciclosporin in the treatment of severe atopic eczema in children: the TREatment of severe Atopic eczema Trial (TREAT). Br J Dermatol. 2018;179(6):1297–306.
356. ISAAC. Worldwide variations in the prevalence of asthma symptoms: the International Study of Asthma and Allergies in Childhood (ISAAC). Eur Respir J. 1998a;12(2):315–35.
357. ISAAC. Worldwide variations in the prevalence of asthma symptoms: The international study of asthma and allergies in childhood (ISAAC). Lancet. 1998b;351:1225–32.
358. Ishizaka K, Ishizaka T. Identification of gamma-E-antibodies as a carrier of reaginic activity. J Immunol. 1967;99(6):1187–98.
359. Isolauri E, Arvola T, Sutas Y, Moilanen E, Salminen S. Probiotics in the management of atopic eczema. Clin Exp Allergy. 2000;30(11):1604–10.
360. Jablonski NG. The evolution of human skin and skin color. Ann Rev Anthropol. 2004;33:1604–10.
361. Jacobi A, Antoni C, Manger B, Schuler G, Hertl M. Infliximab in the treatment of moderate to severe atopic dermatitis. J Am Acad Dermatol. 2005;52(3 Pt 1):522–6.
362. Jacquet L. La pratique dermatologique. In: Besnier E, Brocq L, Jacquet L, editors. La pratique dermatologique, vol. 5; 1904. p. 341.
363. Jaeger T, Rothmaier M, Zander H, Ring J, Gutermuth J, Anliker MD. Acid-coated Textiles (pH 5.5-6.5)—A New Therapeutic Strategy for Atopic Eczema? Acta Derm Venereol. 2015;95(6):659–63.
364. James JM, Burks AW, Roberson PK, Sampson HA. Safe administration of the measles vaccine to children allergic to eggs. N Engl J Med. 1995;332(19):1262–6.
365. Janeway CA Jr, Medzhitov R. Innate immune recognition. Annu Rev Immunol. 2002;20:197–216.
366. Janmohamed SR, Oranje AP, Devillers AC, Rizopoulos D, van Praag MC, Van Gysel D, et al. The proactive wet-wrap method with diluted corticosteroids versus emollients in children with atopic dermatitis: a prospective, randomized, double-blind, placebo-controlled trial. J Am Acad Dermatol. 2014;70(6):1076–82.
367. Jarnagin K, Chanda S, Coronado D, Ciaravino V, Zane LT, Guttman-Yassky E, et al. Crisaborole topical ointment, 2%: a nonsteroidal, topical, anti-inflammatory phosphodiesterase 4 inhibitor in clinical development for the treatment of atopic dermatitis. J Drugs Dermatol. 2016;15(4):390–6.
368. Jensen AO, Svaerke C, Kormendine Farkas D, Olesen AB, Kragballe K, Sorensen HT. Atopic dermatitis and risk of skin cancer: a Danish nationwide cohort study (1977-2006). Am J Clin Dermatol. 2012;13(1):29–36.
369. Johansson SG, Bennich H. Immunological studies of an atypical (myeloma) immunoglobulin. Immunology. 1967;13(4):381–94.
370. Johansson SG, Bieber T, Dahl R, Friedmann PS, Lanier BQ, Lockey RF, et al. Revised nomenclature for allergy for global use: report of the nomenclature review committee of the world allergy organization, october 2003. J Allergy Clin Immunol. 2004;113(5):832–6.
371. Johansson SG, Hourihane JO, Bousquet J, Bruijnzeel-Koomen C, Dreborg S, Haahtela T, et al. A revised nomenclature for allergy. An EAACI position statement from the EAACI nomenclature task force. Allergy. 2001;56(9):813–24.
372. Jones HE, Reinhardt JH, Rinaldi MG. A clinical, mycological, and immunological survey for dermatophytosis. Arch Dermatol. 1973;108(1):61–5.
373. Jones HE, Rinaldi MG, Chai H, Kahn G. Apparent cross-reactivity of airborne molds and the dermatophytic fungi. J Allergy Clin Immunol. 1973;52(6):346–51.
374. Juhlin L, Johansson GO, Bennich H, Hogman C, Thyresson N. Immunoglobulin E in dermatoses. Levels in atopic dermatitis and urticaria. Arch Dermatol. 1969;100(1):12–6.
375. Jutel M, Watanabe T, Klunker S, Akdis M, Thomet OA, Malolepszy J, et al. Histamine regulates T-cell and antibody responses by differential expression of H1 and H2 receptors. Nature. 2001;413(6854):420–5.

376. Kabashima K, Furue M, Hanifin JM, Pulka G, Wollenberg A, Galus R, et al. Nemolizumab in patients with moderate-to-severe atopic dermatitis: Randomized, phase II, long-term extension study. J Allergy Clin Immunol. 2018;142(4):1121–30 e7.
377. Kabashima K, Matsumura T, Komazaki H, Kawashima M, Nemolizumab JPSG. Trial of nemolizumab and topical agents for atopic dermatitis with pruritus. N Engl J Med. 2020;383(2):141–50.
378. Kajihara Y, Murakami M, Imagawa T, Otsuguro K, Ito S, Ohta T. Histamine potentiates acid-induced responses mediating transient receptor potential V1 in mouse primary sensory neurons. Neuroscience. 2010;166(1):292–304.
379. Kalliomaki M, Salminen S, Arvilommi H, Kero P, Koskinen P, Isolauri E. Probiotics in primary prevention of atopic disease: a randomised placebo-controlled trial. Lancet. 2001;357(9262):1076–9.
380. Kang KF, Tian RM. Criteria for atopic dermatitis in a Chinese population. Acta Derm Venereol Suppl (Stockh). 1989;144:26–7.
381. Kaposi M. Erkrankungen der Haut. 2nd ed. Wien; 1891.
382. Kapp A, Papp K, Bingham A, Folster-Holst R, Ortonne JP, Potter PC, et al. Long-term management of atopic dermatitis in infants with topical pimecrolimus, a nonsteroid anti-inflammatory drug. J Allergy Clin Immunol. 2002;110(2):277–84.
383. Karthik A, Subramanian G, Rao CM, Bhat K, Ranjithkumar A, Musmade P, et al. Simultaneous determination of pioglitazone and glimepiride in bulk drug and pharmaceutical dosage form by RP-HPLC method. Pak J Pharm Sci. 2008;21(4):421–5.
384. Kasraie S, Niebuhr M, Baumert K, Werfel T. Functional effects of interleukin 31 in human primary keratinocytes. Allergy. 2011;66(7):845–52.
385. Katagiri K, Arakawa S, Hatano Y, Fujiwara S. Tolerogenic antigen-presenting cells successfully inhibit atopic dermatitis-like skin lesion induced by repeated epicutaneous exposure to ovalbumin. Arch Dermatol Res. 2008;300(10):583–93.
386. Katsarou A, Armenaka M. Atopic dermatitis in older patients: particular points. J Eur Acad Dermatol Venereol. 2011;25(1):12–8.
387. Kawashima M, Tango T, Noguchi T, Inagi M, Nakagawa H, Harada S. Addition of fexofenadine to a topical corticosteroid reduces the pruritus associated with atopic dermatitis in a 1-week randomized, multicentre, double-blind, placebo-controlled, parallel-group study. Br J Dermatol. 2003;148(6):1212–21.
388. Kemeny L, Szabo K. Toll-like receptors link atopic march to the hygiene hypothesis. J Invest Dermatol. 2013;133(4):874–8.
389. Kemp AS. Atopic eczema: its social and financial costs. J Paediatr Child Health. 1999;35(3):229–31.
390. Kerschenlohr K, Darsow U, Burgdorf WH, Ring J, Wollenberg A. Lessons from atopy patch testing in atopic dermatitis. Curr Allergy Asthma Rep. 2004;4(4):285–9.
391. Kerschenlohr K, Decard S, Darsow U, Ollert M, Wollenberg A. Clinical and immunologic reactivity to aeroallergens in "intrinsic" atopic dermatitis patients. J Allergy Clin Immunol. 2003;111(1):195–7.
392. Khattri S, Brunner PM, Garcet S, Finney R, Cohen SR, Oliva M, et al. Efficacy and safety of ustekinumab treatment in adults with moderate-to-severe atopic dermatitis. Exp Dermatol. 2017;26(1):28–35.
393. Kilpelainen M, Koskenvuo M, Helenius H, Terho EO. Stressful life events promote the manifestation of asthma and atopic diseases. Clin Exp Allergy. 2002;32(2):256–63.
394. Kim E, Lee JE, Namkung JH, Kim PS, Kim S, Shin ES, et al. Single nucleotide polymorphisms and the haplotype in the DEFB1 gene are associated with atopic dermatitis in a Korean population. J Dermatol Sci. 2009;54(1):25–30.
395. Kim BS, Sun K, Papp K, Venturanza M, Nasir A, Kuligowski ME. Effects of ruxolitinib cream on pruritus and quality of life in atopic dermatitis: results from a phase 2, randomized, dose-ranging, vehicle- and active-controlled study. J Am Acad Dermatol. 2020;82(6):1305–13.
396. Kimura T, Miyazawa H. The 'butterfly' sign in patients with atopic dermatitis: evidence for the role of scratching in the development of skin manifestations. J Am Acad Dermatol. 1989;21(3 Pt 1):579–80.
397. Kini SP, DeLong LK, Veledar E, McKenzie-Brown AM, Schaufele M, Chen SC. The impact of pruritus on quality of life: the skin equivalent of pain. Arch Dermatol. 2011;147(10):1153–6.
398. Kissling S, Wuthrich B. Follow-up of atopic dermatitis after early childhood. Hautarzt. 1993;44(9):569–73.
399. Kjellman NIM. Atopic disease in seven-year-old children. Incidence in relation to family history. Acta Pediat Scand. 1977;66:465–71.
400. Klaschka F, Ring J. Systemically induced (hematogenous) contact eczema. Semin Dermatol. 1990;9(3):210–5.
401. Kleijnen J, Knipschild P, ter Riet G. Trials of homeopathy. BMJ. 1991;302(6782):960.
402. Klein PA, Clark RA. An evidence-based review of the efficacy of antihistamines in relieving pruritus in atopic dermatitis. Arch Dermatol. 1999;135(12):1522–5.
403. Kleine-Tebbe J, Fuchs T, Klimek L, Kuhr J, Lepp U, Niggemann B, et al. Allergen immunotherapy - a position paper of the German society for allergology and clinical immunology. Pneumologie. 2001;55(9):438–44.
404. Klimek L, Bachert C, Pfaar O, Becker S, Bieber T, Brehler R, et al. ARIA guideline 2019: treatment of allergic rhinitis in the German health system. Allergol Select. 2019;3(1):22–50.
405. Klimek L, Pfaar O, Worm M, Bergmann KC, Bieber T, Buhl R, et al. Allergen immunotherapy in the current COVID-19 pandemic: A position paper of AeDA, ARIA, EAACI, DGAKI and GPA: Position

paper of the German ARIA Group(A) in cooperation with the Austrian ARIA Group(B), the Swiss ARIA Group(C), German Society for Applied Allergology (AEDA)(D), German Society for Allergology and Clinical Immunology (DGAKI)(E), Society for Pediatric Allergology (GPA)(F) in cooperation with AG Clinical Immunology, Allergology and Environmental Medicine of the DGHNO-KHC(G) and the European Academy of Allergy and Clinical Immunology (EAACI)(H). Allergol Select. 2020;4:44–52.
406. Kneipp S. Meine Wasser-Kur. Severus Verlag. 1994.
407. Knobler RM. Photopheresis—Extracorporeal irradiation of 8-MOP containing blood—A new therapeutic modality. Blut. 1987;54(4):247–50.
408. Knobler R, Arenberger P, Arun A, Assaf C, Bagot M, Berlin G, et al. European dermatology forum - updated guidelines on the use of extracorporeal photopheresis 2020 - part 1. J Eur Acad Dermatol Venereol. 2020;34(12):2693–716.
409. Knobler R, Arenberger P, Arun A, Assaf C, Bagot M, Berlin G, et al. European dermatology forum: Updated guidelines on the use of extracorporeal photopheresis 2020 - Part 2. J Eur Acad Dermatol Venereol. 2021;35(1):27–49.
410. Koblenzer CS. Itching and the atopic skin. J Allergy Clin Immunol. 1999;104(3 Pt 2):S109–13.
411. von Kobyletzki G, Freitag M, Herde M, Hoxtermann S, Stucker M, Hoffmann K, et al. Phototherapy in severe atopic dermatitis. Comparison between current UVA1 therapy, UVA1 cold light and combined UVA-UVB therapy. Hautarzt. 1999;50(1):27–33.
412. Kodama A, Horikawa T, Suzuki T, Ajiki W, Takashima T, Harada S, et al. Effect of stress on atopic dermatitis: investigation in patients after the great hanshin earthquake. J Allergy Clin Immunol. 1999;104(1):173–6.
413. Kolesnik M, Franke I, Lux A, Quist SR, Gollnick HP. Eczema in psoriatico: an important differential diagnosis between chronic allergic contact dermatitis and psoriasis in palmoplantar localization. Acta Derm Venereol. 2018;98(1):50–8.
414. Kondo H, Ichikawa Y, Imokawa G. Percutaneous sensitization with allergens through barrier-disrupted skin elicits a Th2-dominant cytokine response. Eur J Immunol. 1998;28(3):769–79.
415. Kong HH, Oh J, Deming C, Conlan S, Grice EA, Beatson MA, et al. Temporal shifts in the skin microbiome associated with disease flares and treatment in children with atopic dermatitis. Genome Res. 2012;22(5):850–9.
416. Kong HH, Segre JA. Skin microbiome: looking back to move forward. J Invest Dermatol. 2012;132(3 Pt 2):933–9.
417. Koppes SA, Brans R, Ljubojevic Hadzavdic S, Frings-Dresen MH, Rustemeyer T, Kezic S. Stratum corneum tape stripping: monitoring of inflammatory mediators in atopic dermatitis patients using topical therapy. Int Arch Allergy Immunol. 2016;170(3):187–93.
418. Korting GW. Zur Pathogenese des endogenen Ekzems. Stuttgart: Thieme; 1954.
419. Kottner J, Hillmann K, Fastner A, Conzade R, Heidingsfelder S, Neumann K, Blume-Peytavi U; ADAPI Study Group. Effectiveness of a standardized skin care regimen to prevent atopic dermatitis in infants at risk for atopy: a randomized, pragmatic, parallel-group study. J Eur Acad Dermatol Venereol. 2022.
420. Koutroulis I, Pyle T, Kopylov D, Little A, Gaughan J, Kratimenos P. The association between bathing habits and severity of atopic dermatitis in children. Clin Pediatr (Phila). 2016;55(2):176–81.
421. Kowalzick L, Kleinheinz A, Weichenthal M, Neuber K, Kohler I, Grosch J, et al. Low dose versus medium dose UV-A1 treatment in severe atopic eczema. Acta Derm Venereol. 1995;75(1):43–5.
422. Kramer U, Behrendt H, Dolgner R, Ranft U, Ring J, Willer H, et al. Airway diseases and allergies in East and West German children during the first 5 years after reunification: time trends and the impact of sulphur dioxide and total suspended particles. Int J Epidemiol. 1999;28(5):865–73.
423. Kramer MS, Chalmers B, Hodnett ED, Sevkovskaya Z, Dzikovich I, Shapiro S, et al. Promotion of breastfeeding intervention trial (PROBIT): a randomized trial in the Republic of Belarus. JAMA. 2001;285(4):413–20.
424. Kramer U, Heinrich J, Wjst M, Wichmann HE. Age of entry to day nursery and allergy in later childhood. Lancet. 1999;353(9151):450–4.
425. Kramer MS, Kakuma R. Maternal dietary antigen avoidance during pregnancy and/or lactation for preventing or treating atopic disease in the child. Cochrane Database Syst Rev. 2003;(4):CD000133.
426. Kramer U, Lemmen CH, Behrendt H, Link E, Schafer T, Gostomzyk J, et al. The effect of environmental tobacco smoke on eczema and allergic sensitization in children. Br J Dermatol. 2004;150(1):111–8.
427. Kramer U, Link E, Oppermann H, Ranft U, Schafer T, Thriene B, et al. Studying school beginners in western and eastern Germany: allergy trends and sensitisations 1991-2000. Gesundheitswesen. 2002;64(12):657–63.
428. Kramer U, Schmitz R, Ring J, Behrendt H. What can reunification of East and West Germany tell us about the cause of the allergy epidemic? Clin Exp Allergy. 2015;45(1):94–107.
429. Kramer U, Weidinger S, Darsow U, Mohrenschlager M, Ring J, Behrendt H. Seasonality in symptom severity influenced by temperature or grass pollen: results of a panel study in children with eczema. J Invest Dermatol. 2005;124(3):514–23.
430. Kreft B, Wohlrab J, Fischer M, Uhlig H, Skolziger R, Marsch WC. Analysis of serum zinc level in patients with atopic dermatitis, psoriasis vulgaris and in probands with healthy skin. Hautarzt. 2000;51(12):931–4.
431. Kreth HW, Hoeger PH. Members of the VZVADsg. Safety, reactogenicity, and immunogenicity of live

attenuated varicella vaccine in children between 1 and 9 years of age with atopic dermatitis. Eur J Pediatr. 2006;165(10):677–83.
432. Kronauer C, Eberlein-Konig B, Ring J, Behrendt H. Inhibition of histamine release of human basophils and mast cells in vitro by ultraviolet A (UVA) irradiation. Inflamm Res. 2001;50(Suppl 2): S44–6.
433. Kronauer C, Eberlein-Konig B, Ring J, Behrendt H. Influence of UVB, UVA and UVA1 irradiation on histamine release from human basophils and mast cells in vitro in the presence and absence of antioxidants. Photochem Photobiol. 2003;77(5): 531–4.
434. Krutmann J, Czech W, Diepgen T, Niedner R, Kapp A, Schopf E. High-dose UVA1 therapy in the treatment of patients with atopic dermatitis. J Am Acad Dermatol. 1992;26(2 Pt 1):225–30.
435. Kunz B, Lüdtke R, Leeber N, Ring J. Test-retest-reliability and validity of the kinesiology muscle test. Complement Ther Med. 2001;9(3):141–5.
436. Kunz B, Oranje AP, Labreze L, Stalder JF, Ring J, Taieb A. Clinical validation and guidelines for the SCORAD index: consensus report of the European Task Force on Atopic Dermatitis. Dermatology. 1997;195(1):10–9.
437. Lack G, Fox D, Northstone K, Golding J, Avon Longitudinal Study of P, Children Study T. Factors associated with the development of peanut allergy in childhood. N Engl J Med. 2003;348(11):977–85.
438. Lacour M, Hauser C. The role of microorganisms in atopic dermatitis. Clin Rev Allergy. 1993;11(4):491–522.
439. Lang CCV, Masenga J, Semango G, Kaderbhai H, Li N, Tan G, et al. Evidence for different immune signatures and sensitization patterns in sub-Saharan African vs. Central European atopic dermatitis patients. J Eur Acad Dermatol Venereol. 2021;35(2):e140–e2.
440. Langan SM. Flares in childhood eczema. Skin Therapy Lett. 2009;14(8):4–5.
441. Langan SM, Irvine AD, Weidinger S. Atopic dermatitis. Lancet. 2020;396(10247):345–60.
442. Langeland T, Fagertun HE, Larsen S. Therapeutic effect of loratadine on pruritus in patients with atopic dermatitis. A multi-crossover-designed study. Allergy. 1994;49(1):22–6.
443. Larko O. Phototherapy of psoriasis - clinical aspects and risk evaluation. Acta Derm Venereol Suppl (Stockh). 1982;103:1–42.
444. Lau S, Falkenhorst G, Weber A, Werthmann I, Lind P, Buettner-Goetz P, et al. High mite-allergen exposure increases the risk of sensitization in atopic children and young adults. J Allergy Clin Immunol. 1989;84(5 Pt 1):718–25.
445. Lau S, Schulz G, Sommerfeld C, Wahn U. Comparison of quantitative ELISA and semi-quantitative Dustscreen for determination of Der p 1, Der f 1, and Fel d 1 in domestic dust samples. Allergy. 2001;56(10):993–5.
446. Lauffer F, Baghin V, Standl M, Stark SP, Jargosch M, Wehrle J, et al. Predicting persistence of atopic dermatitis in children using clinical attributes and serum proteins. Allergy. 2021;76(4):1158–72.
447. Laughter MR, Maymone MBC, Mashayekhi S, Arents BWM, Karimkhani C, Langan SM, et al. The global burden of atopic dermatitis: lessons from the Global Burden of Disease Study 1990-2017. Br J Dermatol. 2021;184(2):304–9.
448. Lee JY, Her Y, Kim CW, Kim SS. Topical corticosteroid phobia among parents of children with atopic eczema in Korea. Annals of dermatology. 2015;27(5):499–506.
449. Lee YL, Su HJ, Sheu HM, Yu HS, Guo YL. Traffic-related air pollution, climate, and prevalence of eczema in Taiwanese school children. J Invest Dermatol. 2008;128(10):2412–20.
450. Lee YA, Wahn U, Kehrt R, Tarani L, Businco L, Gustafsson D, et al. A major susceptibility locus for atopic dermatitis maps to chromosome 3q21. Nat Genet. 2000;26(4):470–3.
451. Leonardi A, Bogacka E, Fauquert JL, Kowalski ML, Groblewska A, Jedrzejczak-Czechowicz M, et al. Ocular allergy: recognizing and diagnosing hypersensitivity disorders of the ocular surface. Allergy. 2012;67(11):1327–37.
452. Leung DY. Infection in atopic dermatitis. Curr Opin Pediatr. 2003a;15(4):399–404.
453. Leung DY. Preface to atopic dermatitis intervention to control the atopic march. J Allergy Clin Immunol. 2003b;112(6 Suppl):S117.
454. Leung DY, Bieber T. Atopic dermatitis. Lancet. 2003;361(9352):151–60.
455. Leung DY, Hirsch RL, Schneider L, Moody C, Takaoka R, Li SH, et al. Thymopentin therapy reduces the clinical severity of atopic dermatitis. J Allergy Clin Immunol. 1990;85(5):927–33.
456. Leung DY, Sampson HA, Yunginger JW, Burks AW Jr, Schneider LC, Wortel CH, et al. Effect of anti-IgE therapy in patients with peanut allergy. N Engl J Med. 2003;348(11):986–93.
457. Lever R, Hadley K, Downey D, Mackie R. Staphylococcal colonization in atopic dermatitis and the effect of topical mupirocin therapy. Br J Dermatol. 1988;119(2):189–98.
458. Lewis-Jones S. Quality of life and childhood atopic dermatitis: the misery of living with childhood eczema. Int J Clin Pract. 2006;60(8):984–92.
459. Lewis-Jones MS, Finlay AY, Dykes PJ. The infants' dermatitis quality of life index. Br J Dermatol. 2001;144(1):104–10.
460. Lindelof B, Sigurgeirsson B, Tegner E, Larko O, Johannesson A, Berne B, et al. PUVA and cancer: a large-scale epidemiological study. Lancet. 1991;338(8759):91–3.
461. Lipozencic J, Wolf R. Atopic dermatitis: an update and review of the literature. Dermatologic clinics. 2007;25(4):605–12, x
462. Liu B, Tai Y, Achanta S, Kaelberer MM, Caceres AI, Shao X, et al. IL-33/ST2 signaling excites sensory neurons and mediates itch response in a mouse model of poison ivy contact allergy. Proc Natl Acad Sci U S A. 2016;113(47):E7572–E9.

463. Loden M, Andersson AC, Lindberg M. Improvement in skin barrier function in patients with atopic dermatitis after treatment with a moisturizing cream (Canoderm). Br J Dermatol. 1999;140(2):264–7.
464. Loden M, Bostrom P, Kneczke M. Distribution and keratolytic effect of salicylic acid and urea in human skin. Skin Pharmacol. 1995;8(4):173–8.
465. Lonne-Rahm SB, Rickberg H, El-Nour H, Marin P, Azmitia EC, Nordlind K. Neuroimmune mechanisms in patients with atopic dermatitis during chronic stress. J Eur Acad Dermatol Venereol. 2008;22(1):11–8.
466. Lord GM, Tagore R, Cook T, Gower P, Pusey CD. Nephropathy caused by Chinese herbs in the UK. Lancet. 1999;354(9177):481–2.
467. Lowe AJ, Leung DYM, Tang MLK, Su JC, Allen KJ. The skin as a target for prevention of the atopic march. Ann Allergy Asthma Immunol. 2018;120(2):145–51.
468. Lu ZR, Park TH, Lee ES, Kim KJ, Park D, Kim BC, et al. Dysregulated genes of extrinsic type of atopic dermatitis: 34K microarray and interactomic analyses. J Dermatol Sci. 2009;53(2):146–50.
469. Lubbe J. Practice experience with topical calcineurin inhibitors. Hautarzt. 2003;54(5):432–9.
470. Ludwig CM, Krase JM, Shi VY. T helper 2 inhibitors in allergic contact dermatitis. Dermatitis. 2021;32(1):15–8.
471. Luger TA. Balancing efficacy and safety in the management of atopic dermatitis: the role of methylprednisolone aceponate. J Eur Acad Dermatol Venereol. 2011;25(3):251–8.
472. Luger TA, Bieber T, Meurer M, Mrowietz U, Schwarz T, Simon J, et al. Therapy of atopic eczema with calcineurin inhibitors. J Dtsch Dermatol Ges. 2005;3(5):385–91.
473. Luger T, Boguniewicz M, Carr W, Cork M, Deleuran M, Eichenfield L, et al. Pimecrolimus in atopic dermatitis: consensus on safety and the need to allow use in infants. Pediatr Allergy Immunol. 2015;26(4):306–15.
474. Luger T, Loske KD, Elsner P, Kapp A, Kerscher M, Korting HC, et al. Topical skin therapy with glucocorticoids—Therapeutic index. J Dtsch Dermatol Ges. 2004;2(7):629–34.
475. Lyakhovitsky A, Barzilai A, Heyman R, Baum S, Amichai B, Solomon M, et al. Low-dose methotrexate treatment for moderate-to-severe atopic dermatitis in adults. J Eur Acad Dermatol Venereol. 2010;24(1):43–9.
476. Lynch MD, Sears A, Cookson H, Lew T, Laftah Z, Orrin L, et al. Disseminated coxsackievirus A6 affecting children with atopic dermatitis. Clin Exp Dermatol. 2015;40(5):525–8.
477. Maarouf M, Hendricks AJ, Shi VY. Bathing additives for atopic dermatitis - a systematic review. Dermatitis. 2019;30(3):191–7.
478. Mackie RM, Husain SL. Juvenile plantar dermatosis: a new entity? Clin Exp Dermatol. 1976;1(3):253–60.
479. Maeda K, Yamamoto K, Tanaka Y, Anan S, Yoshida H. House dust mite (HDM) antigen in naturally occurring lesions of atopic dermatitis (AD): the relationship between HDM antigen in the skin and HDM antigen-specific IgE antibody. J Dermatol Sci. 1992;3(2):73–7.
480. Mailhol C, Lauwers-Cances V, Rance F, Paul C, Giordano-Labadie F. Prevalence and risk factors for allergic contact dermatitis to topical treatment in atopic dermatitis: a study in 641 children. Allergy. 2009;64(5):801–6.
481. Malekzad F, Arbabi M, Mohtasham N, Toosi P, Jaberian M, Mohajer M, et al. Efficacy of oral naltrexone on pruritus in atopic eczema: a double-blind, placebo-controlled study. J Eur Acad Dermatol Venereol. 2009;23(8):948–50.
482. Malisiewicz B, Murer C, Pachlopnik Schmid J, French LE, Schmid-Grendelmeier P, Navarini AA. Eosinophilia during psoriasis treatment with TNF antagonists. Dermatology. 2011;223(4):311–5.
483. Malmontet T, Guarmit B, Gaillet M, Michaud C, Garceran N, Chanlin R, et al. Spectrum of skin diseases in Amerindian villages of the Upper Oyapock, French Guiana. Int J Dermatol. 2020;59(5):599–605.
484. Manenti L, Vaglio A. Gabapentin for uraemic pruritus. Nephrol Dial Transplant. 2005;20(6):1278–9.
485. Mansfield KE, Schmidt SAJ, Darvalics B, Mulick A, Abuabara K, Wong AYS, et al. Association Between Atopic Eczema and Cancer in England and Denmark. JAMA Dermatol. 2020;156(10):1086–97.
486. Mao XQ, Shirakawa T, Yoshikawa T, Yoshikawa K, Kawai M, Sasaki S, et al. Association between genetic variants of mast-cell chymase and eczema. Lancet. 1996;348(9027):581–3.
487. Marchionini A, Hausknecht W. Säuremantel der Haut und Bakterienabwehr. Klin Wochenschr. 1938;17:633–66.
488. Marghescu S. Patch test reactions in atopic patients. Acta Derm Venereol Suppl (Stockh). 1985;114:113–6.
489. Marsh DG, Meyers DA, Bias WB. The epidemiology and genetics of atopic allergy. N Engl J Med. 1981;305(26):1551–9.
490. Marsh DG, Neely JD, Breazeale DR, Ghosh B, Freidhoff LR, Ehrlich-Kautzky E, et al. Linkage analysis of IL4 and other chromosome 5q31.1 markers and total serum immunoglobulin E concentrations. Science. 1994;264(5162):1152–6.
491. Marty P. La relation objectale allergique. Rev Franc Psychoanal. 1958;22:5–35.
492. Matterne U, Bohmer MM, Weisshaar E, Jupiter A, Carter B, Apfelbacher CJ. Oral H1 antihistamines as 'add-on' therapy to topical treatment for eczema. Cochrane Database Syst Rev. 2019;1:CD012167.
493. Matzinger P. Tolerance, danger, and the extended family. Annu Rev Immunol. 1994;12:991–1045.
494. Maurer M, Eyerich K, Eyerich S, Ferrer M, Gutermuth J, Hartmann K, et al. Urticaria: Collegium Internationale Allergologicum (CIA) Update 2020. Int Arch Allergy Immunol. 2020;181(5):321–33.
495. Mayaux MJ, Guihard-Moscato ML, Schwartz D, Benveniste J, Coquin Y, Crapanne JB, et al. Controlled clinical trial of homoeopathy in postoperative ileus. Lancet. 1988;1(8584):528–9.

496. Mayr A, Stickl H, Muller HK, Danner K, Singer H. The smallpox vaccination strain MVA: marker, genetic structure, experience gained with the parenteral vaccination and behavior in organisms with a debilitated defence mechanism (author's transl). Zentralbl Bakteriol B. 1978;167(5-6):375–90.
497. Mayser P, Kupfer J, Nemetz D, Schafer U, Nilles M, Hort W, et al. Treatment of head and neck dermatitis with ciclopiroxolamine cream—results of a double-blind, placebo-controlled study. Skin Pharmacol Physiol. 2006;19(3):153–8.
498. McClanahan D, Wong A, Kezic S, Samrao A, Hajar T, Hill E, Simpson EL. A randomized controlled trial of an emollient with ceramide and filaggrin-associated amino acids for the primary prevention of atopic dermatitis in high-risk infants. J Eur Acad Dermatol Venereol. 2019;33:2087–94.
499. McNally NJ, Phillips DR, Williams HC. The problem of atopic eczema: aetiological clues from the environment and lifestyles. Soc Sci Med. 1998;46(6):729–41.
500. McNally NJ, Williams HC, Phillips DR, Smallman-Raynor M, Lewis S, Venn A, et al. Atopic eczema and domestic water hardness. Lancet. 1998;352(9127):527–31.
501. Mee AS, Brown D, Jewell DP. Atopy in inflammatory bowel disease. Scand J Gastroenterol. 1979;14(6):743–6.
502. Meerwaldt R, Odink RJ, Landaeta R, Aarts F, Brunekreef FB, Gerritsen J, van Aalderen WM, Hoekstra MO. A lower prevalence of atopy symptoms in children with type 1 diabetes mellitus. Clin Exp Allergy. 2002;32:254–5.
503. Meggitt SJ, Gray JC, Reynolds NJ. Azathioprine dosed by thiopurine methyltransferase activity for moderate-to-severe atopic eczema: a double-blind, randomised controlled trial. Lancet. 2006;367(9513):839–46.
504. Meingassner JG, Grassberger M, Fahrngruber H, Moore HD, Schuurman H, Stutz A. A novel anti-inflammatory drug, SDZ ASM 981, for the topical and oral treatment of skin diseases: in vivo pharmacology. Br J Dermatol. 1997;137(4):568–76.
505. Melin L, Frederiksen T, Noren P, Swebilius BG. Behavioural treatment of scratching in patients with atopic dermatitis. Br J Dermatol. 1986;115(4):467–74.
506. Mengeaud V, Phulpin C, Bacquey A, Boralevi F, Schmitt AM, Taieb A. An innovative oat-based sterile emollient cream in the maintenance therapy of childhood atopic dermatitis. Pediatr Dermatol. 2015;32(2):208–15.
507. Mercuriali H. De morbis cutaneis et omnibus corporis humani excrementis tractatus. Venetiis: Aput Iuntas; 1601.
508. Meurer M, Fartasch M, Albrecht G, Vogt T, Worm M, Ruzicka T, et al. Long-term efficacy and safety of pimecrolimus cream 1% in adults with moderate atopic dermatitis. Dermatology. 2004;208(4):365–72.
509. Milgrom H, Berger W, Nayak A, Gupta N, Pollard S, McAlary M, et al. Treatment of childhood asthma with anti-immunoglobulin E antibody (omalizumab). Pediatrics. 2001;108(2):E36.
510. Milingou M, Antille C, Sorg O, Saurat JH, Lubbe J. Alcohol intolerance and facial flushing in patients treated with topical tacrolimus. Arch Dermatol. 2004;140(12):1542–4.
511. Min KD, Yi SJ, Kim HC, Leem JH, Kwon HJ, Hong S, et al. Association between exposure to traffic-related air pollution and pediatric allergic diseases based on modeled air pollution concentrations and traffic measures in Seoul, Korea: a comparative analysis. Environ Health. 2020;19(1):6.
512. Mitchell EB, Askenase PW. Suppression of T cell-mediated cutaneous basophil hypersensitivity by serum from guinea pigs immunized with mycobacterial adjuvant. J Exp Med. 1982;156(1):159–72.
513. Mitschenko AV, Lwow AN, Kupfer J, Niemeier V, Gieler U. Atopic dermatitis and stress? How do emotions come into skin? Hautarzt. 2008;59(4):314–8.
514. Miyagaki T, Sugaya M. Erythrodermic cutaneous T-cell lymphoma: how to differentiate this rare disease from atopic dermatitis. J Dermatol Sci. 2011;64(1):1–6.
515. Mohrenschlager M, Haberl VM, Kramer U, Behrendt H, Ring J. Early BCG and pertussis vaccination and atopic diseases in 5- to 7-year-old preschool children from Augsburg, Germany: results from the MIRIAM study. Pediatr Allergy Immunol. 2007;18(1):5–9.
516. Mohrenschlager M, Ring J. Atopic eczema. Curr Allergy Asthma Rep. 2006;6(6):445–7.
517. Mohrenschlager M, Schafer T, Huss-Marp J, Eberlein-Konig B, Weidinger S, Ring J, et al. The course of eczema in children aged 5-7 years and its relation to atopy: differences between boys and girls. Br J Dermatol. 2006;154(3):505–13.
518. Moller H. Atopic winter feet in children. Acta Derm Venereol. 1972;52(5):401–5.
519. Monroe EW. Efficacy and safety of nalmefene in patients with severe pruritus caused by chronic urticaria and atopic dermatitis. J Am Acad Dermatol. 1989;21(1):135–6.
520. Moret L, Anthoine E, Aubert-Wastiaux H, Le Rhun A, Leux C, Mazereeuw-Hautier J, et al. TOPICOP(c): a new scale evaluating topical corticosteroid phobia among atopic dermatitis outpatients and their parents. PLoS One. 2013;8(10):e76493.
521. Morgan DB. A suggestive sign of allergy. Arch Derm Syphilol. 1948;57(6):1050.
522. Morgenstern V, Zutavern A, Cyrys J, Brockow I, Koletzko S, Kramer U, et al. Atopic diseases, allergic sensitization, and exposure to traffic-related air pollution in children. Am J Respir Crit Care Med. 2008;177(12):1331–7.
523. Mrabet-Dahbi S, Maurer M. Does allergy impair innate immunity? Leads and lessons from atopic dermatitis. Allergy. 2010;65(11):1351–6.
524. Mueller SM, Itin P, Vogt DR, Walter M, Lang U, Griffin LL, et al. Assessment of "corticophobia"

as an indicator of non-adherence to topical corticosteroids: A pilot study. J Dermatolog Treat. 2017;28(2):104–11.
525. Muller SM, Tomaschett D, Euler S, Vogt DR, Herzog L, Itin P. Topical corticosteroid concerns in dermatological outpatients: a cross-sectional and interventional study. Dermatology. 2016;232(4):444–52.
526. Munkvad M. A comparative trial of Clinitar versus hydrocortisone cream in the treatment of atopic eczema. Br J Dermatol. 1989;121(6):763–6.
527. Munzel K, Schandry R. Atopic eczema: psychophysiological reactivity with standardized stressors. Hautarzt. 1990;41(11):606–11.
528. Murata Y, Song M, Kikuchi H, Hisamichi K, Xu XL, Greenspan A, et al. Phase 2a, randomized, double-blind, placebo-controlled, multicenter, parallel-group study of a H4 R-antagonist (JNJ-39758979) in Japanese adults with moderate atopic dermatitis. J Dermatol. 2015;42(2):129–39.
529. Murota H, Kitaba S, Tani M, Wataya-Kaneda M, Katayama I. Effects of nonsedative antihistamines on productivity of patients with pruritic skin diseases. Allergy. 2010;65(7):929–30.
530. Murphy LA, Atherton D. A retrospective evaluation of azathioprine in severe childhood atopic eczema, using thiopurine methyltransferase levels to exclude patients at high risk of myelosuppression. Br J Dermatol. 2002;147(2):308–15.
531. Murray CS, Rees JL. Are subjective accounts of itch to be relied on? The lack of relation between visual analogue itch scores and actigraphic measures of scratch. Acta Derm Venereol. 2011;91(1):18–23.
532. von Mutius E, Braun-Fahrlander C, Schierl R, Riedler J, Ehlermann S, Maisch S, et al. Exposure to endotoxin or other bacterial components might protect against the development of atopy. Clin Exp Allergy. 2000;30(9):1230–4.
533. von Mutius E, Martinez FD, Fritzsch C, Nicolai T, Roell G, Thiemann HH. Prevalence of asthma and atopy in two areas of West and East Germany. Am J Respir Crit Care Med. 1994;149(2 Pt 1):358–64.
534. von Mutius E, Vercelli D. Farm living: effects on childhood asthma and allergy. Nat Rev Immunol. 2010;10(12):861–8.
535. von Mutius E, Weiland SK, Fritzsch C, Duhme H, Keil U. Increasing prevalence of hay fever and atopy among children in Leipzig, East Germany. Lancet. 1998;351(9106):862–6.
536. Nahm DH, Lee ES, Park HJ, Kim HA, Choi GS, Jeon SY. Treatment of atopic dermatitis with a combination of allergen-specific immunotherapy and a histamine-immunoglobulin complex. Int Arch Allergy Immunol. 2008;146(3):235–40.
537. Nakagawa H, Nemoto O, Igarashi A, Saeki H, Kaino H, Nagata T. Delgocitinib ointment, a topical Janus kinase inhibitor, in adult patients with moderate to severe atopic dermatitis: A phase 3, randomized, double-blind, vehicle-controlled study and an open-label, long-term extension study. J Am Acad Dermatol. 2020;82(4):823–31.
538. Nakano T, Shimojo N, Okamoto Y, Ebisawa M, Kurihara K, Hoshioka A, et al. The use of complementary and alternative medicine by pediatric food-allergic patients in Japan. Int Arch Allergy Immunol. 2012;159(4):410–5.
539. Naldi L, Mercuri SR. Chronic pruritus management: a plea for improvement—can itch clinics be an option? Dermatology. 2010;221(3):216–8.
540. Napadow V, Li A, Loggia ML, Kim J, Schalock PC, Lerner E, et al. The brain circuitry mediating antipruritic effects of acupuncture. Cereb Cortex. 2014;24(4):873–82.
541. Nedoszytko B, Reszka E, Gutowska-Owsiak D, Trzeciak M, Lange M, Jarczak J, et al. Genetic and epigenetic aspects of atopic dermatitis. Int J Mol Sci. 2020;21(18):6484.
542. Neri I, Dondi A, Wollenberg A, Ricci L, Ricci G, Piccirilli G, et al. Atypical forms of hand, foot, and mouth disease: a prospective study of 47 Italian children. Pediatr Dermatol. 2016;33(4):429–37.
543. Neuber K, Gerhard C, Held KR, Ring J. Dramatic improvement of nummular eczema after parenteral testosterone substitution in a patient with mixed gonadal dysgenesia. Allergo J. 1993;5:77–8.
544. Neuber K, Schwartz I, Itschert G, Dieck AT. Treatment of atopic eczema with oral mycophenolate mofetil. Br J Dermatol. 2000;143(2):385–91.
545. Nezamololama N, Fieldhouse K, Metzger K, Gooderham M. Emerging systemic JAK inhibitors in the treatment of atopic dermatitis: a review of abrocitinib, baricitinib, and upadacitinib. Drugs Context 2020;9.
546. Niemeier V, Kupfer J, Al-Abesie S, Schill WB, Gieler U. From neuropeptides and cytokines to psychotherapy. Skin diseases between psychoneuroimmunology research and psychosomatic treatment. Forsch Komplementarmed. 1999;6(Suppl 2):14–8.
547. Niggemann B. The role of the atopy patch test (APT) in diagnosis of food allergy in infants and children with atopic dermatitis. Pediatr Allergy Immunol. 2001;12(Suppl 14):37–40.
548. Niggemann B, Reibel S, Roehr CC, Felger D, Ziegert M, Sommerfeld C, et al. Predictors of positive food challenge outcome in non-IgE-mediated reactions to food in children with atopic dermatitis. J Allergy Clin Immunol. 2001;108(6):1053–8.
549. Nishioka K, Yasueda H, Saito H. Preventive effect of bedding encasement with microfine fibers on mite sensitization. J Allergy Clin Immunol. 1998;101(1 Pt 1):28–32.
550. Niwa Y, Sumi H, Akamatsu H. An association between ulcerative colitis and atopic dermatitis, diseases of impaired superficial barriers. J Invest Dermatol. 2004;123(5):999–1000.
551. Novak N. New insights into the mechanism and management of allergic diseases: atopic dermatitis. Allergy. 2009;64(2):265–75.
552. Novak N, Allam JP, Bieber T. Allergic hyperreactivity to microbial components: a trigger fac-

tor of "intrinsic" atopic dermatitis? J Allergy Clin Immunol. 2003;112(1):215–6.
553. Novak N, Bieber T. Allergic and nonallergic forms of atopic diseases. J Allergy Clin Immunol. 2003;112(2):252–62.
554. Novak N, Bieber T, Hoffmann M, Folster-Holst R, Homey B, Werfel T, et al. Efficacy and safety of subcutaneous allergen-specific immunotherapy with depigmented polymerized mite extract in atopic dermatitis. J Allergy Clin Immunol. 2012;130(4):925–31 e4.
555. Novak N, Peng W, Naegeli MC, Galvan C, Kolm-Djamei I, Bruggen C, et al. SARS-CoV-2, COVID-19, skin and immunology - What do we know so far? Allergy. 2021;76(3):698–713.
556. Novak N, Yu CF, Bussmann C, Maintz L, Peng WM, Hart J, et al. Putative association of a TLR9 promoter polymorphism with atopic eczema. Allergy. 2007;62(7):766–72.
557. Novembre E, Cianferoni A, Lombardi E, Bernardini R, Pucci N, Vierucci A. Natural history of "intrinsic" atopic dermatitis. Allergy. 2001;56(5):452–3.
558. Novembre E, Vierucci A. Milk allergy/intolerance and atopic dermatitis in infancy and childhood. Allergy. 2001;56(Suppl 67):105–8.
559. Nowak D, Heinrich J, Jorres R, Wassmer G, Berger J, Beck E, et al. Prevalence of respiratory symptoms, bronchial hyperresponsiveness and atopy among adults: west and east Germany. Eur Respir J. 1996;9(12):2541–52.
560. O'Driscoll J, Burden AD, Kingston TP. Potent topical steroid obtained from a Chinese herbalist. Br J Dermatol. 1992;127(5):543–4.
561. O'Shea JJ, Laurence A, McInnes IB. Back to the future: oral targeted therapy for RA and other autoimmune diseases. Nat Rev Rheumatol. 2013;9(3):173–82.
562. O'Shea JJ, Schwartz DM, Villarino AV, Gadina M, McInnes IB, Laurence A. The JAK-STAT pathway: impact on human disease and therapeutic intervention. Annu Rev Med. 2015;66:311–28.
563. Oetjen LK, Mack MR, Feng J, Whelan TM, Niu H, Guo CJ, et al. Sensory neurons co-OPT classical immune signaling pathways to mediate chronic itch. Cell. 2017;171(1):217–28 e13.
564. Offenbacher M, Sauer S, Hieblinger R, Hufford DJ, Walach H, Kohls N. Spirituality and the International Classification of Functioning, Disability and Health: content comparison of questionnaires measuring mindfulness based on the International Classification of Functioning. Disabil Rehabil. 2011;33(25-26):2434–45.
565. Oh SH, Bae BG, Park CO, Noh JY, Park IH, Wu WH, et al. Association of stress with symptoms of atopic dermatitis. Acta Derm Venereol. 2010;90(6):582–8.
566. Ohtsuka T, Matsumaru S, Uchida K, Onobori M, Matsumoto T, Kuwahata K, et al. Time course of plasma histamine and tryptase following food challenges in children with suspected food allergy. Ann Allergy. 1993;71(2):139–46.
567. Oji V, Eckl KM, Aufenvenne K, Natebus M, Tarinski T, Ackermann K, et al. Loss of corneodesmosin leads to severe skin barrier defect, pruritus, and atopy: unraveling the peeling skin disease. Am J Hum Genet. 2010;87(2):274–81.
568. Oldhoff JM, Darsow U, Werfel T, Katzer K, Wulf A, Laifaoui J, et al. Anti-IL-5 recombinant humanized monoclonal antibody (mepolizumab) for the treatment of atopic dermatitis. Allergy. 2005;60(5):693–6.
569. Olesen AB, Ellingsen AR, Larsen FS, Larsen PO, Veien NK, Thestrup-Pedersen K. Atopic dermatitis may be linked to whether a child is first- or second-born and/or the age of the mother. Acta Derm Venereol. 1996;76(6):457–60.
570. Olesen AB, Ellingsen AR, Olesen H, Juul S, Thestrup-Pedersen K. Atopic dermatitis and birth factors: historical follow up by record linkage. BMJ. 1997;314(7086):1003–8.
571. Olesen AB, Juul S, Birkebaek N, Thestrup-Pedersen K. Association between atopic dermatitis and insulin-dependent diabetes mellitus: a case-control study. Lancet. 2001;357(9270):1749–52.
572. Olesen AB, Juul S, Thestrup-Pedersen K. Atopic dermatitis is increased following vaccination for measles, mumps and rubella or measles infection. Acta Derm Venereol. 2003;83(6):445–50.
573. Oranje AP, de Waard-van der Spek FB. Atopic dermatitis and diet. J Eur Acad Dermatol Venereol. 2000;14(6):437–8.
574. Ordovas-Montanes J, Rakoff-Nahoum S, Huang S, Riol-Blanco L, Barreiro O, von Andrian UH. The regulation of immunological processes by peripheral neurons in homeostasis and disease. Trends Immunol. 2015;36(10):578–604.
575. Ozkaya E. Adult-onset atopic dermatitis. J Am Acad Dermatol. 2005;52(4):579–82.
576. Pacifico A, Iacovelli P, Damiani G, Ferraro C, Cazzaniga S, Conic RRZ, et al. 'High dose' vs. 'medium dose' UVA1 phototherapy in italian patients with severe atopic dermatitis. J Eur Acad Dermatol Venereol. 2019;33(4):718–24.
577. Pajno GB. Sublingual immunotherapy: the optimism and the issues. J Allergy Clin Immunol. 2007;119(4):796–801.
578. Paller A, Eichenfield LF, Leung DY, Stewart D, Appell M. A 12-week study of tacrolimus ointment for the treatment of atopic dermatitis in pediatric patients. J Am Acad Dermatol. 2001;44(1 Suppl):S47–57.
579. Paller AS, Lebwohl M, Fleischer AB Jr, Antaya R, Langley RG, Kirsner RS, et al. Tacrolimus ointment is more effective than pimecrolimus cream with a similar safety profile in the treatment of atopic dermatitis: results from 3 randomized, comparative studies. J Am Acad Dermatol. 2005;52(5):810–22.
580. Palmer CN, Irvine AD, Terron-Kwiatkowski A, Zhao Y, Liao H, Lee SP, et al. Common loss-of-function variants of the epidermal barrier protein filaggrin are a major predisposing factor for atopic dermatitis. Nat Genet. 2006;38(4):441–6.

581. Papoiu AD, Wang H, Coghill RC, Chan YH, Yosipovitch G. Contagious itch in humans: a study of visual 'transmission' of itch in atopic dermatitis and healthy subjects. Br J Dermatol. 2011;164(6):1299–303.
582. Passeron T, Lim HW, Goh CL, Kang HY, Ly F, Morita A, et al. Photoprotection according to skin phototype and dermatoses: practical recommendations from an expert panel. J Eur Acad Dermatol Venereol. 2021;35(7):1460–9.
583. Paternoster L, Standl M, Waage J, Baurecht H, Hotze M, Strachan DP, et al. Multi-ancestry genome-wide association study of 21,000 cases and 95,000 controls identifies new risk loci for atopic dermatitis. Nat Genet. 2015;47(12):1449–56.
584. Paul C, Lahfa M, Bachelez H, Chevret S, Dubertret L. A randomized controlled evaluator-blinded trial of intravenous immunoglobulin in adults with severe atopic dermatitis. Br J Dermatol. 2002;147(3):518–22.
585. Payan DG, Brewster DR, Goetzl EJ. Specific stimulation of human T lymphocytes by substance P. J Immunol. 1983;131(4):1613–5.
586. Penders A. Alopecia areata and atopy. Nederlands tijdschrift voor geneeskunde. 1968;112(6):301–3.
587. Peppers J, Paller AS, Maeda-Chubachi T, Wu S, Robbins K, Gallagher K, et al. A phase 2, randomized dose-finding study of tapinarof (GSK2894512 cream) for the treatment of atopic dermatitis. J Am Acad Dermatol. 2019;80(1):89–98 e3.
588. Pereira MP, Stander S. How to define chronic prurigo? Exp Dermatol. 2019;28(12):1455–60.
589. Peserico A, Stadtler G, Sebastian M, Fernandez RS, Vick K, Bieber T. Reduction of relapses of atopic dermatitis with methylprednisolone aceponate cream twice weekly in addition to maintenance treatment with emollient: a multicentre, randomized, double-blind, controlled study. Br J Dermatol. 2008;158(4):801–7.
590. Pfab F, Huss-Marp J, Gatti A, Fuqin J, Athanasiadis GI, Irnich D, et al. Influence of acupuncture on type I hypersensitivity itch and the wheal and flare response in adults with atopic eczema - a blinded, randomized, placebo-controlled, crossover trial. Allergy. 2010;65(7):903–10.
591. Pfab F, Schalock PC, Napadow V, Athanasiadis GI, Huss-Marp J, Ring J. Acupuncture for allergic disease therapy—the current state of evidence. Expert Rev Clin Immunol. 2014;10(7):831–41.
592. Pfab F, Valet M, Sprenger T, Huss-Marp J, Athanasiadis GI, Baurecht HJ, et al. Temperature modulated histamine-itch in lesional and nonlesional skin in atopic eczema - a combined psychophysical and neuroimaging study. Allergy. 2010;65(1):84–94.
593. Phan C, Beauchet A, Burztejn AC, Severino-Freire M, Barbarot S, Girard C, et al. Biological treatments for paediatric psoriasis : a retrospective observational study on biological drug survival in daily practice in childhood psoriasis. J Eur Acad Dermatol Venereol. 2019;33(10):1984–92.
594. Pion IA, Koenig KL, Lim HW. Is dermatologic usage of coal tar carcinogenic? A review of the literature. Dermatol Surg. 1995;21(3):227–31.
595. von Pirquet C. Allergie. Münch med Wochenschr. 1906;53:1457.
596. Platts-Mills TA, Tovey ER, Mitchell EB, Moszoro H, Nock P, Wilkins SR. Reduction of bronchial hyperreactivity during prolonged allergen avoidance. Lancet. 1982;2(8300):675–8.
597. Platts-Mills TA, Tovey ER, Mitchell EB, Mozarro H. Long-term effects of living in a dust-free room on patients with allergic asthma - reversal of bronchial hyper-reactivity. Monogr Allergy. 1983;18:153–5.
598. Plotz SG, Simon HU, Darsow U, Simon D, Vassina E, Yousefi S, et al. Use of an anti-interleukin-5 antibody in the hypereosinophilic syndrome with eosinophilic dermatitis. N Engl J Med. 2003;349(24):2334–9.
599. Plotz SG, Wiesender M, Todorova A, Ring J. What is new in atopic dermatitis/eczema? Expert Opin Emerg Drugs. 2014;19(4):441–58.
600. Prausnitz C, Küstner H. Studien über die Überempfindlichkeith. Zentralbl Bakteriol. 1921;86:160–9.
601. Prescott SL. Allergy: the price we pay for cleaner living? Ann Allergy Asthma Immunol. 2003;90(6 Suppl 3):64–70.
602. Prinz B, Nachbar F, Plewig G. Treatment of severe atopic dermatitis with extracorporeal photopheresis. Arch Dermatol Res. 1994;287(1):48–52.
603. Proksch E, Jensen JM, Elias PM. Skin lipids and epidermal differentiation in atopic dermatitis. Clin Dermatol. 2003;21(2):134–44.
604. Przybilla B, Holzle E, Enders F, Gollhausen R, Ring J. Photopatch testing with different ultraviolet A sources can yield discrepant test results. Photodermatol Photoimmunol Photomed. 1991;8(2):57–61.
605. Przybilla B, Ring J. Food allergy and atopic eczema. Semin Dermatol. 1990;9(3):220–5.
606. Przybilla B, Ring J, Enders F, Winkelmann H. Stigmata of atopic constitution in patients with atopic eczema or atopic respiratory disease. Acta Derm Venereol. 1991;71(5):407–10.
607. Pugh SM, Rhodes J, Mayberry JF, Roberts DL, Heatley RV, Newcombe RG. Atopic disease in ulcerative colitis and Crohn's disease. Clin Allergy. 1979;9(3):221–3.
608. Purohit A, Duvernelle C, Melac M, Pauli G, Frossard N. Twenty-four hours of activity of cetirizine and fexofenadine in the skin. Ann Allergy Asthma Immunol. 2001;86(4):387–92.
609. Purvis DJ, Thompson JM, Clark PM, Robinson E, Black PN, Wild CJ, et al. Risk factors for atopic dermatitis in New Zealand children at 3.5 years of age. Br J Dermatol. 2005;152(4):742–9.
610. Queille-Roussel C, Raynaud F, Saurat JH. A prospective computerized study of 500 cases of atopic dermatitis in childhood. I. Initial analysis of 250

parameters. Acta Derm Venereol Suppl (Stockh). 1985;114:87–92.
611. Raap M, Rudrich U, Stander S, Gehring M, Kapp A, Raap U. Substance P activates human eosinophils. Exp Dermatol. 2015;24(7):557–9.
612. Raap U, Werfel T, Jaeger B, Schmid-Ott G. Atopic dermatitis and psychological stress. Hautarzt. 2003;54(10):925–9.
613. Rajka G. On definition and framework of atopic dermatitis. Acta Derm Venereol Suppl (Stockh). 1989;144:10–2.
614. Rajka G, Winkelmann RK. Atopic dermatitis and Sezary syndrome. Arch Dermatol. 1984;120(1):83–4.
615. Ravens-Sieberer U, Bullinger M. Assessing health-related quality of life in chronically ill children with the German KINDL: first psychometric and content analytical results. Qual Life Res. 1998;7(5):399–407.
616. Reekers R, Beyer K, Niggemann B, Wahn U, Freihorst J, Kapp A, et al. The role of circulating food antigen-specific lymphocytes in food allergic children with atopic dermatitis. Br J Dermatol. 1996;135(6):935–41.
617. Reich K, Hartjen A, Reich J, Schroder J, Steingrube N, Bresch M, et al. Immunoglobulin E-selective immunoadsorption reduces peripheral and skin-bound immunoglobulin e and modulates cutaneous IL-13 expression in severe atopic dermatitis. J Invest Dermatol. 2019;139(3):720–3.
618. Reich K, Kabashima K, Peris K, Silverberg JI, Eichenfield LF, Bieber T, et al. Efficacy and safety of baricitinib combined with topical corticosteroids for treatment of moderate to severe atopic dermatitis: a randomized clinical trial. JAMA dermatology. 2020;156(12):1333–43.
619. van Reijsen FC, Bruijnzeel-Koomen CA, Kalthoff FS, Maggi E, Romagnani S, Westland JK, et al. Skin-derived aeroallergen-specific T-cell clones of Th2 phenotype in patients with atopic dermatitis. J Allergy Clin Immunol. 1992;90(2):184–93.
620. Reitamo S, Harper J, Bos JD, Cambazard F, Bruijnzeel-Koomen C, Valk P, et al. 0.03% Tacrolimus ointment applied once or twice daily is more efficacious than 1% hydrocortisone acetate in children with moderate to severe atopic dermatitis: results of a randomized double-blind controlled trial. Br J Dermatol. 2004;150(3):554–62.
621. Reitamo S, Ortonne JP, Sand C, Bos J, Cambazard F, Bieber T, et al. Long-term treatment with 0.1% tacrolimus ointment in adults with atopic dermatitis: results of a two-year, multicentre, non-comparative study. Acta Derm Venereol. 2007;87(5):406–12.
622. Reitamo S, Rustin M, Harper J, Kalimo K, Rubins A, Cambazard F, et al. A 4-year follow-up study of atopic dermatitis therapy with 0.1% tacrolimus ointment in children and adult patients. Br J Dermatol. 2008;159(4):942–51.
623. Renner ED, Rylaarsdam S, Anover-Sombke S, Rack AL, Reichenbach J, Carey JC, et al. Novel signal transducer and activator of transcription 3 (STAT3) mutations, reduced T(H)17 cell numbers, and variably defective STAT3 phosphorylation in hyper-IgE syndrome. J Allergy Clin Immunol. 2008;122(1):181–7.
624. Renz H, Becker WM, Bufe A, Kleine-Tebbe J, Raulf-Heimsoth M, Saloga J, et al. In vitro allergy diagnosis. Guideline of the German Society of Asthma and Immunology in conjunction with the German Society of Dermatology. J Dtsch Dermatol Ges. 2006;4(1):72–85.
625. Renz H, Skevaki C. Early life microbial exposures and allergy risks: opportunities for prevention. Nat Rev Immunol. 2021;21(3):177–91.
626. Reuter J, Merfort I, Schempp CM. Botanicals in dermatology: an evidence-based review. Am J Clin Dermatol. 2010;11(4):247–67.
627. Reyes H, Gonzalez MC, Ribalta J, Aburto H, Matus C, Schramm G, et al. Prevalence of intrahepatic cholestasis of pregnancy in Chile. Ann Intern Med. 1978;88(4):487–93.
628. Reynolds NJ, Franklin V, Gray JC, Diffey BL, Farr PM. Narrow-band ultraviolet B and broad-band ultraviolet A phototherapy in adult atopic eczema: a randomised controlled trial. Lancet. 2001;357(9273):2012–6.
629. Ricci G, Patrizi A, Bendandi B, Menna G, Varotti E, Masi M. Clinical effectiveness of a silk fabric in the treatment of atopic dermatitis. Br J Dermatol. 2004;150(1):127–31.
630. Richter R, Ahrens S. In: Fuchs E, Schulz KH, editors. Psychosomatische Aspekte der Allergie. München: Dustri Verlag; 1990.
631. Ridolo E, Martignago I, Riario-Sforza GG, Incorvaia C. Allergen immunotherapy in atopic dermatitis. Expert Rev Clin Immunol. 2018;14(1):61–8.
632. Riedler J, Braun-Fahrlander C, Eder W, Schreuer M, Waser M, Maisch S, et al. Exposure to farming in early life and development of asthma and allergy: a cross-sectional survey. Lancet. 2001;358(9288):1129–33.
633. Rigopoulos D, Gregoriou S, Charissi C, Kontochristopoulos G, Kalogeromitros D, Georgala S. Tacrolimus ointment 0.1% in pityriasis alba: an open-label, randomized, placebo-controlled study. Br J Dermatol. 2006;155(1):152–5.
634. Ring J. Atopic dermatitis: a disease of general vaso-active mediator dysregulation. Int Arch Allergy Appl Immunol. 1979;59(2):233–9.
635. Ring J. Increased vasoactive mediator releasability: a possible pathogenic factor of atopic dermatitis. Int Arch Allergy Appl Immunol. 1981a;66(Suppl 1):156–8.
636. Ring J. Mechanisms of acute allergic reactions (author's transl). MMW Munch Med Wochenschr. 1981b;123(44):1670–4.
637. Ring J. Atopic eczema. Allergy, minimal immunologic deficiency or "immuno-vegetative dysregulation"? Dtsch Med Wochenschr. 1982a;107(13):483–5.
638. Ring J. The psyche and allergy. MMW Munch Med Wochenschr. 1982b;124(13):72–4.

639. Ring J. Successful hyposensitization treatment in atopic eczema: results of a trial in monozygotic twins. Br J Dermatol. 1982c;107(5):597–602.
640. Ring J. Food allergy and other adverse reactions caused by food. Klin Wochenschr. 1984;62(17):795–802.
641. Ring J. 1st description of an "atopic family anamnesis" in the Julio-Claudian imperial house: Augustus, Claudius, Britannicus. Hautarzt. 1985;36(8):470–1.
642. Ring J. Drug intolerance caused by pseudo-allergic reactions. Wien Med Wochenschr. 1989;139(6-7):130–4.
643. Ring J. In: Ruzicka T, Ring J, Przybilla B, editors. Atopy: condition, disease, or syndrome? Berlin: Springer; 1991.
644. Ring J. Allergy in practice. 2005.
645. Ring J. The skin is close to our heart. J Eur Acad Dermatol Venereol. 2019;33(4):627–8.
646. Ring J, Abraham A, de Cuyper C, Kim K, Langeland T, Parra V, et al. Control of atopic eczema with pimecrolimus cream 1% under daily practice conditions: results of a > 2000 patient study. J Eur Acad Dermatol Venereol. 2008;22(2):195–203.
647. Ring J, Alomar A, Bieber T, Deleuran M, Fink-Wagner A, Gelmetti C, et al. Guidelines for treatment of atopic eczema (atopic dermatitis) part I. J Eur Acad Dermatol Venereol. 2012a;26(8):1045–60.
648. Ring J, Alomar A, Bieber T, Deleuran M, Fink-Wagner A, Gelmetti C, et al. Guidelines for treatment of atopic eczema (atopic dermatitis) Part II. J Eur Acad Dermatol Venereol. 2012b;26(9):1176–93.
649. Ring J, Bachert C, Bauer P, Czech W, editors. Whitebook Allergy in Germany. 3rd ed. Munich: Urban Vogel; 2010.
650. Ring J, Brockow K, Abeck D. The therapeutic concept of "patient management" in atopic eczema. Allergy. 1996;51(4):206–15.
651. Ring J, Brockow K, Behrendt H. Adverse reactions to foods. J Chromatogr B Biomed Sci Appl. 2001;756(1-2):3–10.
652. Ring J, Frohlich HH. Wirkstoffe in der dermatologischen Therapie. Berlin: Springer; 1985.
653. Ring J, Kramer U, Schafer T, Behrendt H. Why are allergies increasing? Curr Opin Immunol. 2001;13(6):701–8.
654. Ring J, Landthaler M. Hyper-IgE syndromes. Curr Probl Dermatol. 1989;18:79–88.
655. Ring J, Mohrenschlager M. Allergy to peanut oil—clinically relevant? J Eur Acad Dermatol Venereol. 2007;21(4):452–5.
656. Ring J, Palos E. Psychosomatic aspects of parent-child relations in atopic eczema in childhood. II. Child-rearing style, the family situation in a drawing test and structured interview. Hautarzt. 1986;37(11):609–17.
657. Ring J, Palos E, Zimmermann F. Psychosomatic aspects of parent-child relations in atopic eczema in childhood. I. Psychodiagnostic test procedures in parents and children in comparison with somatic findings. Hautarzt. 1986;37(10):560–7.
658. Ring J, Przybilla B, Ruzicka T. Handbook of atopic eczema. Berlin: Springer; 2006.
659. Ring J, Worm M, Wollenberg A, Thyssen JP, Jakob T, Klimek L, et al. Risk of severe allergic reactions to COVID-19 vaccines among patients with allergic skin diseases - practical recommendations. A position statement of ETFAD with external experts. J Eur Acad Dermatol Venereol. 2021;35(6):e362–e5.
660. Ring J, Zink A, Arents BWM, Seitz IA, Mensing U, Schielein MC, et al. Atopic eczema: burden of disease and individual suffering - results from a large EU study in adults. J Eur Acad Dermatol Venereol. 2019;33(7):1331–40.
661. Roberts IF, West RJ, Ogilvie D, Dillon MJ. Malnutrition in infants receiving cult diets: a form of child abuse. Br Med J. 1979;1(6159):296–8.
662. Roduit C, Frei R, Loss G, Buchele G, Weber J, Depner M, et al. Development of atopic dermatitis according to age of onset and association with early-life exposures. J Allergy Clin Immunol. 2012;130(1):130–6 e5.
663. Roelofzen JH, Aben KK, Oldenhof UT, Coenraads PJ, Alkemade HA, van de Kerkhof PC, et al. No increased risk of cancer after coal tar treatment in patients with psoriasis or eczema. J Invest Dermatol. 2010;130(4):953–61.
664. Roesner LM, Werfel T. Autoimmunity (or not) in atopic dermatitis. Front Immunol. 2019;10:2128.
665. Romanos M, Gerlach M, Warnke A, Schmitt J. Association of attention-deficit/hyperactivity disorder and atopic eczema modified by sleep disturbance in a large population-based sample. J Epidemiol Community Health. 2010;64(3):269–73.
666. Rombold S, Lobisch K, Katzer K, Grazziotin TC, Ring J, Eberlein B. Efficacy of UVA1 phototherapy in 230 patients with various skin diseases. Photodermatol Photoimmunol Photomed. 2008;24(1):19–23.
667. Rosenfeldt V, Benfeldt E, Nielsen SD, Michaelsen KF, Jeppesen DL, Valerius NH, et al. Effect of probiotic Lactobacillus strains in children with atopic dermatitis. J Allergy Clin Immunol. 2003;111(2):389–95.
668. Rosenwasser LJ, Klemm DJ, Dresback JK, Inamura H, Mascali JJ, Klinnert M, et al. Promoter polymorphisms in the chromosome 5 gene cluster in asthma and atopy. Clin Exp Allergy. 1995;25(Suppl 2):74–8; discussion 95-6
669. Rost GA. Allergische Disposition und Status exsudativus. Klin Wochenschr. 1929;8:2009–13.
670. Rothenberg ME, Klion AD, Roufosse FE, Kahn JE, Weller PF, Simon HU, et al. Treatment of patients with the hypereosinophilic syndrome with mepolizumab. N Engl J Med. 2008;358(12):1215–28.
671. Ruzicka T. Atopic eczema between rationality and irrationality. Arch Dermatol. 1998;134(11):1462–9.

672. Ruzicka T, Bieber T, Schopf E, Rubins A, Dobozy A, Bos JD, et al. A short-term trial of tacrolimus ointment for atopic dermatitis. European Tacrolimus Multicenter Atopic Dermatitis Study Group. N Engl J Med. 1997;337(12):816–21.
673. Ruzicka T, Hanifin JM, Furue M, Pulka G, Mlynarczyk I, Wollenberg A, et al. Anti-interleukin-31 receptor A antibody for atopic dermatitis. N Engl J Med. 2017;376(9):826–35.
674. Ruzicka T, Ring J. Enhanced releasability of prostaglandin E2 and leukotrienes B4 and C4 from leukocytes of patients with atopic eczema. Acta Derm Venereol. 1987;67(6):469–75.
675. Rystedt I. Contact sensitivity in adults with atopic dermatitis in childhood. Contact Dermatitis. 1985;13(1):1–8.
676. Rystedt I, Strannegard IL, Strannegard O. Recurrent viral infections in patients with past or present atopic dermatitis. Br J Dermatol. 1986;114(5):575–82.
677. Sahni D, Darley CR, Hawk JL. Glaucoma induced by periorbital topical steroid use—a rare complication. Clin Exp Dermatol. 2004;29(6):617–9.
678. Salob SP, Laverty A, Atherton DJ. Bronchial hyperresponsiveness in children with atopic dermatitis. Pediatrics. 1993;91(1):13–6.
679. Sampson HA. Use of food-challenge tests in children. Lancet. 2001;358(9296):1832–3.
680. Sandilands A, Sutherland C, Irvine AD, McLean WH. Filaggrin in the frontline: role in skin barrier function and disease. J Cell Sci. 2009;122(Pt 9):1285–94.
681. Sanz ML, Maselli JP, Gamboa PM, Oehling A, Dieguez I, de Weck AL. Flow cytometric basophil activation test: a review. J Investig Allergol Clin Immunol. 2002;12(3):143–54.
682. Sapolsky RM. Stress, the aging brain, and the mechanisms of neuron death. Cambridge, MA: MIT Press; 1992.
683. Saurat JH. Eczema in primary immune-deficiencies. Clues to the pathogenesis of atopic dermatitis with special reference to the Wiskott-Aldrich syndrome. Acta Derm Venereol Suppl (Stockh). 1985;114:125–8.
684. Savolainen J, Lammintausta K, Kalimo K, Viander M. Candida albicans and atopic dermatitis. Clin Exp Allergy. 1993;23(4):332–9.
685. Saxon A, Diaz-Sanchez D. Air pollution and allergy: you are what you breathe. Nat Immunol. 2005;6(3):223–6.
686. Schabitz A, Eyerich K, Garzorz-Stark N. So close, and yet so far away: the dichotomy of the specific immune response and inflammation in psoriasis and atopic dermatitis. J Intern Med. 2021;290(1):27–39.
687. Schafer T, Borowski C, Diepgen TL, Hellermann M, Piechotowski I, Reese I, et al. Evidence-based and consented guideline on allergy prevention. J Dtsch Dermatol Ges. 2004;2(12):1030–6, 8
688. Schafer T, Borowski C, Reese I, Werfel T, Gieler U, German Network on Allergy P. Systematic review and evidence-based consensus guideline on prevention of allergy and atopic eczema of the German Network on Allergy Prevention (ABAP). Minerva Pediatr. 2008;60(3):313–25.
689. Schafer T, Breuer K. Epidemiology of food allergies. Hautarzt. 2003;54(2):112–20.
690. Schafer T, Dirschedl P, Kunz B, Ring J, Uberla K. Maternal smoking during pregnancy and lactation increases the risk for atopic eczema in the offspring. J Am Acad Dermatol. 1997;36(4):550–6.
691. Schafer T, Kramer U, Dockery D, Vieluf D, Behrendt H, Ring J. What makes a child allergic? Analysis of risk factors for allergic sensitization in preschool children from East and West Germany. Allergy Asthma Proc. 1999;20(1):23–7.
692. Schafer T, Riehle A, Wichmann HE, Ring J. Alternative medicine in allergies - prevalence, patterns of use, and costs. Allergy. 2002;57(8):694–700.
693. Schafer T, Ring J. Epidemiology of allergic diseases. Allergy. 1997;52(38 Suppl):14–22. discussion 35-6
694. Schafer T, Ring J. The possible role of environmental pollution in the development of atopic dermatitis. In: Williams HC, editor. Atopic dermatitis. Cambridge University Press: Cambridge; 2000. p. 155–68.
695. Schafer T, Staudt A, Ring J. German instrument for the assessment of quality of life in skin diseases (DIELH). Internal consistency, reliability, convergent and discriminant validity and responsiveness. Hautarzt. 2001;52(7):624–8.
696. Schafer T, Vieluf D, Behrendt H, Kramer U, Ring J. Atopic eczema and other manifestations of atopy: results of a study in East and West Germany. Allergy. 1996;51(8):532–9.
697. Schauber J, Oda Y, Buchau AS, Yun QC, Steinmeyer A, Zugel U, et al. Histone acetylation in keratinocytes enables control of the expression of cathelicidin and CD14 by 1,25-dihydroxyvitamin D3. J Invest Dermatol. 2008;128(4):816–24.
698. Schempp C, Emde M, Wolfle U. Dermatology in the Darwin anniversary. Part 1: evolution of the integument. J Dtsch Dermatol Ges. 2009;7(9):750–7.
699. Scheynius A, Johansson C, Buentke E, Zargari A, Linder MT. Atopic eczema/dermatitis syndrome and Malassezia. Int Arch Allergy Immunol. 2002;127(3):161–9.
700. Schlaud M, Atzpodien K, Thierfelder W. Allergic diseases. Results from the German Health Interview and Examination Survey for Children and Adolescents (KiGGS). Bundesgesundheitsblatt Gesundheitsforschung Gesundheitsschutz. 2007;50:701–10.
701. Schmid-Grendelmeier P, Simon D, Simon HU, Akdis CA, Wuthrich B. Epidemiology, clinical features, and immunology of the "intrinsic" (non-IgE-mediated) type of atopic dermatitis (constitutional dermatitis). Allergy. 2001;56(9):841–9.
702. Schmid-Grendelmeier P, Takaoka R, Ahogo KC, Belachew WA, Brown SJ, Correia JC, et al. Position statement on atopic dermatitis in Sub-Saharan Africa: current status and roadmap. J Eur Acad Dermatol Venereol. 2019;33(11):2019–28.

703. Schmitt J, Abraham S, Trautmann F, Stephan V, Folster-Holst R, Homey B, et al. Usage and effectiveness of systemic treatments in adults with severe atopic eczema: first results of the German Atopic Eczema Registry TREATgermany. J Dtsch Dermatol Ges. 2017;15(1):49–59.
704. Schmitt J, Apfelbacher C, Heinrich J, Weidinger S, Romanos M. Association of atopic eczema and attention-deficit/hyperactivity disorder - meta-analysis of epidemiologic studies. Z Kinder Jugendpsychiatr Psychother. 2013;41(1):35–42; quiz -4
705. Schmitt J, Buske-Kirschbaum A, Roessner V. Is atopic disease a risk factor for attention-deficit/hyperactivity disorder? A systematic review. Allergy. 2010;65(12):1506–24.
706. Schmitt JM, Ford DE. Role of depression in quality of life for patients with psoriasis. Dermatology. 2007;215(1):17–27.
707. Schmitt J, Kirch W, Meurer M. Effects of the introduction of the German "Praxisgebuhr" on outpatient care and treatment of patients with atopic eczema. J Dtsch Dermatol Ges. 2009;7(10):879–86.
708. Schmitt J, Schakel K, Folster-Holst R, Bauer A, Oertel R, Augustin M, et al. Prednisolone vs. ciclosporin for severe adult eczema. An investigator-initiated double-blind placebo-controlled multicentre trial. Br J Dermatol. 2010;162(3):661–8.
709. Schmitt J, Schmitt NM, Kirch W, Meurer M. Outpatient care and medical treatment of children and adults with atopic eczema. J Dtsch Dermatol Ges. 2009;7(4):345–51.
710. Schmitt J, Schmitt N, Meurer M. Cyclosporin in the treatment of patients with atopic eczema - a systematic review and meta-analysis. J Eur Acad Dermatol Venereol. 2007;21(5):606–19.
711. Schmitt J, Schwarz K, Baurecht H, Hotze M, Folster-Holst R, Rodriguez E, et al. Atopic dermatitis is associated with an increased risk for rheumatoid arthritis and inflammatory bowel disease, and a decreased risk for type 1 diabetes. J Allergy Clin Immunol. 2016;137(1):130–6.
712. Schneider L, Weinberg A, Boguniewicz M, Taylor P, Oettgen H, Heughan L, et al. Immune response to varicella vaccine in children with atopic dermatitis compared with nonatopic controls. J Allergy Clin Immunol. 2010;126(6):1306–7 e2.
713. Schnopp C, Holtmann C, Stock S, Remling R, Folster-Holst R, Ring J, et al. Topical steroids under wet-wrap dressings in atopic dermatitis—a vehicle-controlled trial. Dermatology. 2002;204(1):56–9.
714. Schnuch A, Lessmann H, Geier J, Frosch PJ, Uter W. Contact allergy to fragrances: frequencies of sensitization from 1996 to 2002. Results of the IVDK*. Contact Dermatitis. 2004;50(2):65–76.
715. Schnyder UW, Klunker W. Phenotypical familial pathological reactions of atopic disorders (constitutional neurodermatitis, bronchial asthma, rhinitis allergica). Hautarzt. 1957;8(11):510–1.
716. Schoni MH, Nikolaizik WH, Schoni-Affolter F. Efficacy trial of bioresonance in children with atopic dermatitis. Int Arch Allergy Immunol. 1997;112(3):238–46.
717. Schopf E, Mueller JM, Ostermann T. Value of adjuvant basic therapy in chronic recurrent skin diseases. Neurodermatitis atopica/psoriasis vulgaris. Hautarzt. 1995;46(7):451–4.
718. Schram ME, Borgonjen RJ, Bik CM, van der Schroeff JG, van Everdingen JJ, Spuls PI, et al. Off-label use of azathioprine in dermatology: a systematic review. Arch Dermatol. 2011;147(4):474–88.
719. Schultz Larsen F, Hanifin JM. Secular change in the occurrence of atopic dermatitis. Acta Derm Venereol Suppl (Stockh). 1992;176:7–12.
720. Schultz Larsen FV, Holm NV. Atopic dermatitis in a population based twin series. Concordance rates and heritability estimation. Acta Derm Venereol Suppl (Stockh). 1985;114:159.
721. Schultze-Werninghaus G. Should asthma management include sojourns at high altitude? Chem Immunol Allergy. 2006;91:16–29.
722. Schut C, Felsch A, Zick C, Hinsch KD, Gieler U, Kupfer J. Role of illness representations and coping in patients with atopic dermatitis: a cross-sectional study. J Eur Acad Dermatol Venereol. 2014;28(11):1566–71.
723. Schut C, Kupfer J. Itch and psyche. Hautarzt. 2013;64(6):414–9.
724. Schut C, Weik U, Tews N, Gieler U, Deinzer R, Kupfer J. Psychophysiological effects of stress management in patients with atopic dermatitis: a randomized controlled trial. Acta Derm Venereol. 2013;93(1):57–61.
725. Schwanitz HJ. Diagnostik und Therapie von Handekzemen. Dtsch Med Wochenschr. 1992;117:343–8.
726. Schwartzbaum J, Seweryn M, Holloman C, Harris R, Handelman SK, Rempala GA, et al. Association between prediagnostic allergy-related serum cytokines and glioma. PLoS One. 2015;10(9):e0137503.
727. Schwarz T. No eczema without keratinocyte death. J Clin Invest. 2000;106(1):9–10.
728. Schwarz A, Grabbe S, Grosse-Heitmeyer K, Roters B, Riemann H, Luger TA, et al. Ultraviolet light-induced immune tolerance is mediated via the Fas/Fas-ligand system. J Immunol. 1998;160(9):4262–70.
729. Schwarz T, Kreiselmaier I, Bieber T, Thaci D, Simon JC, Meurer M, et al. A randomized, double-blind, vehicle-controlled study of 1% pimecrolimus cream in adult patients with perioral dermatitis. J Am Acad Dermatol. 2008;59(1):34–40.
730. Scott IC, Hider SL, Scott DL. Thromboembolism with janus kinase (JAK) inhibitors for rheumatoid arthritis: how real is the risk? Drug Saf. 2018;41(7):645–53.
731. Sediva A, Kayserova J, Vernerova E, Polouckova A, Capkova S, Spisek R, et al. Anti-CD20 (rituximab) treatment for atopic eczema. J Allergy Clin Immunol. 2008;121(6):1515–6. author reply 6-7
732. Seegraber M, Worm M, Werfel T, Svensson A, Novak N, Simon D, et al. Recurrent eczema herpe-

ticum - a retrospective european multicenter study evaluating the clinical characteristics of eczema herpeticum cases in atopic dermatitis patients. J Eur Acad Dermatol Venereol. 2019;34(5):1074–9.
733. Seegraber M, Worm M, Werfel T, Svensson A, Novak N, Simon D, et al. Recurrent eczema herpeticum - a retrospective European multicenter study evaluating the clinical characteristics of eczema herpeticum cases in atopic dermatitis patients. J Eur Acad Dermatol Venereol. 2020;34(5):1074–9.
734. Sheehan MP, Atherton DJ. A controlled trial of traditional Chinese medicinal plants in widespread non-exudative atopic eczema. Br J Dermatol. 1992;126(2):179–84.
735. Sheehan MP, Rustin MH, Atherton DJ, Buckley C, Harris DW, Brostoff J, et al. Efficacy of traditional Chinese herbal therapy in adult atopic dermatitis. Lancet. 1992;340(8810):13–7.
736. Shenefelt PD. Hypnosis in dermatology. Arch Dermatol. 2000;136(3):393–9.
737. Sidbury R, Hanifin JM. Systemic therapy of atopic dermatitis. Clin Exp Dermatol. 2000;25(7):559–66.
738. Siebenwirth J, Lüdtke R, Remy W, Rakoski J, Borelli S, Ring J. Wirksamkeit von klassisch-homöopathischer Therapie bei atopischem Ekzem. Forsch Komplementarmed. 2009;16:315–23.
739. Siegels D, Heratizadeh A, Abraham S, Binnmyr J, Brockow K, Irvine AD, et al. Systemic treatments in the management of atopic dermatitis: a systematic review and meta-analysis. Allergy. 2021;76(4):1053–76.
740. Sigurgeirsson B, Boznanski A, Todd G, Vertruyen A, Schuttelaar ML, Zhu X, et al. Safety and efficacy of pimecrolimus in atopic dermatitis: a 5-year randomized trial. Pediatrics. 2015;135(4):597–606.
741. Silny W, Czarnecka-Operacz M. Specific immunotherapy in the treatment of patients with atopic dermatitis—results of double blind placebo controlled study. Pol Merkur Lekarski. 2006;21(126):558–65.
742. Silverberg JI, Margolis DJ, Boguniewicz M, Fonacier L, Grayson MH, Ong PY, et al. Distribution of atopic dermatitis lesions in United States adults. J Eur Acad Dermatol Venereol. 2019;33(7):1341–8.
743. Silverberg JI, Thyssen JP, Paller AS, Drucker AM, Wollenberg A, Lee KH, et al. What's in a name? Atopic dermatitis or atopic eczema, but not eczema alone. Allergy. 2017;72(12):2026–30.
744. Silverberg JI, Toth D, Bieber T, Alexis AF, Elewski BE, Pink AE, et al. Tralokinumab plus topical corticosteroids for the treatment of moderate-to-severe atopic dermatitis: results from the double-blind, randomized, multicentre, placebo-controlled phase III ECZTRA 3 trial. Br J Dermatol. 2020;184(3):450–63.
745. Simon D, Hosli S, Kostylina G, Yawalkar N, Simon HU. Anti-CD20 (rituximab) treatment improves atopic eczema. J Allergy Clin Immunol. 2008;121(1):122–8.
746. Simons FE. Advances in H1-antihistamines. N Engl J Med. 2004;351(21):2203–17.
747. Simons FE, Johnston L, Simons KJ. Clinical pharmacology of the H1-receptor antagonists cetirizine and loratadine in children. Pediatr Allergy Immunol. 2000;11(2):116–9.
748. Simpson EL, Akinlade B, Ardeleanu M. Two phase 3 trials of dupilumab versus placebo in atopic dermatitis. N Engl J Med. 2017;376(11):1090–1.
749. Simpson EL, Chalmers JR, Hanifin JM, Thomas KS, Cork MJ, McLean WH, et al. Emollient enhancement of the skin barrier from birth offers effective atopic dermatitis prevention. J Allergy Clin Immunol. 2014;134:818–23.
750. Simpson EL, Flohr C, Eichenfield LF, Bieber T, Sofen H, Taieb A, et al. Efficacy and safety of lebrikizumab (an anti-IL-13 monoclonal antibody) in adults with moderate-to-severe atopic dermatitis inadequately controlled by topical corticosteroids: A randomized, placebo-controlled phase II trial (TREBLE). J Am Acad Dermatol. 2018;78(5):863–71 e11.
751. Simpson EL, Imafuku S, Poulin Y, Ungar B, Zhou L, Malik K, et al. A phase 2 randomized trial of apremilast in patients with atopic dermatitis. J Invest Dermatol. 2019;139(5):1063–72.
752. Simpson EL, Lacour JP, Spelman L, Galimberti R, Eichenfield LF, Bissonnette R, et al. Baricitinib in patients with moderate-to-severe atopic dermatitis and inadequate response to topical corticosteroids: results from two randomized monotherapy phase III trials. Br J Dermatol. 2020;183(2):242–55.
753. Simpson EL, Paller AS, Siegfried EC, Boguniewicz M, Sher L, Gooderham MJ, et al. Efficacy and safety of dupilumab in adolescents with uncontrolled moderate to severe atopic dermatitis: a phase 3 randomized clinical trial. JAMA dermatology. 2020;156(1):44–56.
754. Simpson EL, Sinclair R, Forman S, Wollenberg A, Aschoff R, Cork M, et al. Efficacy and safety of abrocitinib in adults and adolescents with moderate-to-severe atopic dermatitis (JADE MONO-1): a multicentre, double-blind, randomised, placebo-controlled, phase 3 trial. Lancet. 2020;396(10246):255–66.
755. Skudlik C, Weisshaar E, Scheidt R, Wulfhorst B, Diepgen TL, Elsner P, et al. Multicenter study "medical-occupational rehabilitation procedure skin—optimizing and quality assurance of inpatient-management (ROQ)". J Dtsch Dermatol Ges. 2009;7(2):122–6.
756. Sonkoly E, Muller A, Lauerma AI, Pivarcsi A, Soto H, Kemeny L, et al. IL-31: a new link between T cells and pruritus in atopic skin inflammation. J Allergy Clin Immunol. 2006;117(2):411–7.
757. Sparber F, De Gregorio C, Steckholzer S, Ferreira FM, Dolowschiak T, Ruchti F, et al. The Skin Commensal Yeast Malassezia Triggers a Type 17 Response that Coordinates Anti-fungal Immunity and Exacerbates Skin Inflammation. Cell Host Microbe. 2019;25(3):389–403 e6.
758. Staab D, Diepgen TL, Fartasch M, Kupfer J, Lob-Corzilius T, Ring J, et al. Age related, structured

educational programmes for the management of atopic dermatitis in children and adolescents: multicentre, randomised controlled trial. BMJ. 2006;332(7547):933–8.
759. Stadler PC, Renner ED, Milner J, Wollenberg A. Inborn error of immunity or atopic dermatitis: when to be concerned and how to investigate. J Allergy Clin Immunol Pract. 2021;9(4):1501–7.
760. Stalder JF, Bernier C, Ball A, De Raeve L, Gieler U, Deleuran M, et al. Therapeutic patient education in atopic dermatitis: worldwide experiences. Pediatr Dermatol. 2013;30(3):329–34.
761. Stalder JF, Fleury M, Sourisse M, Allavoine T, Chalamet C, Brosset P, et al. Comparative effects of two topical antiseptics (chlorhexidine vs KMn04) on bacterial skin flora in atopic dermatitis. Acta Derm Venereol Suppl (Stockh). 1992;176:132–4.
762. Stander S. Atopic dermatitis. N Engl J Med. 2021;384(12):1136–43.
763. Stander S, Luger TA. Itch in atopic dermatitis - pathophysiology and treatment. Acta Dermatovenerol Croat. 2010;18(4):289–96.
764. Stander S, Luger TA. NK-1 antagonists and itch. Handb Exp Pharmacol. 2015;226:237–55.
765. Stander S, Schafer I, Phan NQ, Blome C, Herberger K, Heigel H, et al. Prevalence of chronic pruritus in Germany: results of a cross-sectional study in a sample working population of 11,730. Dermatology. 2010;221(3):229–35.
766. Stander S, Steinhoff M, Schmelz M, Weisshaar E, Metze D, Luger T. Neurophysiology of pruritus: cutaneous elicitation of itch. Arch Dermatol. 2003;139(11):1463–70.
767. Stauder A, Kovacs M. Anxiety symptoms in allergic patients: identification and risk factors. Psychosom Med. 2003;65(5):816–23.
768. Steinhoff M, Neisius U, Ikoma A, Fartasch M, Heyer G, Skov PS, et al. Proteinase-activated receptor-2 mediates itch: a novel pathway for pruritus in human skin. J Neurosci. 2003;23(15):6176–80.
769. Strachan DP. Hay fever, hygiene, and household size. BMJ. 1989;299(6710):1259–60.
770. Strachan DP, Ait-Khaled N, Foliaki S, Mallol J, Odhiambo J, Pearce N, et al. Siblings, asthma, rhinoconjunctivitis and eczema: a worldwide perspective from the International Study of Asthma and Allergies in Childhood. Clin Exp Allergy. 2015;45(1):126–36.
771. Stuetz A, Grassberger M, Meingassner JG. Pimecrolimus (Elidel, SDZ ASM 981)—preclinical pharmacologic profile and skin selectivity. Semin Cutan Med Surg. 2001;20(4):233–41.
772. Suaini NHA, Tan CPT, Loo EXL, Tham EH. Global differences in atopic dermatitis. Pediatr Allergy Immunol. 2021;32(1):23–33.
773. Suarez AL, Feramisco JD, Koo J, Steinhoff M. Psychoneuroimmunology of psychological stress and atopic dermatitis: pathophysiologic and therapeutic updates. Acta Derm Venereol. 2012;92(1):7–15.
774. Suarez-Farinas M, Dhingra N, Gittler J, Shemer A, Cardinale I, de Guzman SC, et al. Intrinsic atopic dermatitis shows similar TH2 and higher TH17 immune activation compared with extrinsic atopic dermatitis. J Allergy Clin Immunol. 2013;132(2):361–70.
775. Subramanian A, Adderley NJ, Gkoutos GV, Gokhale KM, Nirantharakumar K, Krishna MT. Ethnicity-based differences in the incident risk of allergic diseases and autoimmune disorders: a UK-based retrospective cohort study of 4.4 million participants. Clin Exp Allergy. 2021;51(1):144–7.
776. Sulzberger MB, Witten VH. The effect of topically applied compound F in selected dermatoses. J Invest Dermatol. 1952;19(2):101–2.
777. Susitaival P, Hannuksela M. The 12-year prognosis of hand dermatosis in 896 Finnish farmers. Contact Dermatitis. 1995;32(4):233–7.
778. Suvas S. Role of substance p neuropeptide in inflammation, wound healing, and tissue homeostasis. J Immunol. 2017;199(5):1543–52.
779. Synnerstad I, Fredrikson M, Ternesten-Bratel A, Rosdahl I. Low risk of melanoma in patients with atopic dermatitis. J Eur Acad Dermatol Venereol. 2008;22(12):1423–8.
780. Szalus K, Trzeciak M, Nowicki RJ. JAK-STAT inhibitors in atopic dermatitis from pathogenesis to clinical trials results. Microorganisms. 2020;8(11):1743.
781. Szentivanyi A, Heim O, Schultze P. Changes in adrenoceptor densities in membranes of lung tissue and lymphocytes from patients with atopic disease. Ann N Y Acad Sci. 1979;332:295–8.
782. Tackett KJ, Jenkins F, Morrell DS, McShane DB, Burkhart CN. Structural racism and its influence on the severity of atopic dermatitis in African American children. Pediatr Dermatol. 2020;37(1):142–6.
783. Taieb A. Hypothesis: from epidermal barrier dysfunction to atopic disorders. Contact Dermatitis. 1999;41(4):177–80.
784. Taïeb A. In: Wallach D, Tilles G, editors. Histoire de la Dermatologie en France. Toulouse: Privat; 2002.
785. Taieb Y, Baum S, Ben Amitai D, Barzilai A, Greenberger S. The use of methotrexate for treating childhood atopic dermatitis: a multicenter retrospective study. J Dermatolog Treat. 2019;30(3):240–4.
786. Takahashi Y, Murota H, Tarutani M, Sano S, Okinaga T, Tominaga K, et al. A case of juvenile dermatomyositis manifesting inflammatory epidermal nevus-like skin lesions: unrecognized cutaneous manifestation of blaschkitis? Allergol Int. 2010;59(4):425–8.
787. Tan BB, Weald D, Strickland I, Friedmann PS. Double-blind controlled trial of effect of house-dust-mite allergen avoidance on atopic dermatitis. Lancet. 1996;347(8993):15–8.
788. Tanaka M, Aiba S, Matsumura N, Aoyama H, Tabata N, Sekita Y, et al. IgE-mediated hypersensitivity and contact sensitivity to multiple environmental allergens in atopic dermatitis. Arch Dermatol. 1994;130(11):1393–401.

789. Teichert T, Hellwig A, Pessler A, Hellwig M, Vossoughi M, Sugiri D, et al. Association between advanced glycation end products and impaired fasting glucose: results from the SALIA study. PLoS One. 2015;10(5):e0128293.
790. Terada N, Hamano N, Maesako KI, Hiruma K, Hohki G, Suzuki K, et al. Diesel exhaust particulates upregulate histamine receptor mRNA and increase histamine-induced IL-8 and GM-CSF production in nasal epithelial cells and endothelial cells. Clin Exp Allergy. 1999;29(1):52–9.
791. Tey HL, Yosipovitch G. Itch in ethnic populations. Acta Derm Venereol. 2010;90(3):227–34.
792. Thomas KS, Apfelbacher CA, Chalmers JR, Simpson E, Spuls PI, Gerbens LAA, et al. Recommended core outcome instruments for health-related quality of life, long-term control and itch intensity in atopic eczema trials: results of the HOME VII consensus meeting. Br J Dermatol. 2021;185(1):139–46.
793. Thomas KS, Dean T, O'Leary C, Sach TH, Koller K, Frost A, et al. A randomised controlled trial of ion-exchange water softeners for the treatment of eczema in children. PLoS Med. 2011;8(2):e1000395.
794. Thomas J, Wang R, Batra R, Bohner A, Garzorz-Stark N, Eberlein B, et al. Cd23 levels on B cells determine long-term therapeutic response in atopic eczema patients treated with selective ige immune apheresis. J Invest Dermatol. 2020;141(3):681–685.e6.
795. Thurmond RL, Gelfand EW, Dunford PJ. The role of histamine H1 and H4 receptors in allergic inflammation: the search for new antihistamines. Nature reviews Drug discovery. 2008;7(1):41–53.
796. Thyssen JP, de Bruin-Weller MS, Paller AS, Leshem YA, Vestergaard C, Deleuran M, et al. Conjunctivitis in atopic dermatitis patients with and without dupilumab therapy - international eczema council survey and opinion. J Eur Acad Dermatol Venereol. 2019;33(7):1224–31.
797. Thyssen JP, Vestergaard C, Barbarot S, de Bruin-Weller MS, Bieber T, Taieb A, et al. European Task Force on Atopic Dermatitis: position on vaccination of adult patients with atopic dermatitis against COVID-19 (SARS-CoV-2) being treated with systemic medication and biologics. J Eur Acad Dermatol Venereol. 2021;35(5):e308–e11.
798. Thyssen JP, Vestergaard C, Deleuran M, de Bruin-Weller MS, Bieber T, Taieb A, et al. European Task Force on Atopic Dermatitis (ETFAD): treatment targets and treatable traits in atopic dermatitis. J Eur Acad Dermatol Venereol. 2020;34(4):839–45.
799. Tobin D, Nabarro G, Baart de la Faille H, van Vloten WA, van der Putte SC, Schuurman HJ. Increased number of immunoreactive nerve fibers in atopic dermatitis. J Allergy Clin Immunol. 1992;90(4 Pt 1):613–22.
800. Tokura Y. Extrinsic and intrinsic types of atopic dermatitis. J Dermatol Sci. 2010;58(1):1–7.
801. Traidl C, Sebastiani S, Albanesi C, Merk HF, Puddu P, Girolomoni G, et al. Disparate cytotoxic activity of nickel-specific CD8+ and CD4+ T cell subsets against keratinocytes. J Immunol. 2000;165(6):3058–64.
802. Traidl S, Werfel T. Atopic dermatitis and general medical comorbidities. Internist (Berl). 2019;60(8):792–8.
803. Troncone R, Merrett TG, Ferguson A. Prevalence of atopy is unrelated to presence of inflammatory bowel disease. Clin Allergy. 1988;18(2):111–7.
804. Tsai TY, Chao YC, Hsieh CY, Huang YC. Association between atopic dermatitis and autism spectrum disorder: a systematic review and meta-analysis. Acta Derm Venereol. 2020;100(10):adv00146.
805. Tuft L. Importance of inhalant allergens in atopic dermatitis. J Invest Dermatol. 1949;12(4):211–9.
806. Tupker RA, De Monchy JG, Coenraads PJ, Homan A, van der Meer JB. Induction of atopic dermatitis by inhalation of house dust mite. J Allergy Clin Immunol. 1996;97(5):1064–70.
807. Turjanmaa K, Darsow U, Niggemann B, Rance F, Vanto T, Werfel T. EAACI/GA2LEN position paper: present status of the atopy patch test. Allergy. 2006;61(12):1377–84.
808. Turpeinen M. Absorption of hydrocortisone from the skin reservoir in atopic dermatitis. Br J Dermatol. 1991;124(4):358–60.
809. Uberla K, Dirschedl P, Gries A, Kunz B, Letzel H, Oed I, Ring J, Schotten K, Stickl H, Vogl-Voswinckel AE. Die Innenraumbelastung mit SO2 und NOx, allergische Symptome und die Keimbelastung der Gaumenmandeln bei 5 – 6-jahrigen. Projektbericht der Arbeitsgruppe, Gesundheitsmonitoring in der Oberpfalz. Munich: Inst f Med Informationsverarbeitung, Biometrie und Epidemiologie; 1988.
810. Uehara M. Clinical and histological features of dry skin in atopic dermatitis. Acta Derm Venereol Suppl (Stockh). 1985;114:82–6.
811. Uehara M, Amemiya T, Arai M. Atopic cataracts in a Japanese population. With special reference to factors possibly relevant to cataract formation. Dermatologica. 1985;170(4):180–4.
812. Uehara M, Kimura C. Descendant family history of atopic dermatitis. Acta Derm Venereol. 1993;73:62–3.
813. Uehara M, Takada K. Use of soap in the management of atopic dermatitis. Clin Exp Dermatol. 1985;10(5):419–25.
814. Undre NA, Moloney FJ, Ahmadi S, Stevenson P, Murphy GM. Skin and systemic pharmacokinetics of tacrolimus following topical application of tacrolimus ointment in adults with moderate to severe atopic dermatitis. Br J Dermatol. 2009;160(3): 665–9.
815. Ungar B, Pavel AB, Li R, Kimmel G, Nia J, Hashim P, et al. Phase 2 randomized, double-blind study of IL-17 targeting with secukinumab in atopic dermatitis. J Allergy Clin Immunol. 2021;147(1):394–7.
816. Valenta R, Seiberler S, Natter S, Mahler V, Mossabeb R, Ring J, et al. Autoallergy: a pathogenetic fac-

tor in atopic dermatitis? J Allergy Clin Immunol. 2000;105(3):432–7.
817. Van Bever HP, Docx M, Stevens WJ. Food and food additives in severe atopic dermatitis. Allergy. 1989;44(8):588–94.
818. Vandenplas Y. The use of hydrolysates in allergy prevention programmes. Eur J Clin Nutr. 1995;49(Suppl 1):S84–91.
819. Vanslow NA, Yamate M, Adams MS, Callies Q, Arbor A. The increased prevalence of atopic diseases in anhidrotic congenital ectodermal dysplasia. J Allergy. 1970;45:302–9.
820. Verhoef CM, van Roon JA, Vianen ME, Bruijnzeel-Koomen CA, Lafeber FP, Bijlsma JW. Mutual antagonism of rheumatoid arthritis and hay fever; a role for type 1/type 2 T cell balance. Ann Rheum Dis. 1998;57(5):275–80.
821. Verhoeven EW, de Klerk S, Kraaimaat FW, van de Kerkhof PC, de Jong EM, Evers AW. Biopsychosocial mechanisms of chronic itch in patients with skin diseases: a review. Acta Derm Venereol. 2008;88(3):211–8.
822. Vermeulen FM, Gerbens LAA, Schmitt J, Deleuran M, Irvine AD, Logan K, et al. The European TREatment of ATopic eczema (TREAT) Registry Taskforce survey: prescribing practices in Europe for phototherapy and systemic therapy in adult patients with moderate-to-severe atopic eczema. Br J Dermatol. 2020;183(6):1073–82.
823. Vestergaard C, Thyssen JP, Barbarot S, Paul C, Ring J, Wollenberg A. Quality of care in atopic dermatitis - a position statement by the European Task Force on Atopic Dermatitis (ETFAD). J Eur Acad Dermatol Venereol. 2020;34(3):e136–e8.
824. Vestergaard C, Wollenberg A, Barbarot S, Christen-Zaech S, Deleuran M, Spuls P, et al. European task force on atopic dermatitis position paper: treatment of parental atopic dermatitis during preconception, pregnancy and lactation period. J Eur Acad Dermatol Venereol. 2019;33(9):1644–59.
825. Vickers CF. The management of the problem atopic child in 1988. Acta Derm Venereol Suppl (Stockh). 1989;144:23–5.
826. Vieluf D, Wieben A, Ring J. Oral provocation tests with food additives in atopic eczema. Int Arch Allergy Immunol. 1999;118(2-4):232–3.
827. Vieths S, Bieber T. Personalised medicine for the diagnosis and treatment of allergic diseases. Bundesgesundheitsblatt Gesundheitsforschung Gesundheitsschutz. 2013;56(11):1531–7.
828. Vigo PG, Girgis KR, Pfuetze BL, Critchlow ME, Fisher J, Hussain I. Efficacy of anti-IgE therapy in patients with atopic dermatitis. J Am Acad Dermatol. 2006;55(1):168–70.
829. Villarino AV, Kanno Y, O'Shea JJ. Mechanisms and consequences of Jak-STAT signaling in the immune system. Nat Immunol. 2017;18(4):374–84.
830. Vocks E, Borelli S, Busch R, Dungemann H, Ring J. Biometrische Studie zur Wetterabhangigkeit und Wetterempofindlichkeit beim atopischen Ekzem. Akt Dermatol. 2002;28:363–9.
831. Vocks E, Borelli S, Rakoski J. Climatotherapy in atopic dermatitis. Allergologie. 1994;17:208–13.
832. Voorhoorst R, Spieksma-Boezeman MIA, Spieksma FTM. Is a mite (Dermatophagoides sp.) the producer of the housedust allergen? Allergie Asthma. 1964;10:329–34.
833. Vourc'h-Jourdain M, Barbarot S, Taieb A, Diepgen T, Ambonati M, Durosier V, et al. Patient-oriented SCORAD: a self-assessment score in atopic dermatitis. A preliminary feasibility study. Dermatology. 2009;218(3):246–51.
834. Wahn U, Bos JD, Goodfield M, Caputo R, Papp K, Manjra A, et al. Efficacy and safety of pimecrolimus cream in the long-term management of atopic dermatitis in children. Pediatrics. 2002;110(1 Pt 1):e2.
835. Walsh P, Aeling JL, Huff L, Weston WL. Hypothalamus-pituitary-adrenal axis suppression by superpotent topical steroids. J Am Acad Dermatol. 1993;29(3):501–3.
836. Wang H, Diepgen TL. Atopic dermatitis and cancer risk. Br J Dermatol. 2006;154(2):205–10.
837. Wang IJ, Hsieh WS, Wu KY, Guo YL, Hwang YH, Jee SH, et al. Effect of gestational smoke exposure on atopic dermatitis in the offspring. Pediatr Allergy Immunol. 2008;19(7):580–6.
838. Warnecke J, Wendt A. Anti-inflammatory action of pale sulfonated shale oil (ICHTHYOL pale) in UVB erythema test. Inflamm Res. 1998;47(2):75–8.
839. Warner JO. Asthma, allergen avoidance and residence at high altitude. Pediatr Allergy Immunol. 2009;20(6):509.
840. Warschburger P, Busch S, Bauer CP, Kiosz D, Stachow R, Petermann F. Health-related quality of life in children and adolescents with asthma: results from the ESTAR Study. J Asthma. 2004;41(4):463–70.
841. Wassmann A, Werfel T. Atopic eczema and food allergy. Chem Immunol Allergy. 2015;101:181–90.
842. Weidinger S, Baurecht H, Wagenpfeil S, Henderson J, Novak N, Sandilands A, et al. Analysis of the individual and aggregate genetic contributions of previously identified serine peptidase inhibitor Kazal type 5 (SPINK5), kallikrein-related peptidase 7 (KLK7), and filaggrin (FLG) polymorphisms to eczema risk. J Allergy Clin Immunol. 2008;122(3):560–8 e4.
843. Weidinger S, Beck LA, Bieber T, Kabashima K, Irvine AD. Atopic dermatitis. Nat Rev Dis Primers. 2018;4(1):1.
844. Weidinger S, Gieger C, Rodriguez E, Baurecht H, Mempel M, Klopp N, et al. Genome-wide scan on total serum IgE levels identifies FCER1A as novel susceptibility locus. PLoS Genet. 2008;4(8):e1000166.
845. Weidinger S, Klopp N, Rummler L, Wagenpfeil S, Novak N, Baurecht HJ, et al. Association of NOD1 polymorphisms with atopic eczema and related phenotypes. J Allergy Clin Immunol. 2005;116(1):177–84.

846. Weidinger S, Klopp N, Wagenpfeil S, Rummler L, Schedel M, Kabesch M, et al. Association of a STAT 6 haplotype with elevated serum IgE levels in a population based cohort of white adults. J Med Genet. 2004;41(9):658–63.
847. Weidinger S, Mayerhofer A, Raemsch R, Ring J, Kohn FM. Prostate-specific antigen as allergen in human seminal plasma allergy. J Allergy Clin Immunol. 2006;117(1):213–5.
848. Weidinger S, O'Sullivan M, Illig T, Baurecht H, Depner M, Rodriguez E, et al. Filaggrin mutations, atopic eczema, hay fever, and asthma in children. J Allergy Clin Immunol. 2008;121(5):1203–9 e1.
849. Weidinger S, Schafer T, Malek B, von Schmiedeberg S, Schill WB, Ring J, et al. Association between atopy and cryptorchidism. J Allergy Clin Immunol. 2004;114(1):192–3.
850. Weiland SK, von Mutius E, Hirsch T, Duhme H, Fritzsch C, Werner B, et al. Prevalence of respiratory and atopic disorders among children in the East and West of Germany five years after unification. Eur Respir J. 1999;14(4):862–70.
851. Weisshaar E, Diepgen TL, Bruckner T, Fartasch M, Kupfer J, Lob-Corzilius T, et al. Itch intensity evaluated in the German Atopic Dermatitis Intervention Study (GADIS): correlations with quality of life, coping behaviour and SCORAD severity in 823 children. Acta Derm Venereol. 2008;88(3):234–9.
852. Weisshaar E, Grull V, Konig A, Schweinfurth D, Diepgen TL, Eckart WU. The symptom of itch in medical history: highlights through the centuries. Int J Dermatol. 2009;48(12):1385–94.
853. Weisshaar E, Heyer G, Forster C, Handwerker HO. Effect of topical capsaicin on the cutaneous reactions and itching to histamine in atopic eczema compared to healthy skin. Arch Dermatol Res. 1998;290(6):306–11.
854. Weisshaar E, Szepietowski JC, Dalgard FJ, Garcovich S, Gieler U, Gimenez-Arnau AM, et al. European S2k guideline on chronic pruritus. Acta Derm Venereol. 2019;99(5):469–506.
855. Werfel T, Aberer W, Augustin M, Biedermann T, Folster-Holst R, Friedrichs F, et al. Atopic dermatitis: S2 guidelines. J Dtsch Dermatol Ges. 2009;7(Suppl 1):S1–46.
856. Werfel T, Aberer W, Bieber T, Buhles N, Kapp A, Vieluf D, et al. Atopic dermatitis. Version (17 July 2002 - modified final version). J Dtsch Dermatol Ges. 2003;1(7):586–92.
857. Werfel T, Ballmer-Weber B, Eigenmann PA, Niggemann B, Rance F, Turjanmaa K, et al. Eczematous reactions to food in atopic eczema: position paper of the EAACI and GA2LEN. Allergy. 2007;62(7):723–8.
858. Werfel T, Breuer K, Rueff F, Przybilla B, Worm M, Grewe M, et al. Usefulness of specific immunotherapy in patients with atopic dermatitis and allergic sensitization to house dust mites: a multicentre, randomized, dose-response study. Allergy. 2006;61(2):202–5.
859. Werfel T, Heratizadeh A, Niebuhr M, Kapp A, Roesner LM, Karch A, et al. Exacerbation of atopic dermatitis on grass pollen exposure in an environmental challenge chamber. J Allergy Clin Immunol. 2015;136(1):96–103 e9.
860. Werfel T, Layton G, Yeadon M, Whitlock L, Osterloh I, Jimenez P, et al. Efficacy and safety of the histamine H4 receptor antagonist ZPL-3893787 in patients with atopic dermatitis. J Allergy Clin Immunol. 2019;143(5):1830–7 e4.
861. Werfel T, Morita A, Grewe M, Renz H, Wahn U, Krutmann J, et al. Allergen specificity of skin-infiltrating T cells is not restricted to a type-2 cytokine pattern in chronic skin lesions of atopic dermatitis. J Invest Dermatol. 1996;107(6):871–6.
862. Wetzel S, Wollenberg A. Eczema molluscatum in tacrolimus treated atopic dermatitis. Eur J Dermatol. 2004;14(1):73–4.
863. Weymayr C. Scientability - a concept for the handling of homeopathic remedies by EbM. Z Evid Fortbild Qual Gesundhwes. 2013;107(9-10):606–10.
864. Whitlock FA. Psychophysiological aspects of skin disease. London: W.B. Saunders; 1976.
865. Wilkinson JD. Fusidic acid in dermatology. Br J Dermatol. 1998;139(Suppl 53):37–40.
866. Willan R. On cutaneous diseases. London: J. Johnson; 1808.
867. Williams HC. On the definition and epidemiology of atopic dermatitis. Dermatol Clin. 1995;13(3):649–57.
868. Williams HC, Burney PG, Hay RJ, Archer CB, Shipley MJ, Hunter JJ, et al. The U.K. Working Party's Diagnostic Criteria for Atopic Dermatitis. I. Derivation of a minimum set of discriminators for atopic dermatitis. Br J Dermatol. 1994;131(3):383–96.
869. Williams HC, Burney PG, Strachan D, Hay RJ. The U.K. Working Party's Diagnostic Criteria for Atopic Dermatitis. II. Observer variation of clinical diagnosis and signs of atopic dermatitis. Br J Dermatol. 1994;131(3):397–405.
870. Williams HC, Chalmers JR, Simpson EL. Prevention of atopic dermatitis. F1000 Med Rep. 2012;4:24.
871. Wilson SR, The L, Batia LM, Beattie K, Katibah GE, McClain SP, et al. The epithelial cell-derived atopic dermatitis cytokine TSLP activates neurons to induce itch. Cell. 2013;155(2):285–95.
872. Wise F, Sulzberger MB. Yearbook of dermatology and syphilology. Chicago, IL: Year Book Medical; 1933.
873. Wistokat-Wulfing A, Schmidt P, Darsow U, Ring J, Kapp A, Werfel T. Atopy patch test reactions are associated with T lymphocyte-mediated allergen-specific immune responses in atopic dermatitis. Clin Exp Allergy. 1999;29(4):513–21.
874. Wohlrab W. Introduction neurodermatitis and urea. Hautarzt. 1992;43(Suppl 11):1–4.
875. Wollenberg A. Eczema herpeticum. Chem Immunol Allergy. 2012;96:89–95.
876. Wollenberg A, Barbarot S, Bieber T, Christen-Zaech S, Deleuran M, Fink-Wagner A, et al.

Consensus-based European guidelines for treatment of atopic eczema (atopic dermatitis) in adults and children: part I. J Eur Acad Dermatol Venereol. 2018a;32(5):657–82.
877. Wollenberg A, Barbarot S, Bieber T, Christen-Zaech S, Deleuran M, Fink-Wagner A, et al. Consensus-based European guidelines for treatment of atopic eczema (atopic dermatitis) in adults and children: part II. J Eur Acad Dermatol Venereol. 2018b;32(6):850–78.
878. Wollenberg A, Bieber T. Topical immunomodulatory agents and their targets in inflammatory skin diseases. Transplant Proc. 2001;33(3):2212–6.
879. Wollenberg A, Bieber T. Proactive therapy of atopic dermatitis—an emerging concept. Allergy. 2009;64(2):276–8.
880. Wollenberg A, Christen-Zach S, Taieb A, Paul C, Thyssen JP, de Bruin-Weller M, et al. ETFAD/EADV Eczema task force 2020 position paper on diagnosis and treatment of atopic dermatitis in adults and children. J Eur Acad Dermatol Venereol. 2020;34(12):2717–44.
881. Wollenberg A, Howell MD, Guttman-Yassky E, Silverberg JI, Kell C, Ranade K, et al. Treatment of atopic dermatitis with tralokinumab, an anti-IL-13 mAb. J Allergy Clin Immunol. 2019;143(1):135–41.
882. Wollenberg A, Kinberger M, Arents B, et al. European guideline (EuroGuiDerm) on atopic eczema: part I —systemic therapy. J Eur Acad Dermatol Venereol. 2022a;36:1409–31.
883. Wollenberg A, Kinberger M, Arents B, et al. European guideline (EuroGuiDerm) on atopic eczema—part II: non-systemic treatments and treatment recommendations for special AE patient populations. J Eur Acad Dermatol Venereol. 2022b;36:1904–26.
884. Wollenberg A, Reitamo S, Atzori F, Lahfa M, Ruzicka T, Healy E, et al. Proactive treatment of atopic dermatitis in adults with 0.1% tacrolimus ointment. Allergy. 2008;63(6):742–50.
885. Wollenberg A, Thomsen SF, Lacour JP, Jaumont X, Lazarewicz S. Targeting immunoglobulin E in atopic dermatitis: A review of the existing evidence. World Allergy Organ J. 2021;14(3):100519.
886. Wollenberg A, Wetzel S, Burgdorf WH, Haas J. Viral infections in atopic dermatitis: pathogenic aspects and clinical management. J Allergy Clin Immunol. 2003;112(4):667–74.
887. Wollenberg A, Zoch C, Wetzel S, Plewig G, Przybilla B. Predisposing factors and clinical features of eczema herpeticum: a retrospective analysis of 100 cases. J Am Acad Dermatol. 2003;49(2):198–205.
888. Wong RC, Fairley JA, Ellis CN. Dermographism: a review. J Am Acad Dermatol. 1984;11(4 Pt 1):643–52.
889. Worm M, Ehlers I, Sterry W, Zuberbier T. Clinical relevance of food additives in adult patients with atopic dermatitis. Clin Exp Allergy. 2000;30(3):407–14.
890. Worm M, Forschner K, Lee HH, Roehr CC, Edenharter G, Niggemann B, et al. Frequency of atopic dermatitis and relevance of food allergy in adults in Germany. Acta Derm Venereol. 2006;86(2):119–22.
891. Worm M, Henz BM. Novel unconventional therapeutic approaches to atopic eczema. Dermatology. 2000;201(3):191–5.
892. Worm M, Reese I, Ballmer-Weber B, Beyer K, Bischoff SC, Bohle B, et al. Update of the S2k guideline on the management of IgE-mediated food allergies. Allergol Select. 2021;5:195–243.
893. Wright RJ. Stress and atopic disorders. J Allergy Clin Immunol. 2005;116(6):1301–6.
894. Wüthrich B. Neurodermitis atopica sive constitutionalis. Ein pathogenetisches Modell aus der Sicht des Allergologen. Aktuel Dermatol. 1983;9:1–7.
895. Wuthrich B, Schmid-Grendelmeier P. The atopic eczema/dermatitis syndrome. Epidemiology, natural course, and immunology of the IgE-associated ("extrinsic") and the nonallergic ("intrinsic") AEDS. J Investig Allergol Clin Immunol. 2003;13(1):1–5.
896. Wuthrich B, Schmid-Grendelmeier P, Schindler C, Imboden M, Bircher A, Zemp E, et al. Prevalence of atopy and respiratory allergic diseases in the elderly SAPALDIA population. Int Arch Allergy Immunol. 2013;162(2):143–8.
897. Yamaguchi J, Aihara M, Kobayashi Y, Kambara T, Ikezawa Z. Quantitative analysis of nerve growth factor (NGF) in the atopic dermatitis and psoriasis horny layer and effect of treatment on NGF in atopic dermatitis. J Dermatol Sci. 2009;53(1):48–54.
898. Yamamoto M, Haruna T, Ueda C, Asano Y, Takahashi H, Iduhara M, et al. Contribution of itch-associated scratch behavior to the development of skin lesions in Dermatophagoides farinae-induced dermatitis model in NC/Nga mice. Arch Dermatol Res. 2009;301(10):739–46.
899. Yanase DJ, David-Bajar K. The leukotriene antagonist montelukast as a therapeutic agent for atopic dermatitis. J Am Acad Dermatol. 2001;44(1):89–93.
900. Yang Q. Acupuncture treatment of 139 cases of neurodermatitis. J Tradit Chin Med. 1997;17(1):57–8.
901. Yang EJ, Hendricks AJ, Beck KM, Shi VY. Bioactive: A new era of bioactive ingredients in topical formulations for inflammatory dermatoses. Dermatol Ther. 2019;32(6):e13101.
902. Yew YW, Thyssen JP, Silverberg JI. A systematic review and meta-analysis of the regional and age-related differences in atopic dermatitis clinical characteristics. J Am Acad Dermatol. 2019;80(2):390–401.
903. Yosipovitch G, Bernhard JD. Clinical practice. Chronic pruritus. N Engl J Med. 2013;368(17):1625–34.
904. Young SHRJ, Daman HR. Psychobiological aspects of allergic disorders. New York: Praeger; 1986.
905. Yun JW, Seo JA, Jang WH, Koh HJ, Bae IH, Park YH, et al. Antipruritic effects of TRPV1 antagonist in murine atopic dermatitis and itching models. J Invest Dermatol. 2011;131(7):1576–9.

906. Yun JW, Seo JA, Jeong YS, Bae IH, Jang WH, Lee J, et al. TRPV1 antagonist can suppress the atopic dermatitis-like symptoms by accelerating skin barrier recovery. J Dermatol Sci. 2011;62(1):8–15.
907. Zeiser K, Hammel G, Kirchberger I, Traidl-Hoffmann C. Social and psychosocial effects on atopic eczema symptom severity - a scoping review of observational studies published from 1989 to 2019. J Eur Acad Dermatol Venereol. 2021;35(4):835–43.
908. Zhao M, Liang Y, Shen C, Wang Y, Ma L, Ma X. Patient education programs in pediatric atopic dermatitis: a systematic review of randomized controlled trials and meta-analysis. Dermatol Ther (Heidelb). 2020;10(3):449–64.
909. Zink AGS, Arents B, Fink-Wagner A, Seitz IA, Mensing U, Wettemann N, et al. Out-of-pocket Costs for Individuals with Atopic Eczema: A Cross-sectional Study in Nine European Countries. Acta Derm Venereol. 2019;99(3):263–7.
910. Zink A, Gensbaur A, Zirbs M, Seifert F, Suarez IL, Mourantchanian V, et al. Targeting IgE in severe atopic dermatitis with a combination of immunoadsorption and omalizumab. Acta Derm Venereol. 2015;96(1):72–6.
911. Zink A, et al. Pruritus in Germany—a Google search engine analysis. Hasutarzt. 2019;70:21–8. https://doi.org/10.1007/s00105-018-4215-5.
912. Zirbs M, Reindel U, Hermann K, Church MK, Behrendt H, Ring J, et al. Reduced skin reactivity to vasoconstrictor and vasodilator substances in atopic eczema. Eur J Dermatol. 2013;23(6):812–9.
913. Zuberbier T, Edenharter G, Worm M, Ehlers I, Reimann S, Hantke T, et al. Prevalence of adverse reactions to food in Germany - a population study. Allergy. 2004;59(3):338–45.
914. Zurbriggen B, Wuthrich B, Cachelin AB, Wili PB, Kagi MK. Comparison of two formulations of cyclosporin A in the treatment of severe atopic dermatitis. Aa double-blind, single-centre, cross-over pilot study. Dermatology. 1999;198(1):56–60.
915. van Zuuren EJ, Fedorowicz Z, Christensen R, Lavrijsen A, Arents BWM. Emollients and moisturisers for eczema. Cochrane Database Syst Rev. 2017;2:CD012119.

Index

A
Absence, 17, 31, 33, 59, 61, 63, 119, 133, 188
Acid mantle, 91, 137
Acrodermatitis enteropathica, 62
Acupuncture, 176, 177, 180
Acute flare, 138–141, 143, 155, 161, 162, 183
Acute therapy, 117, 139, 140, 154, 156, 157
Acyclovir, 70, 153
Adhesion factor, 92
Adrenergic, 5
Adstringentia, 159
Adult, 5, 11–13, 17–23, 28, 31, 32, 41, 43–45, 59, 61–63, 65–67, 74, 75, 77, 102, 112, 114, 124, 139, 141, 164, 168, 190
Aeroallergens, 43, 102, 118, 119, 121, 132–134, 140, 183
Affection, 31, 41, 43, 45, 109, 110
Air pollutant, 17, 27, 183, 186
Airway disease, 17, 25, 70, 187, 188, 195
Alcohol, 131, 135, 150, 156, 158, 159
Allergen avoidance, 126, 130, 184
Allergen dilution, 119
Allergen exposure, 11, 15, 29, 181, 182
Allergen extract, 119, 122
Allergic diathesis, 4
Allergy
  burden, 31–33, 91, 174
  diagnosis, 118–128
  protective factors, 184
  risk, 65, 151, 186
Alopecia areata, 65
Alternative procedures, 33, 173, 175, 176, 179–180, 187
Ammonium bituminosulfonates, 159
Anaphylaxis, 4, 22, 25, 65, 66, 123, 124, 154, 162, 183
Androgens, 112
Angulus infectiosus, 43
Animal dander allergy, 133
Anthroposophic medicine, 179
Antibiotics, 147, 148, 151–153, 156, 165, 179, 183
Antibody, monoclonal, 168–171
Antiemetics, 157
Antigen recognition, 100–102
Antihistamines, 140, 154–157
Anti-IgE-antibody, 64, 169–170
Anti-IL 4-R-antibody, 168
Anti-interleukin, 168–171
Antimetabolite, 165
Antimicrobial, 83, 91, 151–154, 159, 160, 164
Antimycotic, 147, 151, 153, 154, 156, 165
Antipruritic, 103, 139–141, 148, 157–161, 165, 168, 173
Antiseptic, 91, 122–123, 151–154
Anti-T-cell strategy, 165
Anti-TNF strategies, 170
Anxiety, 24, 107, 108, 111
APT, *see* Atopy patch test (APT)
Arousal, emotional, 112
Arrhythmias, 156
Arthritis rheumatoid, 74, 75, 165, 167, 170, 171
ASIT, *see* Immunotherapy, Allergen-specific
Association study, genome-wide, 82, 83
Astemizole, 156
Asthma bronchiale, 7, 8
Atopic disease, 1, 2, 6, 8–10, 14–16, 18, 23, 25–29, 56, 57, 65–68, 71, 73–75, 77, 83, 86, 103, 119, 130, 133, 181, 183
Atopic winter feet, 45, 46
Atopy
  fold, 54, 56, 59
  ointment, 139
  risk, 27
Atopy patch test (APT), 74, 94, 98, 119–122, 124, 125, 133, 162
Atrophy, 143, 145, 148, 151
Autoantibodies, 96, 100, 101
Autogenic training, 173, 174
Autoimmune disease, 18, 59, 100, 166, 171
Autoimmune phenomenon, 101
Autonomic disturbance, 4, 57, 107, 108
Avoidance, 63, 124, 126, 130–134, 136, 163, 182–184, 186, 187, 190, 195
Avoidance recommendations, 133
Axon reflex, 154
Azathioprine, 165, 166

K. Eyerich, J. Ring, *Atopic Dermatitis - Eczema*, https://doi.org/10.1007/978-3-031-12499-0

B

Baby food, hypoallergenic, 26, 134, 182, 185, 186
Bach flower therapy, 176–179
Bacterial, 68, 69, 73, 76, 86, 91, 151
Balneo PUVA therapy, 161
Bamboo hair, 64, 92
Basic therapeutics, 138, 158, 187
Basic therapy, 130, 132, 134, 148, 151
Basophil activation, 123
Bath ingredients, 26, 138–140
B-cell, 96, 99, 112, 113
Behavioral change, 174
Behavioral therapy, 174–175
Besnier, 4, 6
Betablockade, 4
Bioresonance, 176, 177, 179, 180
Bleach bath, 152
Blue (flower), 176
Blue (light), 160, 161
Blue (patches), 64
Body mass index, correlation, 184
Breast milk, 184
Bufexamac, 159
Burden, socioeconomic, 31, 33

C

Calcineurin inhibitor, topical (TCI), 141, 147–151
Candida infection, 43
Candidate gene, 83, 84, 86
Cannabinoid agonist, 139, 158, 160
Capsaicin, 43, 158
Casein hydrolysate, 185, 186
Cataract, 66, 146, 147
Cat keeping, 27, 119, 133
CD8+ cells, 101
CD63, 123
Cell extracts, 178
Cells, 2, 22, 83, 87, 90, 92, 95–100, 103, 104, 113, 121, 122, 128, 143, 154, 161–163, 166, 170
Cheilitis sicca, 43, 54
Chemokines, 86, 97, 128
Chlorhexidine, 151, 153
Cholinergic, 5, 56, 107, 111, 113
Chronic inflammatory, 2, 11, 59–63, 98
Climate change, 11, 15
Climate therapy, 161, 176, 188–190
Clioquinol, 152, 154
Coal tar, 159
Colonization, microbial, 151, 193
Colorings, 124, 133, 151, 154
Combination effects, 152
Communication therapy, 174
Competence, social, 174
Complication, 35, 62, 68, 70–73, 146–147
Conditioning, 107, 133, 174
Contact allergen, 66, 121, 123
Contact allergy, 4, 45, 50, 62, 66, 75, 76, 119, 120, 122–123, 125, 138, 158
Contact dermatitis, allergic, 9, 13, 50, 52, 59, 61, 62, 66, 76, 123, 166, 178
Contact sensitization, 153
Coombs classification, 6, 7
Corneocyte, 84, 91–93
Corneodesmosome, 92
Cornified envelope, 92
Corticoderm, 146
Cortisone, 123, 145, 176
Costs of disease, 32, 33, 127, 136, 171, 187
Cotinin, 27
Cradle cap (crusta lactea), 3, 49, 50
Cream, 135, 136, 138, 139, 148, 150, 151, 156, 158, 161, 162, 175, 195, 196
Crohn, 65, 67
Cromoglycate, 157
Cross-reaction, 22, 41, 101
Crusta lactea (s. Cradle cap), 50
Crusting, 37, 41, 77
Cure, 175, 188
Cyclosporin A, 148, 165, 166
Cystatin A, 93
Cytokine cluster, 86
Cytokines, 90, 96–100, 105, 163, 165–170, 172
Cytomegalovirus infection (CMV), 73

D

Davos climate, 160, 188, 189
DC, *see* Dendritic cells (DC)
Defense mechanisms, 62, 92
Definition, 4, 6–10, 19, 21, 23, 35, 39, 52, 56, 68, 77, 98, 99, 102, 110, 121, 181, 188
Delayed blanch reaction, 54, 108
Delayed type hypersensitivitiy (DTH), 170
Dendritic cells (DC), 84, 90, 100, 121
Dennie-Morgan atopy fold, 56, 59
Dentition, 64
Dermatitis, 8–10, 52, 62, 63, 136
Dermatomyositis, 59, 63, 171
Dermatophagoides pteronyssinus, 62, 132
Dermatophytes, 153
Dermatosis, 35, 64
Dermographism, white, 54, 57, 59–61, 76, 103, 108
Desensitization, 174
Desmosomes, 92
Desquamation, 91–93, 96–98
Detergents, 137–138, 152
Diabetes mellitus, 31, 73, 74
Diagnosis, 117–119, 123, 124, 126, 127, 130
Diagnostic criteria, 5, 76, 77, 79
Diagnostics, 6, 11, 54, 117–119, 123–130, 139, 177, 189, 190, 193, 195
Diaper dermatitis, 59
Diary, 125
Diathesis, 4, 54, 59, 64, 77, 123
Diet, 26, 33, 63, 133, 176, 182, 184, 186

Differential diagnoses, 18, 35, 45, 48–50, 59–64, 68, 118, 126
Differentiation complex, epidermal (EDC), 83, 96
Dirty neck, 50, 52
"Distraction" techniques, 174
Dog allergy, 133, 182, 186
Dog keeping, 27, 186
Dose, 121, 147, 155, 157, 158, 161–163, 165, 168–171, 174, 178
Dry, 2, 4, 45, 46, 48, 50, 53, 54, 57, 59, 64, 76, 89, 91, 96, 119, 134, 136, 138, 153, 156, 158, 170
DTH, *see* Delayed type hypersensitivitiy (DTH)
Dubowitz syndrome, 59, 63, 64
Dysesthesia, 31, 62, 102, 150
Dyshidrosis, 61
Dyshidrosis lamellosa sicca, 45
Dysplasia, ectodermal, 65
Dysregulation, autonomic, 4, 57, 107, 108

E
Ear piercing, 182
EBV, *see* Epstein-Barr-Virus (EBV)
Ecchymosis, 145
Eczema
  flares, 65, 108, 110, 112, 117, 130, 132, 139–141, 153, 154, 156, 162, 173, 183, 195
  herpeticum, 62, 70, 71, 73, 76, 125, 153, 167
  infantum, 18, 19, 59
  molluscatum, 70
  nail, 45, 46, 53
  overalls, 132
  verrucatum, 70, 73
Eczema academy, 191
Eczema school, 113, 130, 174, 175, 180, 190, 191
EDC, *see* Differentiation complex, epidermal (EDC)
Educational programs, 2, 113, 117, 130, 133, 134, 141, 174, 189–191
Education style, 109, 110
Electroacupuncture, 176, 177, 179
Elicitors, 111, 132, 158, 179
Emla, 158
Emollient, 26, 91, 122, 132, 135, 136, 138–139, 141, 147, 159, 164, 186
Emulsion, 119, 136, 138, 147
Emulsion bath, 138
Encasings, 132
Endogenous eczema, 5, 6
Enteropathy, gluten-sensitive, 65
Environmental allergens, 7, 102
Environmental disease, 4, 5
Eosinophil, 49, 96, 99, 104, 120, 155, 169
Eosinophilia, 60, 61, 170
Epicutaneous tests, 122
Epidemiology, 11–13, 15–29, 195
Epidermis, 3, 24, 25, 38, 54, 83, 84, 86, 89–91, 96, 97, 107, 111, 121, 135, 137, 138, 144, 145, 150, 159–161
Epionychitis sicca, 45
Epstein-Barr Virus (EBV), 73
Erosions, 38, 71, 96
Erythema, 35, 37–39, 43, 45, 60, 63, 77, 96, 97, 160, 162
Erythematous, nummular, 49
Erythroderma, 20, 22, 41, 52, 63, 92, 128
Essential oils, 152
Etheric, 159
European task force on atopic dermatitis (ETFAD), 77, 80, 120, 121
Everolimus, 148
Exacerbation, 25, 26, 37, 59, 67, 68, 70, 71, 112, 113, 121, 123, 124, 126, 132, 133, 145, 147, 151, 153, 154, 172, 189
Excoriation, 41, 43, 46, 49, 53, 77
Exposure, 7, 8, 17, 27, 28, 67, 91, 118, 150, 160, 162, 174, 183, 188
Exposure study, 17, 27, 28, 150
Exsudative diathesis, 4
Extensor side eczema, 20, 48, 77
Extrinsic, 6, 21, 22, 86
Eyebrow, scattering, 54

F
Face, 20, 22, 38, 43, 49–51, 56, 64, 69, 91, 121, 138, 145, 148, 151, 158
Factors, prognostic, 20, 28
Family dynamics, 108–110, 190
Family history, 3, 23, 67, 76, 82, 181, 186
Family studies, 23, 24, 41, 82, 113
Fat, 136
Fatty acid, unsaturated, 171
Fibroblasts, 90, 148
Filaggrin, 2, 4, 20, 54, 55, 63, 81, 83–85, 91–93, 98, 100, 159, 181
Fine particles, 134
Finger nail dystrophy, 53
Finger tip eczema, 46, 54, 55
Fingertip rule, 141
Fish consumption, 184
Fissure, 43, 45, 53
Flexural eczema, 38, 40, 72
Fold, infraorbital, 56, 59
Food additives, 65, 118, 124
Food allergen, 65, 66, 119, 122, 124, 133
Food allergy, 32, 60, 61, 65, 66, 68, 123–125, 157, 169, 185
Food IgG, 177
Foot eczema, 53, 61, 123, 161
Formaldehyde, 130
Fusidic acid, 153

G
Gastroenteritis, eosinophil, 65
Gastrointestinal diseases, 65, 66
Gender, 21, 22, 60
Gene associations, 86

Gene locus, 83
Genetics, 2, 4, 15, 22, 23, 60, 65, 68, 81–86, 91, 93, 100, 102, 114, 117, 193, 195
Genital eczema, 45
Genodermatoses, 18, 59
Gentian violet, 151
German Infant Nutritional Intervention Study (GINI), 26, 185
Gianotti-Crosti syndrome, 48
Glucocorticosteroids, 134, 138, 143–148, 150–153, 156, 158, 160, 164, 178
Glycerol, 138, 139
Graft-versus-host disease, 59, 62
Granuloma gluteale infantum, 145
Grass pollen, 17, 119, 121, 133, 162

H

Hair disease, 65
Hair line, temporal, 54, 57–59
Hair mineral analysis, 177
Halo eyes, 56, 57
Halo periorbital, 54, 56, 59
Hand, 19, 39, 53, 55, 70, 73, 121
Hand eczema, 50, 53, 61, 126–128, 161, 187
Hanifin-Rajka criteria, 76, 79
Hay fever, 1, 7, 12, 15–20, 23, 24, 28, 65, 119, 162, 177, 178
Head and neck dermatitis, 19, 153, 154
Head, excoriation, 43, 46, 49, 53, 77
Hereditary, 7, 63–65, 82
Herpes simplex infection, 62, 68, 70, 76, 153, 167
Herpeticum, eczema, 62, 70, 71, 73, 76, 125, 150, 153, 167
Hertoghe sign, 54, 56, 57, 59, 76
High altitude, 119, 131, 134, 160, 188, 189
Histamine, 4, 103–106, 108, 123, 154, 155, 157, 161, 163, 178
Histamine-H1 antagonists, 106
Histamine receptors, 108, 154
Histiocytosis X, 63
History, 1–10, 22, 25, 41, 54, 76, 77, 109, 110, 118–119, 121, 124, 125, 129, 136, 154, 159, 173, 177, 188, 193
Homeopathy, 176, 178, 180
Hormone, 22, 111, 112
Hostility, 109
House dust mite, 4, 17, 62, 66, 93, 98, 101, 119, 121, 122, 125, 132–134, 140, 162, 163, 183, 188
House dust mite extract, 119
Human immunodeficiency virus (HIV) infection, 71
Humidity, air, 132, 189
Hydrolysate formula, 185
Hygiene hypothesis, 15, 26, 29, 86, 182, 183
Hypereosinophilia syndrome, 64
Hyper-IgE syndrome, 59, 63, 64
Hyperkeratosis, 45, 48
Hyperkeratotic, fissuring, 50
Hyperpigmentation, 44, 50, 52
Hyperreactivity, bronchial, 65
Hypersensitivity, 2, 4, 6–9, 65, 117, 195
Hyposensitization, 162, 178

I

Ichthyosis, 22, 41, 54, 55, 59, 63, 76, 83
Imagination techniques, 174
Immediate-type reaction, 7, 124
Immune defect, 68
Immune deviation, 96
Immune response, 18, 22, 23, 25, 68, 84, 86, 94, 95, 98, 130, 148, 150, 163, 170
Immune response adaptive, 86
Immune stimulation, 11
Immune system, 15, 18, 29, 81, 84, 90, 91, 93, 97, 103, 104, 106, 107, 111, 182
Immunoglobulin E (IgE)
  auto antibody, 100, 101, 105
  production, 8, 9, 57, 86
  receptor high affinity, 86, 87
Immunopathy, 62, 63
Immunophilin, 148, 165
Immunosuppression, 161, 162, 165
Immunotherapy, allergen-specific (ASIT), 162, 163
Immuno tolerance, 184
Impetiginisation, 68
Impetigo, 59, 62, 68
Individual, 2, 3, 7, 19, 20, 25, 31–33, 36, 54, 57, 61, 62, 67, 68, 70, 79, 98, 105, 106, 111, 115, 117, 118, 126, 127, 129–134, 136, 139, 147, 156, 160, 173–175, 179, 187, 190, 191, 193
Indoor air, pollutant, 17
Infant formula, 182, 185, 186
Infections, 15, 17, 22, 25, 45, 60, 64, 70, 71, 73, 76, 94, 111, 125, 150, 152–154, 167, 168, 183
Infectious disease, 18, 24–26, 62, 179, 183
Infiltrate inflammatory, 96
Inflammation, 10, 35, 48, 54, 67, 81, 83, 94, 98, 100–103, 108, 113, 119, 121, 123, 129, 135, 136, 174, 177
Inflammation marker, 21
Inflammatory bowel disease, 65, 67
Inflammatory cells, 21–22, 111, 148, 155, 158
Infliximab, 170
Interdigital eczema, 60–62
Interferon gamma, 74
Interleukin 4, 4, 83, 86, 96, 98, 99, 103, 104, 166, 168
Interleukin 5, 86, 96, 98, 99, 169
Interleukin 10, 97, 166
Interleukin 31, 43, 96, 98, 100, 103–105, 166, 169
Interleukin antibodies, 96, 170
Intertrigo, retro-auricular, 43
Intestinal microbiome, 171
Intradermal test, 119
Intravenous, 70, 140, 143, 153, 156, 168, 171
Intrinsic, 6–10, 21, 22, 99
In vitro allergy diagnostics, 123

Irritant, 50, 68, 130–131, 134, 174, 183, 187, 188
Itch diary, 174
Itch questionnaires, 105
Itch research, 103, 104

J
Jungle hypothesis, 15, 24, 29, 182

K
Kaposi's varicelliform eruption, 70
Keratin filaments, 92
Keratinocyte, 62, 84, 90, 92–99, 103–105, 143, 148, 158, 165
Keratoconus, 66
Keratolytic, 65, 138
Keratosis follicularis (pilaris), 64, 65
Ketotifen, 157
KiGGS study, 12, 14
Kinesiology, 176, 177, 179, 180
KLK7 mutation, 84, 93
Knee flexural eczema, 39

L
Lactobacillus, 26, 171
Langerhans cell, 63, 90, 150, 161
Langerhans histiocytosis, 63
Late-phase reaction (LPR), 119
Leukotriene antagonist, 157
Lewis trias, 154
Lichen
  nitidus, 48
  planus, 35, 95, 96, 102, 127, 128
  simplex chronicus, 4, 39, 59, 62
Lichenification, 9, 20, 22, 37, 39–41, 50–52, 77
Lichenoid, 22, 41, 42, 48, 95, 96
Lid eczema, 43, 44, 56, 63, 66
Life events, 24, 105, 111, 125, 191
Lifestyle, 26–29
Light dermatosis, polymorphic, 67
Light sensitivity, 160
Linear grooves, 54, 55
Lip, dry, 43, 44
Lipid layer, 92
Lip licking eczema, 43
Lipodystrophy, 147
Living on a farm, 24, 27
Living room cleaning, 133
Local anesthetics, 158
Lotio, 135
Lotio alba, 135, 140, 158
Lotion, 135, 158, 159
Lower lip fissure, 44
Lymphocyte, 83, 90, 95–99, 104, 108, 113, 123, 130, 148, 165
Lymphoepithelial Kazal typerelated inhibitor (LEKTI), 64, 83, 84, 93

M
Macrolactams, 148
Major criteria (Hanifin Rajka), 76
Malassezia furfur, 60, 125, 153
Mamillar eczema, 45, 47
Marker, 9, 10, 21, 56, 65, 86, 114, 123, 127–130
Mast cell, 4, 84, 96, 99, 103, 104, 106, 107, 112, 113, 122, 148, 154, 155, 157, 161, 165
Mast cell blocker, 157
Measles, 24, 25, 150, 183
Mediator release, 111, 112
Menthol, 159
Mepolizumab, 169
Metabolic disorders, 63
Methicillin-resistant *Staphylococcus aureus* (MRSA), 151
Methotrexate, 165–166
Minor criteria (Hanifin Rajka), 76
Mite scabies, 62
Model learning, 174
Modified virus Ankara (MVA) vaccine, 25
Moisturizing factor, 83
Molecular genetics, 86, 117, 181
Molluscum contagiosum, 70, 153
Montelukast, 157
Morbus, 47
Mother milk, 184
MRSA, *see* Methicillinresistant *Staphylococcus aureus* (MRSA)
Multicenter International Study On Risk Assessment of Indoor and Outdoor Pollution on Allergy and Eczema Morbidity (MIRIAM) study, 21, 27
Mupirocin, 153
Muscular atrophy, 147
Music therapy, 191
Mutation, 64, 83–86, 91, 93, 114
Mycophenolate mofetil, 166
Mycosis, 63
Mycosis fungoides, 63

N
Naevus, 62, 75
Nail changes, 53
Nasal, 43, 56, 125, 153
Natural moisturizer, 83, 91, 138, 139
Neck, dirty, 50
Neck eczema, 19–20, 41, 49, 52, 69, 77, 131, 153, 154
Neonatal age, 18
Nephrotic syndrome, 66
Nervous system, 5, 56, 89, 106–108, 111, 113, 155, 157, 188–190
Netherton syndrome, 59, 63, 64, 84, 92, 150
Neurodermitis, 4, 6, 24, 77, 106
Neurovegetative, 5
Neutrophil activation, 99
New therapy, 173, 176
Nickel allergy, 75

Nitric oxide, 65
Node, 90, 99, 100, 107, 161
Notalgia paresthetica, 158
N-palmitoyl ethanolamine, 158
Nummular eczema, 39, 49, 112, 128
Nutrition, 15, 17, 26, 33, 111, 117, 124, 134, 182, 184–186, 190

O

Obesity, 184
Occlusion, 140
Octenidine, 151
Ocular changes, 66
Oedema, 99
Oil, 138, 151, 159
Oil bath, 138, 139
Oil-in-water (O/W) emulsion, 136
Ointment, 2, 117, 135, 136, 138–141, 148, 175
Oligosaccharides, 171, 186
Omalizumab, 99, 114, 169, 170
Oozing, 3, 37, 39, 43, 49, 69, 77, 125, 151
Otitis media, 67

P

Paget, 45
Pallor facial, 54, 56, 59
Papiloma virus, human (HPV), 70, 154
Papule, 35, 39, 41, 42, 62, 64, 77, 96, 97, 145
Parasites, 93, 96, 182, 183
Paronychia, 45, 46
Partner problems, 108
Patches, 32, 37, 48, 61
Patch test, 4, 61, 75, 76, 119–126, 132
Patchy pityriasiform lichenoid eczema, 42, 48
Pathophysiology, 3, 23, 48, 61, 63, 105–107, 113, 195
Patient empowerment, 117, 196
Patient exploration, 173
Patient information flyer, 187
Patient management, 117
Peanut oil, 26
Pemphigoid bullous, 59, 62
Peptide antimicrobial (AMP), 84, 168
Periorbital shade, 89
Perlèche, 43
Personality pattern, 105
Pertussis vaccination, 17, 25
Pet keeping, 27, 29, 182, 186, 187
Petrolatum, 119–121, 136
Phase triangle for topical therapy, 135
Phenylketonuria, 59, 63
Phosphodiesterase, inhibitors, 160, 168
Photocarcinogenicity, 150, 165
Photopheresis, 162
Phototherapy, 138, 160, 162, 170
pH value, 91, 93, 136
Phytotherapy, 176–178, 180
Pimecrolimus, 148, 150, 151, 158
Pityriasis
  pityriasis, 52
  rubra pylaris, 52
  versicolor, 73, 94
Placebo, 114, 124, 125, 152, 156, 162, 163, 167–169, 171–173, 177–179
Plantar dermatosis juvenilis, 45
Plaque lichenoid, 48
Plasma cell, 96, 99, 112
Plasmapheresis, 170
Point prevalence, 11, 19, 102
Polidocanol, 158, 160
Pollen avoidance, 133
Pollen count, 134
Pollen exposure, 48, 113
Pollen surface, 28
Pollutant exposure, 29
Polyhexanide, 151, 153
Polyunsaturated fatty acids (PUFA), 26, 171, 184, 185
Pompholyx, 50, 61
Potassium permanganate, 84
Povidone iodine, 151
Powder, 135, 136, 157
Prebiotics, 26
Predilection, 48, 97, 153
Pregnancy, 18, 26, 27, 29, 43, 145, 150, 157, 166, 171, 179, 182–186
Prevalence, 1, 2, 11–19, 21–23, 25–28, 32, 41, 57, 60, 61, 65–68, 71, 73–76, 82, 93, 132, 137, 150, 182–184, 186
Prevention, 26, 37, 117, 130, 132–134, 136, 140, 171, 181–191, 195
Prick test, 21, 119, 121, 122, 124, 129
Primary skin lesion, 35–37
Probiotics, 26, 171–172, 183, 184, 186
Pro-filaggrin, 83
Pro-inflammatory, 37, 93, 94, 97, 103, 148, 154, 166, 183
Protease, 81, 83, 84, 93, 94, 103
Protease-activated receptor (PAR)2, 84
Protease inhibitor, 64, 84, 93
Protein allergens, 7, 21, 119
Protein contact dermatitis, 65
Protein kinase inhibitor
Provocation factors, 2, 130–134, 139, 190
Provocation test, oral, 123–125
Prurigo, 4, 6, 22, 41, 43, 68, 102
Psoralens (PUVA), 160, 161
Psoriasis, 1, 33, 35, 49, 50, 52, 59–61, 65, 74, 75, 101, 102, 105, 111, 126–128, 159, 160, 165, 166, 168, 170–172, 189
Psychological, 105–113, 119, 125, 131, 136, 172, 173, 175, 190, 195
Psychopharmaceuticals, 106, 157, 173
Psychosomatic, 20, 24, 29, 45, 68, 105, 106, 110–112, 125, 172–176, 180, 189, 190, 195
Psychotherapy, 173
Pulpitis sicca, 45, 46
Purpura, thrombocytopenic, 171
Pyjama, 140

Q
Quality control, 187, 190, 191
Quality of life (QOL), 31, 79
Questionnaire, 11, 19, 77, 104, 113, 125

R
Rapamycin, 148
Reactivity, 4, 5, 9, 20, 56, 106–108, 113, 163, 168, 188
Reagin, atopic, 4, 7
Redness, 52, 57, 64, 145
Reflex erythema, 154
Regulatory T cells (Tregs), 97, 108, 161, 166
Rehabilitation, 33, 187, 189, 190
Relaxation techniques, 173–176, 180, 190
Repair activity, 161
Respiratory, 6, 7, 20, 23, 25, 27–29, 43, 56, 57, 60, 61, 65–67, 73, 75, 86, 123, 157
Rhinoconjunctivitis, allergic, 1, 3, 6–8, 10, 15, 16, 43, 56, 65, 66, 68, 75, 126, 129
Risk group, 181, 187
Rituximab, 114, 170
Rodents, 133
Rosacea-like dermatitis, 145–146, 148, 150

S
Saline, 106, 132, 162
Scabies, 45, 47, 59–62, 102, 105
Scaling, 38, 48–50, 52, 54
School beginners, 27
Scoring system for atopic dermatitis (SCORAD), 6, 77, 78
Scratching, 35–37, 39, 45, 56, 59, 61, 105, 106, 108, 119, 140, 151, 160, 174, 175
Scrotal eczema, 45, 47
Sea climate, 188, 189
Seborrhea, 137
Seborrheic dermatitis, 43, 60
Sebostasis, 54, 59
Secondary, 35, 56, 64, 94, 96, 104, 113, 181, 183, 187, 193
Sedation, 156
Self-confidence, 174
Seminal plasma, anaphylaxis, 66
Sensitisation, 17, 130
Sezary syndrome, 63
Sharply margined, 49
Shiny nails, 45
Shock fragment, 4
Shoe, 45, 62, 123
Shower oils, 139
Side effects, 136, 140, 144, 145, 148, 150, 151, 155–157, 161, 162, 164–170
Signal transduction inhibition, 84
Silver nitrate, 152
Silver textiles, 152
Sirolimus, 148
Skin
- barrier function, 22, 54, 64, 92, 130, 134, 139, 151, 173
- care, 26, 32, 130, 134, 136, 139, 147, 195
- changes, 3, 4, 36, 38, 39, 42, 43, 48–50, 52, 55, 59, 62–64, 68, 70, 71, 84, 122
- cleaning, 136–139, 152
- disease, 1, 2, 4, 11, 18, 28, 32, 33, 35, 50, 59, 61–63, 65, 70, 73, 76, 92, 94–98, 102, 106, 108, 109, 111, 112, 117, 125, 127, 128, 137, 143, 144, 147, 160, 162, 166, 172, 173, 175, 176, 187, 188, 195
- function, 111
- roughness, 54
- test, 9, 76, 77, 118–125, 177
- types, 160

Skin associated lymphoid tissue (SALT) Sleeplessness, 56
Smallpox vaccination, 25, 72
Soaps, 136–138
Socioeconomic status, 23, 24, 29, 129
Sodium chloride, 138
Sole, hyperlinearity, 54, 55
Solid food, 184, 186
Solvents, 76, 130
SPINK5, 83, 84, 92, 93
Spreading oil baths, 138
Staphylococcus aureus, 26, 39, 68, 73, 76, 151
Steroid, 123, 143, 145–148, 150, 151, 153, 164, 165, 167–169
Stigmata of atopy, 54–57, 59
Stigmatization, 31, 32, 193
Storage mites, 62, 132–133
Stratum, 84, 90, 92, 93
Stratum corneum, 83, 84, 90–93, 111, 138
Stress, 8, 24, 31, 66, 68, 92, 105, 107–113, 118, 125, 129, 173–175, 190, 195
Striae distensae, 145
Substances, vasoactive, 131
Sulfonates, 137, 159
Sun allergy, 67
Superantigen, 20, 81, 94
Superinfection, 39, 43, 45, 54, 71, 125, 151, 153
Surfactants, 137
Sweating, 76, 107
Symptom, 6, 8, 9, 13, 24, 35–39, 41, 43, 50, 54, 59, 65, 67, 76, 79–81, 96, 99, 102–104, 107–111, 113, 118, 119, 124, 128, 133, 138, 139, 154, 155, 158, 160, 163, 165, 187, 190, 196
Syndets, 137
Syndrome of incombable hair, 65

T
Tacrolimus, 148–151
Tandem therapy, 138, 147, 148
Tapinarof, 159
Tar, 159, 160
T cells, 62, 86, 94–96, 98, 100, 101, 103, 148
- activation, 165
- lymphoma, 52, 61, 63, 162

Tea tree oil, 152
Teleangiectasia, 145
Terfenadine, 156

Terminology, 6–9, 39, 76
Textile silver-coated, 152
T helper cell, 96
Th1-Th2 concept, 4
Therapy, 6, 59, 64, 70, 73, 97, 102, 106, 115, 118, 123, 125, 126, 129–131, 136–140, 145, 147–153, 155–157, 160–171, 173–180, 195
Thymic stromal lymphopoietin (TSLP), 103
Thymus and activation regulated chemokine (TARC), 128, 129
Thymus factors, 178
TLR agonists, 84
TNF receptor antagonist, 170
Tobacco smoke, 15, 27, 29, 130, 183, 186
Tolerance development, 184
Toll-like receptor (TLRs), 84, 86, 94
Topical calcineurin inhibitors (TCI), 140, 141, 147, 148, 151, 158
Topicals, 123, 136, 138, 140, 141, 153
Toxin, 94, 96
Traditional Chinese medicine (TCM), 176–178
Traffic exposure, 28, 29
Transforming growth factor β (TGF-β), 97, 98
Treatment, *see* Therapy
Trichophyton rubrum, 70
Trichorrhexis invaginata, 64
Triclosane, 151, 154
Truck traffic, 28
Tumor necrosis factor (TNF), 170
Twin studies, 82, 93
Type I reaction, 6
Type IV reaction, 7

U
UK working party's diagnostic criteria, 19, 76, 80
Ulerythema ophryogenes, 64
Ultraviolet (UV) exposure, 67
Unconventional procedures, 176–179, 190
Unguentum emulsificans aquosum, 139
Urea, 138, 139, 158, 165

V
Vaccination, 15, 24–26, 70, 148, 150, 153–154, 168, 179, 183
Vaccination complication, 70
Vacuum cleaning, 133
Vascular dilatation, 111, 154
Ventilation, 183
Visual analog scale (VAS), 77, 105
Vitiligo, 67
Volatile organic compounds (VOCs), 15, 130
Vulvar eczema, 47

W
Warts, 70, 73
Water content, 189
Water hardness, 137
Water-in-oil emulsion, 136, 151
Water loss, transepidermal (TEWL), 54, 83
Weather changes, 188
Wheal, 37, 154
Wiskott-Aldrich syndrome, 63, 64
Wool hypersensitivity, 130
World Allergy Organization (WAO) definition of allergy, 8

Z
Zinc deficiency, 59, 62
Zinc lotion, 135

GPSR Compliance

The European Union's (EU) General Product Safety Regulation (GPSR) is a set of rules that requires consumer products to be safe and our obligations to ensure this.

If you have any concerns about our products, you can contact us on ProductSafety@springernature.com

In case Publisher is established outside the EU, the EU authorized representative is:

Springer Nature Customer Service Center GmbH
Europaplatz 3
69115 Heidelberg, Germany

Batch number: 10731385

Printed by Printforce, the Netherlands